ENPC

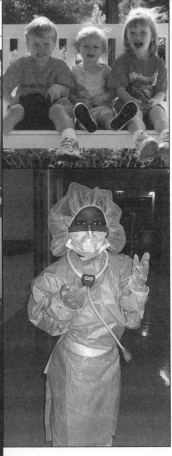

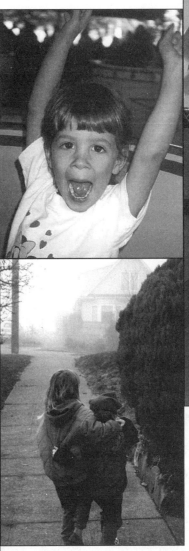

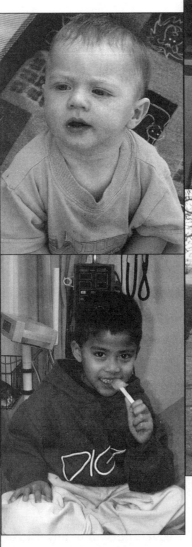

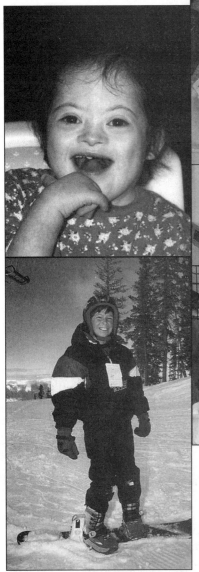

Emergency Nursing Pediatric Course

Third Edition
Revised Printing

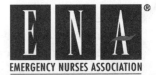

ENA®
EMERGENCY NURSES ASSOCIATION

PROVIDER MANUAL

Printed in the United States of America

ISBN 0-935890-82-3

The official Emergency Nursing Pediatric Course of the Australian College of Emergency Nursing (Australia)

The official Emergency Nursing Pediatric Course of the National Emergency Nurses' Affiliation, Inc. (NENA) (Canada)

The official Emergency Nursing Pediatric Course of the Dutch Trauma Nursing Foundation (STNN) (The Netherlands)

The official Emergency Nursing Pediatric Course of the Swedish Association of Trauma Nurses (RST) (Sweden)

TABLE OF CONTENTS

ACKNOWLEDGMENTS

The Emergency Nurses Association (ENA) would like to extend its appreciation to the 2002-2004 ENPC Revision Work Group for the revision and implementation of the third edition of the *Emergency Nursing Pediatric Course*.

Editor

Harriet S. Hawkins, RN, CCRN
Resuscitation Education Coordinator
Children's Memorial Hospital
Chicago, IL

Work Group Members (Section Editors and Authors)

Beth N. Bolick, RN, MS, PCCNP, CCRN
Assistant Professor/Nurse Practitioner
Department of Women's and Children's Health Nursing
Rush University
Chicago, IL

Nancy Denke, RN, MSN, FNP-C
Nurse Practitioner–Emergency Department
Staff Development Coordinator for Critical Care
Poudre Valley Hospital
Fort Collins, CO

Cindy Garlesky, MSN, ARNP, CEN
Pediatric Pain Specialist
Miami Children's Hospital
Miami, FL

Pamela R. Williams, RN, CPN, CEN, CLNC
Research Coordinator
Sisters of Charity
Providence Hospitals
Columbia, SC

Kathy Woloshyn, RN, BN
Educator Specialty Programs
Health Sciences Centre
Winnipeg, Manitoba, Canada

Additional Contributing Authors

Angela S. Black, RN, BSN
Emergency Department Clinical Educator
Children's Memorial Hospital
Chicago, IL

Bridget A. Cain, RN, BSN
Clinical Nurse Manager
Children's Memorial Hospital
Chicago, IL

Kim M. Dell'Angelo, PhD
Pediatric Psychologist
Loyola Stritch School of Medicine
Ronald McDonald Children's Hospital
Maywood, IL

Renee A. Plendl, RN, BSN
Clinical Nurse Manager
Children's Memorial Hospital
Chicago, IL

Rebecca Steinmann, RN, MS, CCNS, CEN, CCRN
Clinical Educator, Emergency Department
Children's Memorial Hospital
Chicago, IL

Barbara Weintraub, RN, MPH, MSN, PCCNP, CEN
Coordinator, Pediatric Emergency Services
Northwest Community Hospital
Arlington Heights, IL

Kimberly Woods-McCormick, RN, MS
Staff Development Coordinator
Poudre Valley Health System
Fort Collins, CO

A special thanks to the following work group members who made previous editions of ENPC possible.

1998 Task Force

Pam Baker, RN, BSN, CCRN, CEN

Nancy Eckle, RN, MSN, CEN, CNS

Kathy Haley, RN, BSN, CEN

Harriet Hawkins, RN, CCRN

Beth Nachtsheim, RN, MS, PCCNP

Reneé Semonin-Holleran, RN, PhD, CEN, CCRN, CFRN

1992 Task Force

Lisa Bernardo, RN, MSN, PhD

Jan Fredrickson, RN, MSN, CPNP

Janice Rogers, RN, MS, CS

Reneé Semonin-Holleran, RN, PhD, CEN, CCRN, CFRN

Donna Thomas, RN, MSN, CEN

Pam Baker, RN, BSN, CCRN, CEN was the Director of Trauma and Pediatric Services in 1992 and 1998. She worked tirelessly to bring to fruition a course that would improve the care of children. It is to Pam's memory that we dedicate this edition of the Emergency Nursing Pediatric Course.

The following individuals provided images used in the development of the ENPC Provider Manual and Instructor's Supplement.

Beth Bolick

Nancy Denke

Cindy Garlesky

Dale Gibbons

Cindy Goguen

Harriet Hawkins

Patricia Kunz Howard

Donna Massey

Julie Anne Missyabit

Jean A. Proehl

Barbara Remillard

Kathy Robinson

Kelley Rumsey

Carole Rush

Jehan Villalon

Barbara Weintraub

Pam Williams

Mary Ellen (Mel) Wilson

Kathy Woloshyn

PREFACE

While trauma is the leading cause of death in children, acute illness is also a source of unnecessary pediatric death. Emergency care visits by infants, children, and adolescents account for more than 31 million ED visits each year. It is estimated that one pediatric patient per second seeks care in the United States. The majority of children seeking care are seen in general emergency departments. Pediatric patients account for 34% of all emergency department visits in the United States. Injuries account for 43% and illness accounts for 57% of all emergency care visits in the pediatric population. Fortunately severe, life-threatening illness is still relatively infrequent. However, to lessen the morbidity and mortality of children, emergency nurses must be knowledgeable about preventative strategies for injury and disease, as well as triage assessment and categories, nursing assessment, and the appropriate interventions for children requiring emergency care.

In response to requests by the ENA's membership for a greater focus on the pediatric patient, the ENA Pediatric Committee was formed in 1991. One of the charges of this new committee was to assess the need for a pediatric emergency nursing course. A needs assessment done at the 1991 ENA Scientific Assembly overwhelmingly supported the need for such a course.

The first Emergency Nursing Pediatric Course (ENPC) was published in 1993 with the first revision completed in 1998. This third edition continues in the same tradition which is to improve the care of the pediatric patient in the emergency care setting and to increase the skill and confidence of emergency nurses who care for children worldwide. First, you will notice the use of pediatric patient throughout the manual. This term better reflects the age continuum of the pediatric population from infants to toddlers to adolescents.

Next, many changes have been made in this revision to ensure that it reflects current pediatric emergency care. New chapters, such as *Children with Special Health Care Needs*, have been added. The *Pediatric Trauma* and *Resuscitation* skills stations have been combined into one station, *Management of the Ill or Injured Pediatric Patient*, to reflect the continuity in assessment regardless of presentation. The *Pediatric Considerations* skills station, now *Pediatric Clinical Interventions*, has been expanded.

In addition, ENA has been working for the past year with other organizations who also offer pediatric life support education, such as the American Academy of Pediatrics and the American Heart Association, to ensure continuity of terms, i.e., spinal stabilization vs. spinal immobilization, and information across these courses, i.e., definitions of respiratory distress and failure.

ENA has worked very closely with the American Heart Association in order to fulfill the requirements to offer the Pediatric Advanced Life Support (PALS) renewal option during an ENPC. For more information, talk with your ENPC Course Director.

Lastly, ENPC continues to grow internationally. Not only is ENPC offered in Australia and Canada, nurses in Sweden and the Netherlands can now attend ENPC in their countries.

The ENPC represents the hard work, collaboration, and dedication of many people and continues to receive overwhelming support nationally and internationally.

SAMPLE QUESTIONS

1. An unresponsive 2-year-old child was found by his mother with a bottle labeled "Elavil 50 mg" by his side. Which piece of information is important to obtain from his mother?

   A. The size of the medication bottle.

   B. The expiration date of the medication.

   C. The number of pills left in the bottle.

   D. The person for whom the medication was prescribed.

   Reference: Chapter 18, Poisonings

2. A nurse providing crisis intervention to the family of a seriously ill child can best keep the family informed of the child's condition by:

   A. Placing them in a secluded room.

   B. Referring to their child as "the patient."

   C. Telling the family how they should feel.

   D. Appointing one staff member to communicate with them.

   Reference: Chapter 20, Crisis Intervention

3. A 16-month-old child was an unrestrained front seat passenger in a motor vehicle crash. The chest x-ray reveals multiple rib fractures. These findings suggest what type of injury?

   A. Minor surface injury.

   B. Significant underlying injury.

   C. Significant surface injury.

   D. Minor underlying injury.

   Reference: Chapter 11, Pediatric Trauma

4. Which piece of information is most important to know prior to transferring a patient to another facility?

   A. Documentation of the family's health insurance coverage.

   B. Pertinent family health history.

   C. Confirmation of acceptance from the receiving hospital.

   D. Confirmation of a medical diagnosis.

   Reference: Chapter 21, Stabilization and Transport

5. A 10-year-old child who was struck by a car has a distended, tense abdomen. The child's heart rate is 144 beats/minute, respirations 24 breaths/minute, and blood pressure 120/80 mm Hg. Capillary refill is more than 3 seconds, and skin is pale and cool. The patient's signs and symptoms suggest

   A. Obstructive shock.

   B. Distributive shock.

   C. Hypovolemic shock.

   D. Cardiogenic shock.

   Reference: Chapter 11, Pediatric Trauma

6. A school-aged child is about to receive stitches. To evaluate his understanding of the procedure, you tell him:

   A. "Young people your age have questions about getting stitches. What are your questions?"

   B. "Don't cry while you are getting the stitches. Be brave like a man."

   C. "You will probably receive 10 stitches. Do you have any questions before we restrain you?"

   D. "Does your cut hurt? Would you like your mommy to hold you?"

   Reference: Chapter 17, Procedural Preparation and Sedation

7. What is the preferred site for intraosseous access in the infant?

   A. Lateral malleolus

   B. Iliac crest

   C. Proximal femur

   D. Anteromedial tibia

   Reference: Chapter 8, Vascular Access

8. An important consideration in the assessment of pain for an adolescent patient is that they:

   A. May deny or minimize their pain when friends visit for fear of losing control.

   B. Have difficulty localizing or describing the pain.

   C. Are unable to use the 1 to 10 scale to report their pain.

   D. Feel that the pain is a punishment for something they did wrong.

   Reference: Chapter 12, Pediatric Pain Assessment and Management

9. An 8-month-old infant with pneumonia has severe intercostal and substernal retractions, weak muscle tone, lethargy, and gray skin color. The infant's condition does not improve after bag-mask ventilation. The next step in treatment is most likely to be:

    A. Administration of epinephrine.

    B. Supplemental warming measures.

    C. Rapid sequence intubation.

    D. Administration of albuterol.

Reference: Chapter 6, Respiratory Distress and Failure

10. Which combination of medications is best to have prepared for a pediatric resuscitation?

    A. Dopamine and sodium bicarbonate.

    B. Epinephrine and glucose.

    C. Naloxone and lidocaine.

    D. Pentothal and vecuronium.

Reference: Chapter 7, Shock

11. A 20-day-old infant has a 1-week history of not eating well. The infant has a weak cry and is jittery. Which laboratory test is indicated?

    A. Arterial blood gas.

    B. Finger-stick glucose.

    C. Complete blood count with differential.

    D. Toxicology screen.

Reference: Chapter 14, The Neonate

12. Which intervention should be performed next if tactile stimulation, positioning, drying, and blow-by oxygen administration do not increase a newborn's heart rate?

    A. Chest compressions.

    B. Umbilical vein cannulation.

    C. Endotracheal intubation.

    D. Bag-mask ventilation.

Reference: Chapter 14, The Neonate

13. A 10-kg child has deep partial-thickness burns over 35% of the total body surface area. Which evaluation parameter indicates that fluid resuscitation is adequate?

    A. Heart rate of 160 beats/minute.

    B. Respiratory rate of 34 breaths/minute.

    C. Blood pressure of 80/60 mm Hg.

    D. Urine output of 11 ml/hour.

Reference: Chapter 11, Pediatric Trauma

14. A 7-year-old female sustains a minor head injury and did not lose consciousness. She does not respond to commands and groans in response to questions. Which action will quickly determine if her behavior indicates a serious head injury?

    A. Review her medical record for pre-existing developmental problems.

    B. Obtain a head computerized tomography scan.

    C. Conduct a developmental screening test.

    D. Ask the parents if her behavior is unusual.

Reference: Chapter 11, Pediatric Trauma

15. An 8-month-old child presents with purpura, irritability, and a rectal temperature of 39.4°C (102.9°F). An intervention of high priority is:

    A. Encouraging the caregiver to hold and comfort the child.

    B. Monitoring for signs and symptoms of increased intracranial pressure (ICP).

    C. Collecting urine for toxicology screen.

    D. Encouraging oral fluids and food.

Reference: Chapter 15, Childhood Illnesses

16. The Pediatric Assessment Triangle is used to:

    A. Identify all life-threatening conditions that the child presents with.

    B. Perform a complete head-to-toe assessment on the child.

    C. Assess the status of the child's airway only upon arrive in the ED.

    D. Determine the severity of the child's illness or injury using the "across-the-room" assessment.

Reference: Chapter 5, Triaging the Pediatric Patient

17. The caregivers of a 6-year-old boy who is brought to the emergency department for abdominal pain should first be asked:

    A. "Are his immunizations current?"

    B. "Has anything happened to him at school recently?"

    C. "What is the reason for the child's visit and how long has he been ill?"

    D. "Has he been complaining of a sore throat or earache?"

Reference: Chapter 5, Triaging the Pediatric Patient

18. A 9-month-old infant is crying loudly through the nursing assessment, and the caregiver is becoming distraught. The nurse should ask the caregiver to:

A. Read a story to the infant

B. Offer the infant a pacifier.

C. Return when the infant is consoled.

D. Ignore the infant's behavior.

Reference: Chapter 3, From the Start — Dealing with Children

19. During an intubation attempt, the child's heart rate drops to 40 beats/minute. Which intervention is indicated?

A. Ask the physician to stop the intubation attempt and perform bag-mask ventilation.

B. Apply cricoid pressure and establish intravenous access.

C. Inform the physician of the heart rate and ask the physician to intubate faster.

D. Administer blow-by oxygen and begin chest compressions.

Reference: Chapter 7, Shock

20. A 6-week-old infant is pale, has marked substernal retractions, expiratory grunting, and poor muscle tone. The emergency nurse should first:

A. Obtain intravenous access.

B. Apply a pulse oximeter.

C. Obtain a chest x-ray.

D. Administer 100% oxygen.

Reference: Chapter 6, Respiratory Distress and Failure

21. The best method to open the airway in an injured child is:

A. Placing the head and neck in hyperextension.

B. Using the jaw thrust maneuver.

C. Placing the head and neck in flexion.

D. Using the head tilt maneuver.

Reference: Chapter 4, Initial Assessment

22. A 4-year-old child with a history of the flu has a heart rate of 80 beats/minute, respirations of 16 breaths/minute, and capillary refill of more than 3 seconds. The proper sequence for nursing interventions would be:

A. Position the airway, administer 100% oxygen, obtain venous access, and administer 20 ml/kg of an isotonic solution.

B. Administer 100% oxygen, obtain venous access, administer 0.1 mg/kg of epinephrine 1:10,000, and prepare for endotracheal intubation.

C. Position the airway, provide bag-mask ventilation, provide synchronized cardioversion, and provide supplemental warmth.

D. Administer 100% oxygen, prepare for a venous cutdown, administer 20 ml/kg of an isotonic solution, and obtain a chest x-ray.

Reference: Chapter 7, Shock

23. A 3-year-old is transported by prehospital personnel after being struck by a car. The parents are en route. The child is screaming and uncooperative. Which is the best approach while conducting the secondary survey?

A. Hold the child to comfort him.

B. Wait for the parent's arrival.

C. Observe for behavioral pain cues.

D. Use a doll to demonstrate the examination.

Reference: Chapter 3, From the Start — Dealing with Children

24. Which ocular finding is associated with child maltreatment?

A. Glaucoma.

B. Conjunctivitis.

C. Iritis.

D. Retinal hemorrhage.

Reference: Chapter 13, Child Maltreatment

25. A pregnant 18-year-old woman arrives at the emergency department about ready to deliver a full-term infant. She states that she noticed a large amount of dark green fluid the last time she went to the bathroom. During the delivery, the nurse should prepare to:

A. Dry and warm the infant as soon as is it delivered.

B. Stimulate and ventilate the infant immediately after delivery.

C. If needed, suction only after the birth is complete.

D. Administer blow-by oxygen and rub the back immediately after delivery.

Reference: Chapter 14, The Neonate

ENPC SAMPLE QUESTIONS
Answer Key

1.C	6.A	11. B	16. D	21. B
2.D	7.D	12. D	17. C	22. A
3.B	8.A	13. D	18. B	23. C
4.C	9.C	14. D	19. A	24. D
5.C	10. B	15. B	20. D	25. C

OVERALL COURSE OBJECTIVES

On completion of this course, the learner should be able to:

1. Describe the characteristics of life-threatening illness and injury in children.

2. Identify the anatomic and physiologic characteristics of children as a basis for signs and symptoms.

3. Identify the most frequent causes of illness or injury in children.

4. Describe the assessment of pediatric patients with illness or injury.

5. Plan the specific interventions needed to manage the pediatric patient with illness or injury.

6. Evaluate the effectiveness of nursing interventions related to patient outcomes.

7. Identify health promotion strategies related to the pediatric population.

PSYCHOMOTOR SKILL STATION OBJECTIVES

On completion of this course, the learner should be able to:

1. Demonstrate a standardized, systematic, and organized approach to assessment, planning, intervention, and evaluation.

2. Perform a primary and secondary assessment.

3. Identify an appropriate plan of care.

4. Set priorities for nursing interventions based on assessment data.

5. Implement appropriate interventions.

6. Evaluate pediatric patient response to interventions.

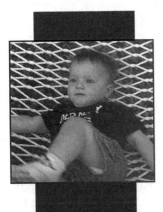

chapter 1

THE EMERGENCY NURSING PEDIATRIC COURSE

Introduction

According to the Child and Adolescent Emergency Department Visit Databook,[1] children under 18 years of age account for approximately 34% of all emergency department (ED) visits, with children under three years representing the largest group. Although the majority of ED visits by children are for nonemergent problems, every ED has the potential to receive a child in need of lifesaving intervention. Schoenfeld and Baker reviewed 80,000 pediatric ED visits to the Children's Hospital of Philadelphia and found that only 201 (0.0025%) needed resuscitation. Of these, only 58% required intubation, and only 30% required Pediatric Advanced Life Support resuscitation protocol drugs.[2] These statistics from a pediatric facility make it easy to see why many emergency care providers lack confidence when providing resuscitative care to children. Critically ill children typically present initially not with full arrest but with prearrest conditions, the most common of which are respiratory distress and compensated shock. The ability to recognize and treat these pre-arrest states is paramount to improving outcomes. All emergency health care providers must be prepared to provide immediate emergency care and appropriate referral for definitive pediatric care.[3,4] Over the last three decades an increasing level of commitment to the improvement of emergency care for children has been demonstrated by

- Creation of pediatric committees by nursing and medical organizations

- Emergence of pediatric emergency medicine and nursing as recognized subspecialties of pediatric care with a corresponding increase in nurses and physicians specializing in pediatric emergency care

- Establishment of professional organizations that provide a forum for pediatric emergency care practitioners

- Development and dissemination of national pediatric emergency care and resuscitation educational programs

- Funding of pediatric emergency medicine residencies and fellowship programs

- Availability of board certification in pediatric emergency medicine offered jointly by the American Board of Pediatrics and the American Board of Emergency Medicine

- Significant increases in the publication of pediatric emergency care textbooks (in both nursing and medicine), research, and clinical articles

- Ongoing funding of the Emergency Medical Services for Children (EMSC) grant program

The scope of emergency nursing practice encompasses nursing assessment, intervention, and evaluation of patients of all ages and all acuity levels. The Emergency Nurses Association (ENA) supports the development of standards to ensure adequate and safe emergency care for children with injuries and illnesses. In response to the needs of children and emergency nurses, ENA developed the Emergency Nursing

Pediatric Course (ENPC) in 1991. ENPC provides nurses and other health care providers with a standardized, internationally disseminated pediatric educational program to enhance their knowledge, skill, and expertise in the care of children.

ENA has continued to respond to the needs of children through (1) monitoring and proposing legislation, (2) identifying issues related to pediatric emergency care, (3) collaborating with other organizations to enhance the emergency care of children, and (4) developing educational resources for emergency nurses who care for children. This chapter describes the role of the emergency nurse in pediatric emergency care and the structure of the ENPC.

The Role of the Emergency Nurse in Pediatric Emergency Care

The evolution of pediatric emergency care as a separate and recognized discipline has been a catalyst for improvement in the emergency care of infants, children, and adolescents. Nurses perform a pivotal role in all phases of pediatric emergency care.

Physiologic baselines and responses to illness or injury in the child differ from the adult. Anatomic and physiologic characteristics as well as emotional, psychosocial, and cognitive responses differ among age groups. These factors are compounded by the fact that children are representative of a smaller percentage of the total population seen in emergency care settings. Generally, emergency nurses have a lower experience level in providing care for children, especially pediatric patients with a life-threatening illness or injury.

To lessen the morbidity and mortality of children, the emergency nurse must be able to quickly recognize and intervene for the pediatric patient in crisis. Knowledge essential for the emergency nurse includes growth and development, pediatric triage/acuity level identification, pediatric assessment and intervention techniques, common pediatric disease and injury processes, and prevention strategies as they relate to the infant, child, and adolescent.[3] In order to provide care to the ill or injured child, the nurse must know not only normal physiologic parameters but also normal behavior patterns. The pediatric patient often presents with subtle symptoms, and the ability to recognize changes from the norm can be key to assessment. Nurses should take every opportunity to observe children of various ages and stages of development. This knowledge is vital when looking at a pediatric patient. Core level and continuing education are necessary for the development and maintenance of competence in emergency pediatric care.

Nurses who provide emergency care to children must ensure that policies and procedures specific to the pediatric patient are developed to guide and maintain consistency in the delivery of emergency care. Additionally, supplies and equipment in a wide array of sizes must be available and functional to provide emergency interventions for children from birth to adolescence.

Promoting Injury and Illness Prevention

The greatest challenge to improving the care of children is to advance injury and disease prevention strategies in both the home and community.[5] Due to the episodic nature of emergency care, a single patient encounter may be the only opportunity the nurse has to affect the health practices of a family. Therefore, nurses must be cognizant of their role in the prevention of childhood illness and injury. Early identification of children at risk is an important element in primary prevention of illness, injury, and child maltreatment. Evaluation of risk factors and the formulation of practical intervention strategies are actions that may enhance or influence family health practices. Each encounter with a child and family provides an opportunity for education, counseling, and anticipatory guidance. Nurses must maintain an awareness of local community resources and work with the hospital team to provide appropriate medical and social service referrals.

Emergency nurses also have the opportunity to participate in endeavors directed at injury and/or illness prevention. The activities may include involvement in public and professional education, legislative efforts for injury control and prevention and regionalization of pediatric emergency care services, child advocacy, and injury/illness prevention initiatives. ENA and the ENA Institute for Injury Prevention/EN CARE have multiple injury prevention resources available.

Participation in Programs to Enhance Emergency Medical Services for Children

In 1984, Congress adopted legislation authorizing the establishment of the EMSC grant program. The purpose of this ongoing grant program is to reduce pediatric morbidity and mortality through expanding access to and improving the quality of emergency medical services for children. EMSC is jointly operated by the Maternal and Child Health Bureau (MCHB) and the Health Resource and Services Administration (HRSA) of the U.S. Department of Health and Human Services in collaboration with the National Highway Traffic and Safety Administration (NHTSA).[6] EMSC provides grants to support the development and implementation of EMSC projects across the country. Educational materials, training programs, pediatric protocols, and pediatric emergency care systems have been funded through EMSC. Through the collaboration of physicians, nurses, and prehospital providers with pediatric expertise, EMSC grants have provided education and training for providers in all phases of emergency care. Information and assistance to those interested in issues related to emergency medical services for children is available through the EMSC resource center at www.ems-c.org.

The Emergency Nursing Pediatric Course

Purpose

The purpose of ENPC is to present core-level knowledge and psychomotor skills associated with implementing the nursing process in the care of children from birth through adolescence. The psychomotor skill stations facilitate initial integration of psychomotor abilities in a setting that simulates pediatric patient situations. It is the intent of ENPC to enhance the nurse's ability to rapidly and accurately assess the pediatric patient's responses to the illness or injury event. It is anticipated that the use of the knowledge and skills learned in ENPC will ultimately contribute to a decrease in the morbidity and mortality associated with pediatric emergencies. Learning is a continuum—a dynamic process—and it is hoped that the ENPC Provider Manual will be used as a reference not only for the course but also for future care.

Summary

Millions of children require emergency care each year. The provision of competent emergency care for children must become an inherent part of our emergency care system. The delivery of emergency care to the pediatric patient requires specialized knowledge, training, equipment and planning. The ENA believes that the knowledge and psychomotor skills as identified in the ENPC will assist professional nurses to systematically assess the pediatric patient and to intervene or assist with interventions in a manner that will decrease pediatric mortality and morbidity.

References

1. Weiss, H. B., Mathers, L. J., Forjuoh, S. N., & Kinnane, J. M. (1997). Child and adolescent emergency department visit databook. Pittsburgh, PA: Center for Violence and Injury Control, Allegheny University of Health Services.
2. Schoenfeld, P. S., & Baker, M. D. (1993). Management of cardiopulmonary and trauma resuscitation in the pediatric emergency department. *Pediatrics, 91*(4), 726-729.
3. Emergency Nurses Association. (2001). Educational recommendation for nurses providing pediatric emergency care [Position statement]. Des Plaines, IL: Author.
4. American Academy of Pediatrics. (2001). Care of children in the emergency department: Guidelines for preparedness [Policy statement]. Retrieved October 30, 2003 from http://www.aap.org/policy/re069904.html
5. Rivara, F. P., & Grossman, D.C. (1996). Prevention of traumatic deaths to children in the United States: How far have we come and where do we need to go? *Pediatrics, 97*(6, Pt 1), 791-797.
6. Weintraub, B. (1997). Emergency medical services for children. *Journal of Emergency Nursing, 23*, 274-275.

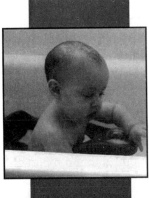

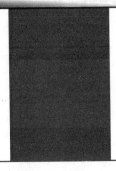

chapter 2

EPIDEMIOLOGY

Objectives

On completion of this chapter, the learner should be able to:

1. Identify characteristics of pediatric patients seen in the emergency department (ED).

2. Describe the characteristics of life-threatening illnesses in children.

3. Discuss the impact of pediatric injuries on pediatric morbidity and mortality.

4. State topics for injury prevention teaching based on the child's age.

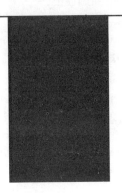

Introduction

The needs of children were generally overlooked during the development of emergency medical services (EMS). It was not until the mid-1970s that the prehospital and hospital-based emergency care needs of children began to be addressed.[1] Pediatric emergencies are influenced by the unique anatomic features, immature physiology, and variable developmental achievements of children.[2] These factors affect the types of illnesses and injuries that occur in the pediatric population and the associated clinical presentation. This chapter describes the characteristics of the pediatric population and the epidemiology of pediatric emergencies.

Characteristics of the Pediatric Population (United States)

Factors influencing the characteristics of the pediatric population treated in emergency care settings include episodic care, changes in health care systems, access to pediatric tertiary care, advances in health care practices, and socioeconomic and community conditions.[3] Pediatric patients account for 34% of all ED visits in the United States. Injuries account for 43% of all emergency care visits and falls are the leading cause of injury in the pediatric population.[4]

Access to Pediatric Health Care Services

- Not all communities have pediatric hospitals or pediatric specialty services. Children may have to be transferred to

another facility with pediatric tertiary care services or a pediatric trauma center for definitive care.

- Many children's hospitals and large metropolitan hospitals maintain facilities and personnel to treat complex, rare, and life-threatening pediatric emergencies. The presence of a pediatric center affects the pediatric census in general EDs in the same service area. Consequently, personnel in general EDs may have significantly less exposure to children with serious illnesses or injuries.

- Managed care plans and health maintenance organizations (HMOs) in the United States have typically included cost containment and utilization management features. A child may be enrolled in a plan that does not provide for care at a children's hospital or a community hospital with a pediatric ED or other pediatric services. Many HMO plans include some gatekeeping function that limits access to emergency care. Managed care restrictions often require complex phone calls and documentation for approval of emergency care visits.[3,5]

Continued Use of the Emergency Department as a Primary Source of Episodic Health Care

- Children who lack access to primary and well-child health care are more likely to utilize emergency care services. The ED is often the easiest and least-restricted entry into the health care delivery system, especially for those who are uninsured. Recent data indicates that children under the age of 18 in the United States account for almost 40% of those living in poverty.[6] The transient lifestyle often associated with poverty results in many children having no established relationship with a primary care provider.

- Restrictions or limitations in the operating hours of primary care providers' offices and clinics often force caregivers to seek care at other sites. Lack of available care and actual or perceived inaccessibility of primary care providers have also been identified as factors in the use of the ED for nonurgent problems.[7]

Referral Patterns of Primary Care Providers (PCP)

- Many physicians are reluctant to handle complex pediatric patients, especially in the office or clinic setting; therefore children are often referred to an ED for evaluation and treatment.[8] Unlike offices or clinics an ED provides 24-hour availability of diagnostic facilities and access to experienced physicians and nurses.
- A combination of full office schedules, lack of open appointments, and a problem that is considered medically urgent by the PCP may influence gatekeeping decisions and result in referral or approval of nonurgent ED visits.[7]

Children with Special Health Care Needs

- It is estimated that in the United States there are 12 million children with special health care needs, encompassing 18% of the pediatric population. Children with special health care needs are those who have or are at increased risk for a chronic physical, developmental, behavioral, or emotional conditions and require health and related services of a type or amount beyond that required by children generally.[9]
- Because of technology and the advancements in health care, these children have become frequent users of emergency care representing about 24% of all pediatric ED visits.[10]
- Special needs children have complicated medical problems and are dependent on technology such as oxygen, home ventilators, and long-term central venous access devices. They are often at greater risk for the development of emergent conditions, such as respiratory failure and sepsis.

Violence Against Children

- Violence against children occurs in both the family and community environments. Inflicted injury has had a significant impact on pediatric morbidity and mortality, as well as on the types of injuries pediatric patients sustain.

- In the year 2000, three million referrals were made in the United States regarding suspected child maltreatment, with approximately 33% of these allegations being substantiated.[11] Despite improved recognition and reporting of child maltreatment, a significant number of cases remain unreported.
- Although child maltreatment victimization rates have been decreasing, the rate of fatality associated with child maltreatment continues to increase. In 2000, there were 1.71 deaths per 100,000 children reported in the United States. This rise may be reflective of better maltreatment reporting. Younger children are the most vulnerable to intentional injury, and children less than one year of age accounted for 44% of child fatalities.[11]
- The United States has the highest reported youth homicide and suicide rates of the industrialized countries. Exposure to violence in the community, through media portrayals, and in combination with other social experiences may increase the risk for youth involvement with violence. Access to firearms, substance abuse, and involvement in antisocial or violent groups are factors that increase a child's risk for entanglement in violent situations.[12,13]
- Gang activity and influences are increasingly evident in inner city, suburban, and rural areas. Violence affiliated with gang activity is extremely volatile and is often associated with illegal drugs, turf wars, and weapons. As a result, children are often the victims of penetrating trauma related to gang activities as either a participant or an innocent bystander.

Nonimmunized and Underimmunized Children

In 1999, 78.4% of children had received a complete immunization series.[6] This rate of immunization shows significant progress compared to the 1994 immunization compliance of 67.5% of children less than 3 years of age. However, regional outbreaks of rubella, rubeola, pertussis, and other preventable illnesses have been directly related to inadequate immunization. Children who contract one of these highly communicable diseases may develop emergent complications or present in the emergency department for acute care in response to the illness.

Infrequent Use of Prehospital EMS

Less than 10% of EMS requests are for children.[14] Caregivers often choose to transport their critically or seriously ill or injured child to an ED by private vehicle rather than waiting for EMS response. Consequently, emergent pediatric patients routinely present to the ED without the benefit of prehospital care and initial stabilization.

Epidemiology (United States)

Data from the Child and Adolescent Emergency Department Visit Databook has provided the best information regarding the epidemiology of pediatric emergencies to date.[4] Determining the precise incidence and prevalence of pediatric emergency illness and injury remains complicated by a number of factors:[2]

- Age definitions for pediatrics are not standardized. The American Academy of Pediatrics defines pediatrics as a continuum from birth through adolescence (0 to 21 years).
- ED data are not consistently reported by age category.
- Qualitative and quantitative data accurately documenting indicators, such as delayed or missed diagnosis, are difficult to obtain.
- Statistics regarding children with emergencies are limited.
- The number of children with emergency conditions who are treated by primary care providers and in urgent care facilities is not well known.[6]
- There is no nationally standardized reporting system for pediatric emergencies.[2]

In 1998, approximately 5,300 hospitals reported providing emergency services.[15] Emergency care visits by infants, children, and adolescents account for more than 31 million ED visits each year in the United States.[4,15] Children under 3 years of age represent 30% of pediatric emergency care visits. It is estimated that one pediatric patient per second seeks care in the United States.[4]

Because of the limited number of pediatric EDs, the majority of children seeking emergency care are seen in general emergency departments.[2] Therefore, all emergency health care providers must be familiar with the signs and symptoms of a life-threatening illness or injury as well as subtle signs of deterioration in the pediatric patient. Recognition of such conditions can be difficult for those who lack pediatric training and experience.[15] Accurate assessment is essential to rapidly provide the pediatric patient with the appropriate interventions and stabilization.

Pediatric Illness

The frequency of emergency visits for pediatric illness varies significantly according to the age group, season, and time of day. ED usage by pediatric patients tends to be higher during evening hours and the winter months.[16] Caregivers often use EDs because onset or worsening of pediatric illness most often occurs during times when primary care availability is most limited.[17,18]

No published data have substantiated significant misuse of EDs for well-child care. In general, caregivers use EDs because they are worried about their child's health and are poorly supported by primary health care.[3]

In one study, pediatric patients presented for emergency care most frequently for complaints of fever (11%), cough (4%), vomiting (3%), earache (3%), and facial laceration (3%). Otitis media was the leading medical diagnosis (9%), followed by upper respiratory illness (5%), gastroenteritis (3%), acute pharyngitis (3%), and asthma (2%).[4]

Although fewer children die from acute illness than from injury, illness accounts for many more hospitalizations. Approximately 57% of all ED visits by children are due to illness.[4] Severe, life-threatening illness is still relatively infrequent when compared to the incidence of all acute illness in children. Thirty-six percent of children who presented to the ED with an illness were classified as urgent-emergent.[4] Characteristics of life-threatening illnesses in children may include a combination of the following.

- Initial subtle signs of illness that progress to a condition that requires emergent intervention
- Relatively rapid in onset with precipitous deterioration
- Frequent involvement of the respiratory system or central nervous system
- Require rapid intervention
- Necessitate care at a pediatric tertiary care center

Pediatric Hospitalizations Due to Illness

Eight percent of medically related pediatric ED visits required hospitalization.[4] The top three primary diagnostic groupings for these children included (1) respiratory symptoms, (2) symptoms and ill-defined conditions, and (3) digestive. Respiratory illnesses accounted for 27% of the admissions in children under 15 years of age.[2,4] Other common admission diagnoses included infectious/parasitic problems and mental health disorders.[4]

Pediatric Deaths Due to Illness

The number of children who die before reaching 1 year of age is reflected in the infant mortality rate. In 1999, there were 7.0 infant deaths per 1,000 live births.[19] Congenital anomalies and premature birth accounted for the majority of deaths in the neonatal period. Sudden infant death syndrome (SIDS) is the third leading cause of death in infancy and the primary cause of infant death outside of the neonatal period accounting for approximately 2,500 infant deaths annually.[19,20] Other leading causes of illness-related pediatric death include malignant neoplasms, congenital anomalies, heart disease, respiratory illnesses, influenza and pneumonia, cerebrovascular illnesses, and septicemia.[20] After 12 months of age, injury becomes the leading cause of death in the pediatric population.[2,20]

Pediatric Trauma

Trauma has a greater impact on pediatric morbidity and mortality than any other disease. Injury accounts for approximately 43% of emergency department visits by children. The greatest number of injury-related visits was in children 0 to 2 and 18 to 20 years of age. The highest rate of injury, 21.1/100 persons, was in the 15- to 17-year-old age group. Of injury-related visits, facial lacerations accounted for the greatest percentage. Other frequent injury-related causes included injury to the head, neck, or face (5%), upper extremity laceration (5%), injury to hand or finger (3%), and head or neck laceration (3%). The majority of the injury-related visits were considered minor, with an injury severity score of < 3 (84%).[4]

Most pediatric injuries occur at home. Common causes of injury in children include

- Falls
- Being struck by or against an object
- Cutting and piercing
- Unspecified motor vehicle traffic
- Bites and stings[4]

As in the adult population, the prevalence of injury-related ED visits is higher for males than females.[2,4] Specific injury events and injuries sustained vary among age groups. These variations are related to differences in cognitive, perceptual, motor, and language abilities as well as to physical development.[21] Variation in developmental maturity, in combination with a proximity to high-risk surroundings or behaviors, can increase the child's risk for some injury events.

Falls are the leading cause of unintentional injury for children. Children 14 years of age or younger account for 21% of all fall-related emergency department visits.[21] More than 2.5 million children are treated in EDs annually for falls. Due to developmental level, motor skills, and curiosity, children less than 10 years of age are at greatest risk for fall-related injury.[21]

Being struck by or against an object encompasses many different mechanisms of injury.

Motor vehicle-related injury is a leading cause of unintentional injury and death among children and adolescents.[4,21] Children as occupants in motor vehicles as well as pedestrians and bicyclists are at risk for

injury. In 2001, more than 800,000 children between 1 and 20 years of age were injured in motor vehicle-related crashes, the vast majority as passengers.[22]

In addition to age and developmental abilities, the child's environment and typical activities are factors affecting the child's risk for injury. Annually, there are a significant number of pediatric injuries and deaths involving nursery furnishings, toys, recreational equipment, and playground apparatus.[21,22]

Pediatric Deaths Due to Injury

Trauma is the leading cause of death in children greater than 1 year of age, accounting for more than one-half of all pediatric deaths annually.[22] Motor vehicle crashes are the leading cause of unintentional injury-related deaths in children of all age groups. In children less than 12 years of age, motor vehicle crashes are responsible for one out of every three injury-related deaths.[22] Adolescents and children less than 4 years of age are at highest risk for unintentional injury-related death.[21,22]

Child maltreatment is the leading cause of injury-related death in children 4 years of age or younger.[11] In the United States, fatal child maltreatment occurs at a rate of 1.71 out of every 100,000 children. Severe head trauma is the primary cause of death from child maltreatment.[11]

Cost of Pediatric Injury

In 2000 more than 14 million pediatric patients sustained injuries significant enough to require medical treatment.[21] An estimated 4 billion dollars is spent annually for injury-related pediatric ED visits.[4] Each year, 4% of the pediatric patients treated in an ED for an injury will require hospitalization.[4] The health care costs for these children exceed $4 billion in ED visit medical costs alone.[4]

Characteristics of the Pediatric Population (Canada)

- Canada is a large and varied landmass characterized by population bases scattered across the country from small northern outpost communities of 50 families to very large urban centers of greater than 1 million families. Children living in these communities have diverse ethnic origins. Aboriginal children, birth to 19 years, make up 44% of their native population and 28% of the national population. They are more likely to be of low income, live in rural areas, and due to genetic, socioeconomic and geographic factors, experience certain types of illness more so than their nonaboriginal peers.[23] A key characteristic is the increase in proportion of immigrants from visible minority backgrounds. Of the immigrants arriving in Canada within the last 10 years, approximately one in two was of Asian descent.[24]

- Another unique characteristic of Canadian culture is the fact that Canada has two official languages: English and French. The proportion of families now speaking nonofficial languages is beginning to rise, thus reflecting an increase in immigration and a revitalization of the aboriginal language within their communities. The diversity of culture and language puts a strain on the health care system to ensure that the modalities of care are offered in an environment and manner that is understood and clearly advocates for the child.

Access to Pediatric Health Care Services

- Though access to pediatric health care services differs somewhat from province to province, access to specialized pediatric care is uniform throughout Canada. Children with complex special needs are referred to pediatric centers with the ability and expertise to manage their care. General pediatrics is seen throughout the country at medical centers, EDs, and family physician and pediatrician offices.
- Children living in isolated northern communities have limited direct access to specialized care. These children require referral to larger metropolitan centers, often requiring air transport services. Unpredictable weather conditions and inaccessibility to specialized services can lead to challenges in management for these children. Families with children with special health care needs often find it necessary to move to urban areas where services and programs are more accessible.[24]
- One of the technologies entering the health care field is telehealth. Through the use of audio/video conferencing, consulting physicians can seek information and assistance for a higher level of expertise and either manage the child within the community hospital or seek assistance in emergency stabilization while the transport team is en route.

Continued Use of the ED as a Primary Source of Episodic Health Care

- In 1996, the Canadian national poverty rate for children under 18 years of age rose to between 18 and 27%. Children living in poverty may encounter barriers to healthy development through poor living conditions and inadequate nutrition, increasing their risk of negative health outcomes.[25,26]

- Access to primary health care may be limited due to variables including knowledge deficit regarding health promotion and prevention of illness, physician shortages, transient lifestyles leading to inconsistent care, and inability to afford associated costs.

Violence Against Children

- In 1998, there were an estimated 21.52 investigations of child maltreatment per 1,000 children in Canada. Forty-five percent of these were substantiated and included abuse in categories of physical and sexual abuse, neglect, and emotional maltreatment.[27]
- Of the 8,344 children admitted due to injury purposely inflicted by another person in 1999/2000, 16% of them were between the ages of 10 and 19 and 4% were less than 10 years old.[27]
- Thirty four percent of the physical abuse cases investigated in Canada were found to be substantiated, the majority being related to inappropriate punishment.[27]

Nonimmunized and Underimmunized Children

Immunization rates for infants and young children are very high in Canada. In 1995-96, immunization rates for diphtheria, pertussis, and tetanus; polio; and measles, mumps, and rubella ranged between 83% and 96%. Although the immunization rate for *H. Influenza type b* (Hib) was lower during the same time period (74.9%), it has steadily increased indicating a greater public and professional awareness of the vaccine. Only anecdotal cases of Hib are now being reported.[28]

Routine immunization schedules now include Hepatitis B, pneumococcal, and meningococcal vaccines.[29] Rapid changes in immunization practice are reflected in guidelines and goals established by the National Advisory Committee on Immunization and include goals to decrease the incidence of Hib and eliminate measles infections. Following recent outbreaks of measles, a second vaccine was added to the immunization schedule resulting in a decrease in incidence to fewer than 400 cases per year.[28,29,30]

Epidemiology (Canada)

Pediatric Illness and Injury

- In 1997, the leading cause of hospitalization in children less than 10 years of age was due to respiratory disease. Other causes of hospitalization in children were related to unintentional injuries and diseases of the digestive system.[31]

- The leading cause of death in Canadian children less than 20 years of age was unintentional injuries. The highest percentage of these occurred in children between the ages of 15 to 19 years. Other causes of death include cancer, congenital anomalies, and death related to suicide.[31]
- Persons under the age of 20 years accounted for 18% of all injury admissions in 1999-2000. The most common causes of injury admissions in this age group were unintentional falls (39%) and motor vehicle collisions (18%). Other leading causes of injury admissions were being struck by an object/person or falling object and cycling-related incidents.[31]
- The highest number of falls occurred in children between the ages of 5 to 9 years. The most common type of fall was from one level to another (40%). This included 1,927 falls from playground equipment, which comprised 14% of falls in this age group.[31]
- Most of the injuries sustained were orthopedic in nature, largely involving upper or lower extremities. Other injuries included intracranial injuries and skin wounds.
- Pediatric trauma or critically ill children require a high level of care or a tertiary trauma center to provide the expertise and resources to manage their treatment. Many provinces in Canada have only one or two major pediatric centers to care for these critically ill or injured children. Due to Canada's large land regions these children require emergent air transport and specialized teams to deliver them to an appropriate facility in a timely and expedient manner.
- Children less than 20 years of age comprised 22% of all admissions related to motor vehicle crashes. In 1999-2000 the highest number of injury related deaths in this same age group was due to motor vehicle crashes.[31]
- Almost one half (49%) of injury admissions were due to cycling injuries in persons less than 20 years of age. This same age group accounted for over one half of unintentional drowning in 1999-2000. This was the highest percentage of all age groups.[31]

Trends in the Health of Canada's Youth

Over the past decade there has been a worldwide increase in the incidence of childhood obesity. An estimated 25% of America's youth are considered to be obese, representing a 20% increase in prevalence over the past 10 years. In Canada, the rate of childhood obesity tripled between 1981 and 1996.[32]

Sedentary lifestyles, video games, computers and television, consumption of fast food, and unhealthy eating are all contributing factors. Approximately 28% of Canadians 12 to 14 years old and 66% of Canadian youth aged 15 to 19 years are considered physically inactive. Obese children are at risk for high cholesterol and triglyceride levels, type 2 diabetes, hypertension, orthopedic problems, and psychological problems. Once considered an adult disease, the prevalence of type 2 diabetes is increasing at an alarming rate in youth, with up to 45% of children newly diagnosed with diabetes having nonimmune-mediated disease. An increased proportion of Canadian aboriginals, African Americans, American Indians, and Asians have type 2 diabetes, with average age of onset in children being between 12 to 14 years of age.[32]

Characteristics of the Pediatric Population (Australia)

Factors influencing the characteristics of the pediatric population treated in emergency care settings include episodic care, changes in health care systems, access to pediatric tertiary care, advances in health care practices, and socioeconomic and community conditions.[3]

Access to Pediatric Health Care Services

- Not all communities have pediatric hospitals or pediatric specialty services. Children may have to be transferred to a facility with pediatric tertiary care services or pediatric trauma center for definitive care.
- Many children's hospitals and large metropolitan hospitals maintain facilities and personnel to treat complex, rare, and life-threatening pediatric emergencies. The presence of a pediatric center affects the pediatric census in general EDs in the same service area. Consequently, personnel in general EDs may have significantly less exposure to children with serious illnesses or injuries. Many hospitals in Australia offer services to both the pediatric and adult population, and consequently a wide range of skills and knowledge is required to prepare for possible pediatric populations.

Continued Use of the Emergency Department as a Primary Source of Episodic Health Care

- Use of hospital service and consultations with doctors are strongly age related. A survey on National Health conducted by the Australian Bureau of Statistics from February to November 2001 indicated that 1 in 4 children aged less than 5 years had consulted a doctor in the previous 2 weeks either by a general practitioner or an ED. The proportion of children consulting a doctor was the lowest for those aged 14 to 15 years.[33]

- Children who lack access to primary and well-child health care are more likely to utilize emergency care services. The ED is often the easiest and least restricted entry into the health care delivery system. Recent data indicates that 12.8% of children under the age of 14 years in Australia are living in poverty.[34] The transient lifestyle associated with poverty results in many children having no established relationship with a primary care provider.
- Restrictions or limitations in the operating hours of primary care provider's offices and clinics often force caregivers to seek care at other sites. Lack of available care and actual or perceived inaccessibility of primary care providers have also been identified as factors in the use of the emergency department for nonurgent problems.[7]

Referral Patterns of Primary Care Providers

Many primary care physicians are reluctant to handle complex pediatric patients, especially in the office or clinic setting. Therefore, children are referred to an emergency department for evaluation and treatment.[8] Unlike offices or clinics, an ED provides 24-hour availability of diagnostic facilities and access to experienced physicians and nurses.

Higher Survival Rates and a Greater Number of Children with Chronic Illness

- Although death rates in the early decades of the 20th century probably reflected the occurrence of illness reasonably well, the rarity of death among children now means that death rates do not reflect the burden of illness and disability affecting the children and youth.[35]
- Population data on disability in childhood is not readily available but suggests increases in both incidence and prevalence due to an increased survival of high-risk newborns and of children with established disability.[35] Children with special health care needs are those who have or are at increased risk for a chronic physical, developmental, behavioral, or emotional conditions and require health and related services of a type or amount beyond that required by children generally.[9] Because of technology and the advancements in health care, these children have become frequent users of emergency care, representing 24% of all pediatric emergency department visits.[10] These children have complicated medical problems dependent on medical technology such as oxygen, home ventilators, and long-term central venous access devices. These children are often at greater risk for the development of emergent conditions such as respiratory failure and sepsis.

Violence Against Children

Violence against children occurs in both the family and community environments. Inflicted injury has had a significant impact on pediatric morbidity and mortality, as well as the types of injuries pediatric patients sustain.

In 2000-2001 the number of reported abused or neglected children in Australia was 115,471, which is more than double the 1988-1989 figure of 42,468.[36] Despite improved recognition and mandatory reporting of child maltreatment, a significant number of cases remain unreported. Younger children are the most vulnerable to intentional injury and children less than 4 years of age accounted for 19 out of 60 fatal assaults in New South Wales (32%) for the years 1996-1999.[37]

In Australia about 6% of all child deaths classified as being from external causes were homicides. This average has remained constant for the last 15 years at 11 deaths per year, which is 1.1 per 100,000 children aged 1 to 4 years.[38] Exposure to violence in the community, through media portrayals, and in combination with other social experiences, may increase the risk for youth involvement with violence. Access to firearms, substance abuse and use, and involvement in antisocial or violent groups are factors that increase a child's risk for entanglement in violent situations.[12,13] In Australia there has been an increase in gang activity and gang influences in the inner-city, suburban, and rural areas. Violence affiliated with gang activity is extremely volatile and is often associated with illegal drugs, "turf wars," and weapons. As a result, children are increasingly the victims of trauma, as either a participant in or an innocent bystander to gang activities.

Nonimmunized and Underimmunized Children

- Recent surveys conducted in Australia indicated that most children ages 0 to 6 years were fully immunized against each of the diseases in the National Health and Medical Research Connection (NHMRC) recommended Childhood Immunization Schedule. These immunization levels have risen since the previous surveys in 1995.
- Children in the 0 to 12 months age groups had a high level of immunization declining to a moderate level for children ages 5 to 6 years. For example, 95% of children less than 6 months of age were fully immunized against diphtheria and tetanus but only 60% of children ages 5 to 6 years were fully immunized.[39]

Infrequent Use of Prehospital Emergency Medical Services

Caregivers often choose to transport their critically or seriously ill or injured child to an ED by private vehicle rather than waiting for emergency medical services to respond. Consequently, emergent pediatric patients routinely present to the ED without benefit of prehospital care.

Epidemiology (Australia)

The exact epidemiology of pediatric emergencies is not known. Determining the precise incidence and prevalence of pediatric emergency illness and injury is complicated by a number of factors.

- Age definitions for pediatrics are not standardized. Australia defines pediatrics as a continuum from birth through adolescence, or 0 to 18 years of age. EDs often categorize pediatric patients as those between 0 and 14 years.
- ED data are not consistently reported by age category.
- Qualitative and quantitative data that accurately document indicators, such as delayed or missed diagnosis, are difficult to obtain.
- Statistics regarding children with emergencies are seriously limited.
- The number of children with emergency conditions who are treated by primary care providers and in urgent care facilities is unknown.
- There is no nationally standardized reporting system for pediatric emergencies. Because of the limited number of pediatric EDs, the majority of children seeking emergency care are treated in general EDs. Therefore, all emergency health care providers must be familiar with the signs and symptoms of a life-threatening illness or injury as well as subtle signs of deteriorating conditions in children. Recognition of such conditions can be difficult for those who lack pediatric training and experience. Accurate assessment is essential to rapidly providing the child with the appropriate interventions and stabilization.

Pediatric Illness

The frequency of pediatric illness varies significantly according to the age group, season, and time of day. ED usage by pediatric patients tends to be higher during evening hours and the winter months.[16] Caregivers often use EDs because onset or worsening of pediatric illness most often occurs during times when primary care availability is most limited.[17,18] No published data has substantiated significant misuse of EDs for well-child care. In general, caregivers use EDs because they are worried about their child's health and are poorly supported by primary health care.[3]

In Australia pediatric patients presented for emergency care most frequently for complaints of fever, cough, vomiting, earache, asthma, upper respiratory illness, and gastroenteritis. Although fewer children die from acute illness than from injury, illness accounts for many more hospitalizations. Severe, life-threatening illness is still relatively infrequent when compared to the incidence of all acute illness in children.

Characteristics of life-threatening illnesses in children may include a combination of the following.

- Initial subtle signs of illness that progress to a condition that requires emergent intervention
- Relatively rapid in onset with precipitous deterioration
- Frequent involvement of the respiratory system or central nervous system
- Require rapid intervention
- Necessitate care at a pediatric tertiary care center

Pediatric Hospitalizations Resulting from Illness

The top three primary diagnostic groupings for admitted children included (1) respiratory, (2) digestive, and (3) ill-defined conditions such as fever. Respiratory illnesses accounted for a large percentage of the admissions in children under 15 years of age.[2,4] Other common admission diagnoses included infectious/parasitic problems and mental health disorders.[4]

Pediatric Deaths Resulting from Illness

Current infant and child death rates in Australia are low by international standards at less than 2% of all deaths reflected in the Australian Bureau of Statistics review of sociodemographic characteristic for the years 1982 to 1996.[40]

The estimated child death rate for indigenous children (1 to 4 years of age) for the years 1994 to 1996 was 4.5 times higher than that for nonindigenous children at 131 deaths per 100,000. This may reflect the poor socioeconomic environment in which most indigenous children live.[38]

The number of children who die before reaching 1 year of age is reflected in the infant mortality rate. The number of deaths decreases significantly with the increasing age of infants.

About 35% of infant deaths occurred on the day of birth. An additional 16% had occurred by the end of the first week. A total of 62% of infant deaths occurred in the neonatal period. The remaining 38% of deaths occurred in the postnatal period, with the proportion of deaths declining steadily over this period. In general, infant mortality rates were higher for males then females by about 27%.[38]

Birth-related conditions and congenital anomalies account for the majority of deaths in the neonatal period. SIDS is the second leading cause of death in the postneonatal period and the primary cause of all deaths annually. Over the 15-year period, 1982 to 1996, the average death rate from SIDS declined by 57% from 189 deaths per 100,000 in 1982 to 1986 to 81 in 1992. Other leading causes of illness-related pediatric death include heart disease, pneumonia, septicemia, stroke, meningitis, infection with the human immunodeficiency virus, and cancer. After 1 year of age, however, injury becomes the leading cause of death in the pediatric population.

Pediatric Trauma

Trauma has a greater impact on pediatric morbidity and mortality than any other disease. Unintentional injuries, poisoning, and violence (external causes) accounted for about 46% of all deaths among children (1982 to 1996).

In Australia, the highest incidence of deaths from drowning occurs in the childhood years. Suicide and transport deaths begin during adolescence. Deaths from motor vehicle crashes continue to decline; in 2000 there were 26 deaths per 100,000 in males and 9 deaths per 100,000 in females. Death rates from drowning also decreased from 8 per 100,000 in 1982 to1986 to 5 per 100,000 in 1992 to1996.[33]

About 6% of all child deaths classified as being due to external sources were homicides. This has remained at around 11 per year, with an average homicide rate of 1.1 per 100,000 in children ages 1 to 4 years.[38]

The most prevalent pediatric injuries include minor traumas, such as sprains, lacerations, contusions, fractures, and mild head injury. However children are also at risk for disabling and life-threatening injuries. Common causes of injury in children include

- Falls
- Motor vehicle crashes
- Being struck by a motor vehicle (pedestrians and bicyclists)
- Bicyclists crashes and collisions
- Drowning
- Thermal sources
- Poisoning
- Sports and recreational activities

- Suffocations or choking
- Penetrating events such as gunshots, stabbing, cutting, piercing
- Child maltreatment

As in the adult population, the prevalence of injury-related emergency department visits is higher for males than females.[2,4] Specific injury events and injuries sustained do vary among age groups. These variations are related to the differences in cognitive, perceptual, motor, and language abilities among age groups as well as physical development.[21] The variation in developmental maturity, in combination with the child's proximity to high-risk surroundings or high-risk behaviors, can increase his or her risk for some injury events.

Falls are the leading cause of unintentional injury for children. In Australia children 14 years of age or younger account for 38% of all fall-related emergency department visits.[37] Due to developmental level, motor skills, and curiosity, children less than 10 years of age are at greatest risk for fall-related injury.[21]

Being struck by or against an object encompasses many different mechanisms of injury.

In the United States and Australia motor vehicle-related injury is a leading cause of unintentional injury and death among children and adolescents.[4,21] Children as occupants in motor vehicles as well as pedestrians and bicyclists are at risk for injury. During the period 1982 to 1996 about a third of all child deaths from external causes were due to motor vehicle crashes (approximately 64 deaths per year).[39]

Fires, flames, and scalds continue to be a factor in pediatric deaths. During 1995, one third of all deaths due to a house fire in Australia occurred in children younger than 15 years of age. Approximately 16% of deaths from fire were children 0 to 4 years of age.[38]

In addition to age and developmental abilities, the child's environment and typical activities are factors affecting the child's risk for injury. Annually, a significant number of pediatric injuries and deaths involve nursery furnishings, toys, recreational equipment, and playground apparatus. Sports and occupational injuries are also evident in the pediatric population, with the greatest number occurring in the adolescent age group.

Pediatric Deaths Resulting from Injury

Trauma is the leading cause of death in children older than 1 year of age, accounting for almost one half of all pediatric deaths annually. Motor vehicle crashes accounted for about a third of all child fatalities.[38]

Severe head trauma is the primary cause of death from child maltreatment.[11]

In 1995, 16 Australian children 0 to 4 years of age and seven children 5 to 9 years of age died from homicide or child maltreatment.[41]

The rate of suicide of Australian males 15 to 24 years of age has remained consistent since the 1980s. There were approximately 25.2 deaths per 100,000 population reported in 1995 due to suicide. Overall, the death rate in males from suicide was four times the death rate in females.[41]

Characteristics of the Pediatric Population (the Netherlands)

The Netherlands is one of the smallest countries of the mainland of Europe. There are about 16 million inhabitants, 3 million of which are immigrants. The western part of the country consists of large urban centers, and children living in these communities have diverse ethnic origins caused by immigration from all over the world, mostly from Turkey, Morocco, and Surinam. The eastern part is less crowded and has more rural areas.

Access to Pediatric Health Care Services

- The Netherlands has 144 general hospitals, 8 of which are university based. There are also 4 children's hospitals, all located in the western part of the country.
- Access to specialized pediatric care is uniform throughout the Netherlands. General pediatrics is seen throughout the country at pediatrician offices, at family physician offices, and in EDs of the general hospitals. Children with complex special needs are referred to pediatric centers with the ability and expertise to manage their care. Because the country is small, is crowded, and distances are short, air transport services are only used for flying in a special advanced life support team.

Continued Use of the ED as a Primary Source of Episodic Health Care

- Restrictions or limitations in the operating hours of primary care providers often force caregivers to seek care at other sites. Lack of available care or trust in the family physician have also been identified as factors in the use of the EDs for nonurgent problems.
- Although the Dutch national poverty rate is low, the ED is the easiest and least-restricted entry in the health care delivery system, especially for those who are uninsured. Most children in the Netherlands have an established relationship with a primary health care provider but in the future this may change. The expectation is that there will be a shortage of family physicians in 2005.

Violence Against Children

- Violence against children occurs throughout the whole country, in both family and community environments.
- Scientific investigation has shown that every year 50,000 to 80,000 children (or 1 in every 10 children) in the Netherlands are victims of child maltreatment. At least 45 children die every year as a result of maltreatment. Despite improved recognition and reporting of child maltreatment, a significant number of cases remain unreported.
- In 2001, 23,000 referrals were made regarding suspected child maltreatment (physical or sexual abuse, neglect, emotional maltreatment) with approximately 35% of these allegations being substantiated. One to four referrals are related to emotional maltreatment.

Nonimmunized and Underimmunized Children

- Immunization rates for infants and young children are very high in the Netherlands—97% in the first year of life—with 90% of children receiving a complete immunization series. Three percent of the population is not immunized for religious reasons.
- Routine immunization schedules now include diphtheria, pertussis, tetanus, polio, measles, mumps, and rubella. In 1993 immunization for *H. influenzae type b* (Hib) was introduced, and in 2003 the meningococcal C vaccine were added. Rapid changes in immunization practice are reflected in guidelines and goals established by the Ministry of Welfare and Health Affairs.

Epidemiology (the Netherlands)

Pediatric Illness and Injury

The epidemiology of pediatric emergencies and determining the precise incidence and prevalence of pediatric emergency illness or injury remains complicated by a number of factors.

- Age definitions for pediatrics are not standardized.
- ED data are not consistently reported by each age category. The number of children with emergency conditions who are treated by primary health care providers is not well known.
- There is no nationally standardized reporting system for pediatric emergencies. The numbers on ED treatments are based on the Dutch Injury Surveillance System (LIS). LIS records statistics of people treated at EDs of about 15 hospitals in the Netherlands. These hospitals form a representative sample of the

general and university hospitals in the Netherlands with a continuously staffed ED. This enables extrapolation of the registered numbers to national figures, provided the numbers are large enough. Although only a selection of hospitals provide their data, it provides a random sample of all Dutch hospitals with a 24 hours/day accessible ED. Due to this, it is possible to calculate the numerical data on a national level.

- The number of hospital admissions is based on the Dutch Information System on Hospital Care and Day Nursing (LMR) by Prismant, which collects registration information on all persons admitted to a hospital in nearly all hospitals in the Netherlands. The external causes of injuries and poisoning are coded following the ICD-9 coding.

Because of the limited number of pediatric EDs, the majority of children seeking emergency care are seen in general EDs. Therefore, all emergency health care providers must be familiar with the signs and symptoms of a life-threatening illness or injury as well as subtle signs of deterioration in the pediatric patient.

In general, every year about 320,000 children, ages 0 through 18 years, are treated at an ED due to injuries caused by accidents, violence, or intentional self-harm. The prevalence of ED treatments is higher for males (58 %) than females (42 %). In addition, every year 25,000 children of this age group are admitted to the hospital.

Age 0 to 4 years

- Every year in the Netherlands 68,000 children of less than 4 years of age are treated at an ED due to injuries caused by accidents, violence, or intentional self-harm. The majority of these injuries are caused by home and leisure accidents, and about 9 % are caused by traffic accidents.
- Forty-one percent of the injuries involve injuries to the head. Injuries to the arms account for 33 %, and injuries to the legs account for 16 %. Furthermore 1,600 (2 %) children were treated in the ED due to poisoning.
- Every year 7,200 of these injured children are admitted to the hospital; 17 % are due to injuries involving a fracture, and 15 % are due to a brain injury without a skull fracture.
- The majority of deaths in this age group are due to infectious diseases and disorders originating in the perinatal period. Metabolic (endocrine) and respiratory diseases are other causes.

Age 5 to 14 years

- Every year about 170,000 children age 5 through 14 years are treated in an ED due to injuries caused by accidents, violence, or intentional self-harm. More than half (53 %) of the victims were injured due to a home and leisure accident, one third (32 %) by a sports accident, and 13 % due to a traffic accident.
- Half of the injuries involve injuries to the arms; 27 % involve injuries to legs.
- Annually 11,000 injured children in this age group are admitted to the hospital, 52 % for injuries involving a fracture, and 12 % with injuries involving the brain (without fracture of the skull).
- In this age group, disorders of the central nervous system (including head trauma) are the major causes of death, followed by the respiratory, metabolic, and cardiovascular diseases. Also in this age group, males are more often involved than females.

Age 14 to 18 years

- The largest number of ED treatments due to accidents, violence, or intentional self-harm are in this age group, 83,000 a year.
- One third (33 %) of the victims are injured due to a home and leisure accident, 29 % are injured due to a sports accident, and 23 % of the victims are injured due to a traffic accident.
- Most of the injuries involve injuries of the arms (41 %) and the legs (33); 16 % involve injuries of the head. In this age group 1,100 (1 %) of the victims are treated in the ED due to poisoning.
- Every year 6,600 early and middle adolescents of 14 through 18 years of age are admitted to the hospital, 38 % due to injuries involving fractures and 13 % due to injuries involving the brain (without a skull fracture).
- In this age group the same causes of death are found as the former group; however, psychiatric disorders (including suicide) are number 5 on this list instead of infectious diseases in the younger age group.

Trends in the Health of Dutch Youth

As is occurring in the rest of the world, the Dutch are seeing an increase in the incidence of childhood obesity. Sedentary lifestyles, video games, computers and television, consumption of fast food, alcohol, and drugs are all contributing factors.

This report was compiled using data from the following resources.

- Statistics Netherlands/Welfare and Health Yearbooks 2001/2002

- The Consumer Safety Institute/ED treatment and hospital admission due to accidents, violence, or intentional selfharm in children from 0-18 years, J.Haagsma, Sept. 2003.
- Information Statistics Netherlands available on Internet
  - www.rivm.nl
  - www.cbs.nl
  - www.prismant.nl (Dutch Information System on Hospital Care and Day Nursing)
  - www.consumentenveiligheid.nl (Dutch Injury Surveillance System)

Health Promotion

Measures to prevent childhood illnesses and injuries have a positive impact in reducing the incidence and cost associated with pediatric illnesses, injury, and death. Despite recent trends that illustrate improved immunization compliance, outbreaks of previously eradicated diseases have been seen over the past few years. Although a reduction in overall incidence is present, injury continues to plague the pediatric population. Some sources estimate that 90% of unintentional injuries could be avoided with prevention activities. For every dollar spent on a child safety restraint device, 32 dollars are saved in direct and indirect injury costs.[21]

Emergency nurses need to provide health promotion and injury prevention strategies to the patients and families they care for. Examples of methods that may prove successful in reducing childhood illness and injury are listed in **Table 2-1**.

Health promotion and injury prevention are essential aspects of the continuum of care. Educating pediatric patients and their families will make a difference in future outcomes.

Summary

This chapter describes characteristics of the pediatric population and the incidence of pediatric illness and injury. Epidemiology provides a foundation for understanding the health care needs of children and their families. Health promotion and injury prevention are essential aspects of the continuum of care. Educating pediatric patients and their families will make a difference in future outcomes.

References

1. Haller, J. A., Shorter, N., Miller, D., Colombani, P., Hall, J., & Buck, J. (1983). Organization and function of a regional trauma center. Does system management improve outcomes? *Journal of Trauma, 23*(8), 691–696.
2. Dieckmann, R. A. (1997). Epidemiology of pediatric emergency care. In R. A. Dieckmann, D. H. Fiser, & S. M. Selbst (Eds.), *Illustrated textbook of pediatric emergency and critical care procedures* (pp. 3-6). St. Louis, MO: Mosby-Year Book.
3. American Academy of Pediatrics. (2000). Access to pediatric emergency care. *Pediatrics, 105*(3), 647–654.
4. Weiss, H.B., Mathers, L. J., Forjuoh, S. N., & Kinnane, J. M. (1997). *Child and adolescent emergency department visit databook.* Pittsburgh, PA: Center for Violence and Injury Control, Allegheny University of Health Services.
5. American Academy of Pediatrics. (2000). Guiding principles for managed care arrangements for the healthcare of newborns, infants, children, adolescents, and young adults (RE9932). *Pediatrics, 105*(1), 132–135.
6. Centers for Disease Control and Prevention. (2001). *CDC Fact Book 2000/2001.* Retrieved on February 6, 2003 from http://www.cdc.gov/maso/factbook/Fact%20Book.pdf
7. Kini, N. M. & Strait, R. T. (1998). Nonurgent use of the pediatric emergency department during the day. *Pediatric Emergency Care, 14*(1), 19–21.

Table 2-1 Methods Successful in Reducing Childhood Illness and Injury

- Use teachable moments to discuss age-appropriate home safety measures.
- Remind children and parents to use child safety restraints at time of discharge.
- Encourage pool fencing laws.
- Display prevention materials in waiting and treatment areas.
- Present injury prevention programs in your community.
- Discuss measures to prevent the spread of contagious diseases, such as frequent handwashing and proper disposal of soiled diapers.

- Provide caregivers with information about immunization schedules and where they may be obtained.
- Inquire about nutritional intake and physical activity levels at health care visits.
- Promote healthy eating habits and regular physical activity and provide education, referrals, and information on diet and exercise.
- Assist caregivers in the identification of appropriate community resources and provide referrals as appropriate.

8. Altieri, M., Bellet, J., & Scott, H. (1990). Preparedness for pediatric emergencies encountered in the practitioner's office. *Pediatrics, 85*(5), 710–714.

9. McPherson, M., Arango, P., Fox, H., Lauver, C., McManus, M., Newacheck, P. W., et al. (1998). A new definition of children with special health care needs. *Pediatrics, 102*(Pt 1),137–140.

10. Adirim, T. (Ed.). (in press). *Special children's outreach and prehospital education.* Emergency Medical Services and Children with Special Health Care Needs Project. Washington, DC: Children's National Medical Center.

11. National Clearinghouse on Child Abuse and Neglect Information. (2002, April). Summary of key findings from calendar year 2000. *National Child Abuse and Neglect Data System (NCANDS).* Retrieved February 6, 2003 from http://www.calib.com/nccanch/pubs/factssheets/canstats.cfm

12. American Academy of Pediatrics. (1999). The role of the pediatrician in youth violence prevention in clinical practice and at the community level. *Pediatrics, 103*(1), 173–181.

13. American Academy of Pediatrics. (1998). Three-year study documents nature of television violence. *AAP News.* Retrieved February 6, 2003 from http://www.aap.org/advocacy/shifrin898.htm

14. Durch, J. S. & Lohn, K. N. (1993). Risking our children's health: A need for emergency care. In J. S. Durch & K. N. Lohn (Eds.), *Emergency medical services for children. Division of health care services, Institute of medicine* (pp. 38–65). Washington, DC: National Academy Press.

15. Athey, J., Dean, M., Ball, J., Wiebe, R., & Melese-d'Hospital, I. (2001). Ability of hospitals to care for pediatric emergency patients. *Pediatric Emergency Care, 17*(3), 170–174.

16. Krauss, B., Harakal, T., & Fleisher, G. R. (1991). The spectrum of frequency of illness presenting to a pediatric emergency department. *Pediatric Emergency Care, 7*(2), 67–71.

17. Pachter, L., Ludwig, S., & Groves, A. (1991). Night people: Utilization of a pediatric emergency department during the night. *Pediatric Emergency Care, 7*(1), 12–14.

18. Nelson, D. S., Walsh, K., & Fleisher, G. (1992). Spectrum and frequency of pediatric illness presenting to a general community hospital emergency department. *Pediatrics, 90*(Pt 1), 5–10.

19. Federal Interagency Forum on Child and Family Statistics. (2002). *America's children: Key national indicators of well-being, 2002.* Washington, DC: U.S. Government Printing Office.

20. National Center for Injury Prevention and Control. (2001). *10 leading causes of death, United States, 2000, all races, both sexes.* Retrieved February 6, 2003 from http://webapp.cdc.gov/cgi-bin/broker.exe

21. National Safe Kids Campaign. (1999). *Fact sheets: Childhood injury facts 1999.* Washington, DC: National Safe Kids Campaign. Retrieved February 6, 2003 from http://www.safekids.org/tier3_cd.cfm?content_item_id=1030&folder_id=540

22. National Center for Injury Prevention and Control. (2002). *Unintentional mv-occupant nonfatal injuries and rates per 100,000. 2001, United States, all races, both sexes, ages 1 to 20.* Retrieved February 6, 2003 from http://www.cdc.gov/ncipc/wisqars

23. Ng, E. (1996). Disability among Canada's Aboriginal peoples in 1991. *Health Reports, 8*(1), 25–32.

24. Chen, J., Ng, E., & Wilkins, R. (1996). The health of Canada's immigrants in 1994–1995. *Health Reports, 7*(4), 33–45.

25. Statistics Canada. (1998). The nation series, complete edition, 1996 census. In *The health of Canada's children: A CICH profile* (3rd ed.). Ottawa, Canada: Canadian Institute of Child Health.

26. Statistics Canada. (1998). Low income persons. 1980–1997. In *The health of Canada's children: A CICH profile* (3rd ed.). Ottawa, Canada: Canadian Institute of Child Health.

27. Health Canada. (2001). *Canadian incidence study of reported child abuse and neglect: Final report.* Retrieved February 6, 2003 from http://www.hc-sc.gc.ca.

28. Health Canada Population and Public Health Branch. (2002). *Canadian immunization guide comparison of diseases and vaccines* (6th ed.). Retrieved February 6, 2003 from http://www.hc-sc.gc.ca29.

29. Health Canada Population and Public Health Branch. (2002). *The Canadian immunization guide recommended immunizations for infants, children and adults.* Retrieved February 6, 2003 from http://www.hc.sc.gc.ca

30. Health Canada. (1999). Canadian national report on immunization, 1998. Pediatrics & child health, Vol. 4, Supplement C. In *The health of Canada's children: A CICH profile* (3rd ed.). Ottawa, Canada: Canadian Institute of Child Health.

31. National Trauma Registry. (2002). *Report of hospital injury admissions.* Ottawa, Canada: Canadian Institute for Health Information.

32. Canadian Pediatric Society. (2002). Healthy active living for children and youth. *Pediatrics & Child Health, 7*(5), 339–345. [Electronic version]. Retrieved August 29, 2002 from www.cps.ca

33. Australian Bureau of Statistics. (2002). *National health survey of results–Australia 4364.0.* Retrieved August 29, 2002 from: http://www.abs.gov.au

34. Harding, A. & Szukalska, A. (1998, November 26). *A portrait of child poverty in Australia in 1995–1996.* Paper presented at the 6th Australian Institute of Family Studies Conference, Melbourne.

35. Stanley, F. J. (2001). Child health since Federation. *Australian Bureau of Statistics Year Book.* Retrieved August 29, 2002 from http://www.abs.gov.au/Ausstats/ABS.

36. Australians Against Child Abuse. (2002). *What is child abuse?* Retrieved August 29, 2002 from http://www.aaca.netlink.com.au/whatis/

37. NSW Commission for Children and Young People. (2002). *NSW child death review team.* Retrieved August 29, 2002 from http://www.kids.nsw.gov.au/publications/cdrt2000.html

38. Australian Bureau of Statistics. (2002). *Causes of infant and child deaths – Australia 43980.* Retrieved August 29, 2002 from http://www.abs.gov.au

39. Australian Bureau of Statistics. (2002). *Australian social trends 2002 health – National summary tables.* Retrieved August 29, 2003 from http://www.abs.gov.au

40. Australian Bureau of Statistics. (2002). *Australian social trends 2002 health – Mortality & morbidity: Infant mortality.* Retrieved August 29, 2002 from http://www.abs. gov.au

41. Bordeaux, S., & Harrison, J. (1998). Injury mortality in Australia 1995. *Australian Injury Prevention Bulletin, 17.*

chapter 3

FROM THE START — DEALING WITH CHILDREN

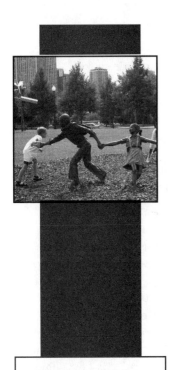

Objectives

On completion of this chapter, the learner should be able to:

1. Discuss basic anatomic and physiologic characteristics of children that may affect their response to illness and injury.

2. Describe key growth and development characteristics of infants, toddlers, preschoolers, school-aged children, and adolescents.

3. Identify age-appropriate techniques to facilitate assessment and intervention through case-scenario presentation.

4. Delineate specific nursing interventions for the pediatric patient based on developmental stages.

Vignette: You are called to a room to assist with a 4-year-old who was brought in via prehospital providers after falling from a second-story window. His cervical spine is stabilized, and he is immobilized on a backboard. The Pediatric Assessment Triangle reveals that his color is pale, he appears in no respiratory distress, and he is quietly crying and does not respond to verbal commands (his eyes are tightly closed). Prehospital providers stated that he was verbal en route until he saw bleeding from lacerations and abrasions on his arms and legs.

What can you do to facilitate the assessment of this preschooler?

Introduction

Childhood—it is a dynamic state of change. It is the very change that brings joy and challenge to every parent but also brings fear and anxiety into the hearts of many health care providers! Health care providers caring for children need to understand basic growth and development in order to provide age-appropriate assessments and plans of care required to care for the pediatric patient.

Each stage of childhood brings about unique changes in anatomic, physiologic, and developmental characteristics that will affect assessments and interventions. Each stage necessitates a different approach. Health care providers must also recognize the unique characteristics in caring for children with special health care needs. Chapter 16 provides additional information regarding children with special health care needs. The purpose of this chapter is to highlight pediatric developmental changes and describe specific approaches to the pediatric patient that will facilitate their effective assessment.

The Child and the Family

The family plays an integral role in the growth and development of children. But first we must define what a family is. The family has been defined differently over the years in terms of roles and responsibilities, structure and function, and biological and genetic relationships, just to name a few. Most significantly when referring to children, families comprise a group of individuals (at least one adult) living in the same house or nearby who take care of one another and provide support and direction for the children.[1] However the family is defined—single families, blended families, foster families, adopted families, extended families—all have common concerns regarding their ill or injured child. The identification of "Mom" and "Dad" may be extended to individuals within the family unit who function in the role.

The parents and other caregivers play an essential role in a child's health care experience.[2] This factor alone differentiates caring for children as compared to adults. The child is not the only patient who requires attention. The family unit must be considered during every interaction with a child, especially if the child is seriously ill or injured. Communicating effectively with the parents is of critical importance to enable obtaining the history and consent for treatment.[2]

The family's response to a child's illness or injury will directly influence how the child responds. The child's and the family's response may be influenced by many of the factors listed in **Box 3-1**.[2,3,5]

Natural parental instincts sometimes evoke strong emotional responses to situations involving their children. Parental responses are affected by a number of emotional factors including guilt, fear, disbelief, anger, and loss of control.[2,5] A parent's own anxiety and reaction may negatively affect his or her ability to comfort the child, to understand information communicated to them, to participate in decision making regarding the child's care, and to recall information required for discharge.[2]

Cultural and religious traditions and values influence family function and health care beliefs and practices, as well as the family and child's response to an illness or injury. Health-related cultural perceptions and the perceived meaning of health and illness affect approaches to treatment and help-seeking behaviors.[6] During the assessment period, it is helpful to elicit information regarding their birth country, the length of time they have lived in this country, the language spoken at home, and information regarding use of home remedies, including over-the-counter and prescription medications, herbal and natural supplements, and health care practices.[3] Health care providers must be aware of cultural differences that can create communication barriers. These cultural differences include eye contact, personal space, and the use of touch and conversation style.[7]

Because of the diversity of society, the health care provider is often confronted not only by an ill or injured child, but also with a range of diverse beliefs related to health and healing practices. The process of performing a cultural assessment is an approach that health care providers can utilize to facilitate understanding of the family's lifestyle, beliefs, and decision-making processes. Failure to recognize how culture influences health and illness can contribute to ineffective and culturally biased care.[26] Six key elements, as shown in **Box 3-2**, facilitate the process of becoming culturally competent.[26]

When caring for children and families from various cultural backgrounds, it is important to identify health care patterns and beliefs that may be a factor in treatment interventions or discharge planning.[8,26] The information obtained from the cultural assessment is essential in the provision of culturally competent care. Assessment of the views and beliefs of the child and family facilitates

---

Box 3-1 Factors that influence child's and family's responses to illness and injury[2,3,4]

- The child's age and developmental stage
- The actual and perceived severity of the situation
- The severity of the physical pain
- Any previous experiences with the health care system
- Previously developed coping skills
- Their cultural beliefs and practices regarding health, illness, pain, and death
- Presence of language barriers
- The presence or availability of support systems
- The current events within the family unit
- The suddenness or expectedness of the situation

Box 3-2 Key elements to facilitate becoming culturally competent[26]

- Actively work on changing your view of the world and reframe thinking about groups with different thoughts and beliefs.
- Increase knowledge about the cultural groups within your community.
- Identify core cultural issues within these cultural groups (such as style of communication, personal space, and family relationships).
- Identify core cultural issues within these cultural groups related to health, health care practices, and illness beliefs.
- Develop a trusting relationship with empathy, understanding, and respect.
- Discuss and adapt interventions that are culturally acceptable to the family and medically beneficial (not harmful) to the patient.

Box 3-3 Sample questions to identify religious and cultural beliefs[8,9]

- Why do you think your child has this problem? The family may believe the illness is caused by Karma, evil, or offended spirits, or have demonic origins.
- Why did it start when it did?
- In your home country, who would you see about this problem, and who would treat the child? Family may see a healer or a family elder. What kind of treatment would be done, and who would administer the treatment?
- How long do you think this illness or problem will last?
- What treatments have you (or your healer) tried at home or in the past?
- What results do you hope your child will receive from the treatments? What treatment do you think your child should receive?
- Do you plan to continue to use those treatments, or are there treatments you will use along with those prescribed in the emergency department?
- Will your healer (or others involved) work with us to make your child well?

treatment and discharge planning, incorporation of cultural practices, and negotiation of culturally acceptable modifications to the discharge plan.[6,26] If the family's approach or practices may be harmful to the child, the health care providers can approach these issues and provide the family with information concerning the implications of those customs. The detail and depth of the cultural assessment will be dependent on the situation and the needs of the child and family. **Table 3-1** provides a practice model for assisting emergency care providers in their approach to cultural diversity and cultural assessment.[6]

Box 3-3 contains a series of questions that may assist the emergency nurse in identifying religious and cultural beliefs related to a child's illness and the family's usual health care routines, including folk-healing practices.[8,9]

Sensitivity to the issues of culture and religion is essential in the emergency care of the pediatric patient. It is impossible for the emergency care team to have knowledge of all types of cultural and religious diversity. Therefore, the use of a diversity model approach is an integral part of the nursing process.

Family-Centered Care

The family is a constant in the child's life and must be able to provide comfort and support to the child during emergency care. The development of a family-supportive environment is an important component of providing family-centered care. In the emergency department (ED), family-centered care incorporates supporting and encouraging family participation and presence during all phases of care.[3] Family participation and involvement in the child's health care promotes collaborative relationships among the health care professional, the patient, and the family. Facilitating family presence during invasive procedures or resuscitation situations is a core component of family-centered care practices. Core components to family-centered care include the following.

- Treating the patients and families with dignity and consideration
- Communicating information without bias
- Encouraging family participation that enhances control and autonomy[10]

Family members of critically ill patients have identified that their most important needs include

- Being present with the patient
- Being helpful to the patient

Table 3-1 Diversity Practice Model[6]

Definition	Application to Assessment
Assumptions: The act of taking for granted or supposing that a thought or idea is true.	*Assumptions are often based on limited experience, bias, or generalizing.* What are my assumptions, and what are they based on?
Beliefs and behaviors: Beliefs are shared ideas about how a group operates. Behaviors are the ways a group conducts itself.	*All patients must be treated with the same respect and dignity, regardless of their diversity.* How do your assumptions compare to what you believe about certain groups?
Communication: The two-way sharing of information that results in an understanding between the receiver and the sender.	*An early assessment must be made regarding the patient's ability to comprehend what is being said.* As communication begins, the emergency care provider's body language must be one of acceptance and respect.
Diversity: The way in which people differ and the effect that differences have on the response to health care.	*There is a wide variety of symptom management among diverse groups.* How does the patient's diversity affect their response to health/illness or the emergency care provider's response to the patient?
Education and ethics: Gaining knowledge about a cultural group and recognizing that ethical issues may be viewed differently by different culturally diverse groups	*The development of a cultural reference manual or collection of reference materials on cultural practices and health beliefs are indispensable in the emergency department (ED).* Criteria for evaluation of staff competency must be developed with periodic evaluation.

- Being informed and updated on the patient's condition
- Being comforted and supported by family members and by health care providers
- Feeling that the patient received the best care possible[10]

Family Presence

The Emergency Nurses Association (ENA),[10] American Association of Critical-Care Nurses (AACN), and numerous physician groups support the option of family presence during invasive procedures and resuscitation. The practice of allowing family presence during invasive procedures and resuscitation is a component of family-centered care.

Research and practice reflect this support. In one study involving pediatricians, findings indicated that those with more frequent contact with seriously ill children were more likely to accept parental presence during cardiopulmonary resuscitation and that the exposure to parental presence during resuscitation increased the probability of allowing parental presence in future resuscitations.[27] In a study from the United Kingdom, 100% of pediatric critical care nurses and 68% of pediatric critical care physicians indicated that parental presence during resuscitation should be a choice.[28] A recent study surveying AACN and ENA members revealed that nearly one-half of the participants indicated that their departments permitted the option of family presence during invasive procedures or resuscitation, even though few institutions have written policies or guidelines regarding family presence.[31]

Before a family member is offered the option to be present during the invasive procedure or resuscitation, a health care provider must assess if the family can cope with the situation. If a family member appears out of control or too emotional, they may be distracting and disruptive to the health care providers caring for the child. In this case, it may not be advisable to offer the opportunity for family presence. A designated member of the staff who functions to support the family and serve as a patient and parent advocate should remain with the family independent of their decision to be present with the child.[25]

The option to remain present during invasive or resuscitation procedures must be the choice of the caregiver.[11,12,30] If the caregiver chooses not to stay with the child, respect that decision and continue to provide appropriate support and explanations.[12] If the caregiver chooses to remain with the child, the health care team must ensure that the caregiver is provided with the following.

- Clear explanations of the procedure(s) and the child's expected responses

- Instruction on strategies to use to facilitate the child's coping with the procedure, as appropriate
- Assessment in relation to his or her support needs
- Emotional support and ongoing explanations by designated staff during resuscitation measures
- Support by staff, as needed, during other invasive procedures

Prior to escorting a family member(s) into the room of a child being resuscitated, the health care provider supporting the family must prepare them for what they will hear, see, and smell.[25] Inform the family of where they should remain while in the room and, if possible, facilitate the opportunity to touch the child. The health care provider supporting the family should offer ongoing narration of activates in a soft, calm, and directive voice. Focus on the child's responses and changes in condition. Should the resuscitation efforts not result in positive changes in the child's condition, the health care provider supporting the family must remember that their role is to support family presence and to avoid being drawn into the "doing" role that emergency providers are accustomed to during critical situations and resuscitation.

Historically family members have been excluded from participation and presence during invasive procedures or resuscitation[31] so encouraging family presence during these events is controversial for some health care providers. Many are concerned that family presence will hinder caring for the patient, that it will be distracting to the members of the team providing care and that it will increase stress amongst the team.[13,31] Contrary to this belief, studies that have been published so far do not confirm these findings.

The Process of Growth and Development

Although growth and development occur simultaneously, they are distinct and separate processes. Patterns of growth and development are predictable, directional, and sequential in nature. They are multifaceted processes that involve and are affected by genetic, nutritional, and environmental factors. Disturbances in these factors may alter the process of growth and development in a child. The sequential nature of growth and development remains the same in normally developing children.[14] Factors that affect growth and development include heredity, neuroendocrine processes, gender, chronic disease, environment hazards, seasonal variances, prenatal influences, nutrition, socioeconomic status, and relationships with significant others.[15]

The term growth refers to the increase in the number of cells and results in an increase in physical size.[15] Growth rates are similar in all cultures, but key differences in race, ethnicity, and gender can be identified.[7] These changes can be plotted on growth charts specific for boys and girls and age range (including head circumference, height, and weight, and body mass index). **Table 3-2** reviews the anatomic and physiologic features of children.

Development refers to the gradual and successive increase in abilities or skills along a predetermined path (often referred to as developmental milestones or tasks).[15] Development is generally age specific and reflects neuro-

Table 3-2 Anatomic and Physiologic Features of Children with Clinical Implications

Assessment	Pediatric Features	Clinical Implications
Airway	Large tongue relative to size of oropharynx	Common cause of airway obstruction; resolved with repositioning of airway.
	Obligate nose breathers	Infants under 4 months can appear to be in respiratory distress from nasal congestion; resolved by keeping nasal passages clear of secretions.
	Smaller airway diameter	Small amounts of blood, mucus, edema, or small foreign objects can easily obstruct airway and increase resistance to airflow.
	Cricoid cartilage narrowest area	Provides an anatomical seal for uncuffed or cuffless endotracheal tubes in children less than 8 years of age.
	Larynx more anterior and cephalad	Increased risk for aspiration causing airway obstruction.
	Cartilaginous larynx	Increased risk for compression of airway with hyperflexion or hyperextension resulting in airway obstruction.
	Short neck, short trachea	Easily dislodge endotracheal tube of intubated patient with head movement; also increases risk for right mainstem intubation.
Breathing	Compensatory mechanisms less effective	Although children in respiratory distress may initially increase both their work of breathing and respiratory rate, they tire easily, resulting in rapid decompensation.
	Higher metabolic rate	Results in a more rapid respiratory rate and less efficient use of oxygen and glucose. Additionally, other symptoms, such as fever and anxiety may further increase metabolic rate.
	Respiratory rate varies with age	Normal respiratory rate is inversely related to age; rates are higher in infants and decrease with age. Children with sustained respiratory rates (RR) over 60 are at risk for respiratory arrest. A slow or irregular RR in an acutely ill infant or child is an ominous sign.[17]
	Thin chest wall	Breath sounds are easily transmitted; for example, breath sounds may be auscultated over a pneumothorax.
	Cartilaginous sternum and ribs and resultant compliant chest wall	Children in respiratory distress often display retractions; if severe, can result in inability to generate adequate tidal volume.
	Poorly developed intercostal muscles	Children rely on diaphragm for respirations; resolved by maintaining a sitting position to promote diaphragmatic excursion.
	Diaphragm positioned flat	Anything that impinges on movement of diaphragm from above (asthma) or below (abdominal distention) impedes diaphragm function and respirations.
	Ribs horizontally oriented	Prevents increasing tidal volume when stressed; therefore, respiratory rate is increased.
	Fewer smaller alveoli	Fewer alveoli, therefore less surface area for gas exchange.
Circulation	Increased circulating blood volume. Infant: 90 ml/kg; child 80 ml/kg; adult 70 ml/kg.	Small amounts of blood loss can lead to circulatory compromise.
	Rapid heart rate	Normal ranges vary with developmental stage.
	Myocardium less compliant with less contractile mass and limited stroke volume	Cardiac output (CO) is maintained by increasing heart rate (HR) rather than stroke volume (SV). CO = HR X SV. The CO falls quickly with HR > 200 beats per minute or bradycardia. Tachycardia is an early sign of shock.
	Infants have higher cardiac output than adults	This provides for increased oxygen demand but depletes cardiac output reserve; times of increased stress such as hypothermia or sepsis may lead to rapid deterioration.

Table 3-2 cont. Anatomic and Physiologic Features of Children with Clinical Implications

Assessment	Pediatric Features	Clinical Implications
	Strong compensatory mechanisms maintain cardiac output for long periods of time. Rapid deterioration occurs when compensatory mechanisms are exhausted.	Compensatory mechanisms will shunt blood to vital organs and away from periphery. Skin temperature, skin color, and capillary refill will be affected. Hypotension is a late sign of circulatory compromise as children may remain normotensive until 25% of volume is lost.[17]
	Higher percentage body water for body weight	Can become dehydrated more rapidly.
	Immature renal function in infants	Dehydration can occur rapidly in infants due to their inability to concentrate urine. Need to monitor output closly. Normal urine ouput is 1-2cc/kg/hr.
	Neonates have poorly developed sympathetic nervous system.	Neonates sensitive to parasympathetic stimulation, such as suctioning and defecating, and may have a bradycardic response.
Disability (Neurological)	Immature reflexes present at birth.	Babinski and Moro reflexes are normal findings.
	Anterior fontanel closes between 12 to 18 months.	Gradual increases in intracranial pressure can be accommodated by increasing skull size.
	Level of consciousness	Greatly affected by adequate ventilation and oxygenation.
	Babinski reflex normal until child begins to walk.	Presence of Babinski in walking child is an abnormal finding.
	Flexion is the normal body posture of an infant.	Useful assessment finding indicating normal neurological function.
	Infants have an immature autonomic nervous system.	Body temperature control due to environmental changes is limited.
Exposure	Infants less than 3 months are unable to produce heat through shivering and must burn brown fat for thermogenesis; known as nonshivering thermogenesis.	This process increases metabolic rate and increases use of oxygen and glucose.
	Infants and children have a higher body surface area (BSA) to weight ratio. Significant heat loss occurs from the skin on the infant's large head.	Ill and injured infants and children are at increased risk for hypothermia. Hypothermia may result in respiratory depression, impaired peripheral oxygen delivery, irritability of heart, metabolic acidosis, hypoglycemia, coagulopathy, and alteration in level of consciousness.
Additional differences	Body weight changes with age. Weight estimate (pounds): 2 times birth weight (BW) by 6 months; 3 times BW by 1 year; 7 times BW by 7 years; 14 times BW by 14 years. Weight estimate (kg) = 8 + 2 (age in years).	Accurate estimates necessary for administration of fluids and medications. When possible, all pediatric patients should be weighed on admission. If weight is not available, use standardized length-based resuscitation tapes that estimate weight based on length.
	High metabolic rate with limited glycogen stores	Increases use of glucose/glycogen storage and increases risk for hypo-glycemia.
	Greater insensible fluid loss	Insensible fluid losses occur through respiration and skin losses. Children have a greater maintenance fluid requirement, which is calculated per kg and adjusted to their condition.
	Incomplete bone calcification	Absence of fractures (even in long bones) does not rule out injury to other structures.
	Medications are metabolized differently in children	All medications are based on kilogram weight.
	Children have a proportionally larger and heavier head as compared to body size, which contributes to a higher center of gravity.	Children are at high risk for head injury. They tend to fall headfirst during a fall.
	Infants have weak neck muscles combined with a large heavy head.	Infants less than 1 year of age and less than 20 lbs must be rear facing in their car seat.

logical, emotional, and social maturation. Although there is cross-cultural similarity in the sequence and timing of developmental milestones, culture exerts an all-pervasive influence on the developing child.[7]

General Approach to the Pediatric Patient

Remembering these basic caveats will assist all health care providers in working with the pediatric patient and their family.

- Establish a child-friendly environment using bright colors, paintings, mobiles, and cartoons.
- Allow the caregiver to remain with the child whenever possible.
- Address the child by his or her name. Ask the child or caregiver what name to use when addressing the child.
- Communicate with the family using nonmedical terminology, especially when talking about planned interventions, treatments, and findings.
- Observe the level of consciousness, activity level (interaction with environment and caregiver), position of comfort, skin color, respiratory rates and effort, and degree of discomfort before touching the child.
- Provide privacy.
- Compare assessment findings with the caregivers' description of their child's normal behavior (i.e., eating and sleeping habits, activity level, and level of consciousness).
- Be honest with the child and caregiver. Provide explanations at the child's developmental level.
- Speak in a calm, empathetic, and directive tone.
- Parents require reassurance and explanations of the situation and the anticipated plan of treatment.
- Acknowledge positive behavior, encourage the child during the procedure, and praise the child afterward. Provide rewards such as stars, stickers, and bandages.
- Allow the child to make simple age-appropriate choices and to participate in their care. Examples include asking the child which arm to measure their muscle (blood pressure) and then providing directions to insufflate the blood pressure cuff.
- Encourage play.
- Use diversion and distraction. Encourage them to blow bubbles and blow the hurt away, to sing their favorite songs (and sing with them), to picture their favorite place, and describe in detail with their senses.
- Give them permission to express their feelings. Tell them it is okay to cry. Sympathy is essential.
- Assess for pain using age-appropriate assessment tools

and guidelines. Identify the child's typical response to pain. Most pain states are characterized by a global pattern of physiologic arousal, which can result in increased heart rate, increased blood pressure, and increased respiratory rate and depth. However, if pain has persisted for several hours or days, these responses are often modified, and cardiovascular and respiratory measurements may be normal.

- Be cautious about what you say in the presence of an apparently unconscious child.
- Health promotion teaching must be tailored to the child's potential risks and needs associated with the child's current developmental level and upcoming developmental changes. Anticipatory guidance should also be provided and include well care and injury and illness prevention. Health promotion education and anticipatory guidance applicable to all age groups may include the following points.
  - The importance of establishing and maintaining a medical home with a primary care provider (PCP) for the child. For children without a PCP, provide information for referrals to PCPs or provide information to obtain health care.
  - Review immunization status of the child. Identify community resources for obtaining low- or no-cost immunizations. Refer to Appendix A for current Childhood Immunization Schedule.
  - The health risks associated with the child's exposure to secondhand smoke, particularly if the child has any allergies, frequent upper respiratory problems, or hyperactive airway disease
  - The use of hand washing to prevent the spread of infections and the need to reduce contacts when a viral or bacterial infection is present
  - Injury prevention focused on risks associated with child's developmental level, including home safety, the use of appropriate child restraints for cars, seat belts, helmets, and other protective equipment. Convey to parents that preventable injuries are the leading cause of death and disability in children.
  - Tips for choosing age-appropriate toys. Suggest the use of the choke tube or toilet paper roll to judge toys that are too small for children less than 3 years of age.
  - Provide the National Poison Center contact number- 1-800-222-1222. Telephone stickers and information are available by calling the toll-free number.
  - Child abuse prevention and community domestic violence resources
  - Parenting information and community resources including The National Safe Kids Campaign® and cardiopulmonary resuscitation courses.

Communicating with children takes knowledge, thoughtfulness, and practice. In any health care setting and particularly in the emergency setting, the child is often frightened by the surroundings, the strangers, and the reason for which they are there. The initial interaction with the pediatric patient needs to acknowledge psychosocial characteristics of the child's development, particularly the common fears and emotions. Understanding these characteristics will promote more effective interactions and accurate assessment of the child. Refer to Appendix B for Childhood Development and **Table 3-3** for a review of common fears and emotions of children in the ED setting.[2,15]

Neonate (birth to 28 days of age)

For additional information, see Chapter 14.

Psychosocial Development

- Following birth, neonates may sleep for the next 2 to 3 days to recover from the trauma of birth.
- Neonates will indiscriminately visually follow anyone meeting their basic needs.[32]
- Parent uses stimulation to play with neonate (such as looking at neonate at close proximity, talking and singing, cradling and rocking infant).[32]
- Pleasure is demonstrated by a quieting attitude.[32]
- Crying is the primary language to express need or displeasure.
- Behavior is reflexive in nature (e.g., sucking, swallowing, rooting, grasping, and crying).[14,32]

Anatomic and Physiologic Characteristics

- The neonate loses between 5 to 10 % of its birth weight (BW) by the third or fourth day of life. Most neonates will return to their BW by the tenth day of life.
- The preterm infant is considered a neonate until the expected due date is reached plus 28 days.

- Neonatal reflexes should be symmetrical. Arm and leg recoil to a state of complete flexion is symmetric. Primary reflexes present at birth include the sucking, rooting, grasping, startle, Moro, and Babinski.[32]
- Flexion is the normal posture, with the extremities pulled close to the chest and abdomen.
- Most neonates are awake and crying for 1 to 4 hours a day. The other hours of the day comprise varying sleep patterns and alert inactivity.[4]
- Breasts in both genders may be enlarged with white liquid (witch's milk) for up to 2 weeks due to maternal estrogen. Females may have some vaginal discharge.
- BSA to weight ratio is three times that of the adult; therefore, heat loss is of great concern.
- Neonates are vulnerable to hypoglycemia due to their limited glycogen stores.

Approaching the Neonate

- Observe the infant for general appearance and condition, skin color, and work of breathing before touching the neonate. Neonates will usually cry when disturbed.
- Assessment should progress from the toe to head direction.
- Neonates are unconcerned about strangers and respond to soothing voices and warm gentle hands.

Infants (1 to 12 months of age)

Psychosocial Development

- Infancy is a period of rapid physical and psychosocial growth and development. Infants are dependent on caregivers to meet their needs.
- Infants understand and experience the world through their bodies. Being held, cuddled, rocked, or comforted with familiar touch and smells soothes infants and develops their sense of trust.[33]

Table 3-3 Common Fears and Emotions in the ED Setting[1,2,3]

Stage of development	Common fears and emotions in the emergency setting
Infant	Pain and discomfort, unfamiliarity with environment, loud sounds, being handled by strangers, separation from caregiver, disruption in feeding and sleeping
Toddlers 1 to 3 years	Pain and discomfort, separation from caregiver, being handled by strangers, darkness, sudden or loud noises, loss of control, loss of mobility
Early childhood (Preschooler) 3 to 5 years	Pain and discomfort often misinterpreted, fear of injury and insides leaking out, unfamiliar environment increases imagination and fear of monsters and ghosts, the dark
School-age 5 to 12 years	Pain and discomfort, feel guilty and responsible for event, darkness, especially in unfamiliar environment, staying alone, appearing physically different from friends
Adolescents	Extreme self-consciousness, loss of autonomy, change in body image, feeling of hopelessness (with chronic illness), anger, separation from peer group and social isolation, appearing physically different from friends

- Common fears, especially for older infants, include separation anxiety and stranger anxiety. Infants' relationship with primary caregivers is crucial for their sense of well-being.
- Infants explore objects by sucking, chewing, and biting. The more mobile, older infant has an increased risk for injury by poisoning, foreign body aspiration, falls, and drowning.

Anatomic and Physiologic Characteristics
- 50th percentile weight is 3.5 to 10 kg.
- Infants are obligate nose breathers for the first several months of life. Blocked or partially blocked nasal passages may cause respiratory distress.
- Infants breathe predominately using abdominal muscles. Any pressure on the diaphragm from above or below can impede respiratory effort.
- The metabolic rate in infants is approximately two times the adult rate. This results in an increased need for oxygen and glucose (calories).
- The infant's circulating blood volume is 90 ml/kg. Volume losses that may be perceived as insignificant can cause circulatory compromise. Volume losses occur primarily due to inadequate intake, vomiting and diarrhea, increased insensible losses, or hemorrhage.
- Infants in the first few months of life have immature renal function. The kidneys cannot efficiently concentrate the urine to conserve water. Normal urine output is 2 ml/kg/hr.
- In infants, the autonomic nervous system is not fully developed. The ability to control body temperature in response to environmental changes is limited.
- Although the central nervous system remains immature, by 6 to 8 weeks, infants can fix on and follow objects placed in front of them.

Approaching Infants
- Approach the infant slowly, gently, and calmly. Loud voices and rapid movements may frighten the infant.
- Assess the infant while he or she is held by the caregiver, whenever possible, to decrease separation anxiety.
- Provide comfort by rocking, swaying, swaddling, and singing to the infant. Up to about 7 months of age, the infant can be comforted by strangers as long as their basic needs are met. Stranger anxiety varies among infants and is dependent on the variety of caregivers in the child's life and individual temperament.
- Vary the sequence of the assessment with the infant's activity level. If the infant is calm and quiet, obtain the respiratory rate and auscultate the lungs at the beginning of the assessment.[18]

- Complete the most distressing (touching) components of the exam last. When examining the infant, warmed hands and stethoscope are less distressing.
- Provide opportunity for self-comforting measures by encouraging access to hand for sucking and use of pacifiers.[3,33]
- Avoid insertion of intravenous lines into the infants' favored extremities whenever possible, as they may want to suck their finger(s), thumb, or hand.
- Provide distraction and diversion during treatments and procedures.
- Explain to the caregivers that the infant will cry once the procedure is initiated. Unlike other age groups, young infants make no link between approaching stimulus and pain.

Anticipatory Guidance and Health Promotion for Neonates and Infants
- Encourage caregivers to lessen the risk for injury within the home by shortening window shade cords and covering electrical outlets.
- Place the infant on its back to sleep.
- If using pacifiers, purchase those with one-piece construction of looped handle.
- Provide age-appropriate injury prevention pamphlets such as those provided by The National Safe Kids Campaign®, the ENA, and the American Academy of Pediatrics (AAP).
- Instruct caregivers to transport infants safely in infant carriers when traveling in motor vehicles and by aircraft. The safest location for the infant car seat is rear facing in the rear seat. Provide airbag information including injury risk associated with air bag deployment and car seats.
- Encourage caregivers with older infants and toddlers to select shopping carts with seat belts attached to the seat section and to avoid children riding in the basket or standing.
- Discourage caregivers from using baby walkers. Walker use increases mobility and access to dangerous objects. This places infants at risk for injury due to falls and the ability to reach potentially dangerous items on tables, counters, and stove tops. Encourage parents to use stationary play stations, such as playpens and highchairs.[19,33]
- Provide poison center information, and encourage caregivers to survey the home for potential hazards and remove them before the infant becomes mobile.
- Review the recommended routine immunizations with the family.[33] If the infant's immunization record is available and the infant is behind schedule, administer needed immunizations and document on the

immunization record. Provide appropriate vaccine information. Be prepared to discuss the risks and benefits, contraindications, and possible reactions.

- Infants explore with their mouth, which places them at greater risk for foreign body airway obstruction. Encourage caregivers to keep small objects from infants. Educate the family on the use of a "choke tube" or toilet paper roll to safely measure toys and objects that are too small for the young child to handle and play. The choke tube is a commercially available safety measure that is intended to simulate the size of a child's airway in relationship to the size of object that a small child can handle safely.

Toddlers (1 to 3 years of age)

Psychosocial Developmental

- Toddlers are in a stage of rapid physical and psychological growth and development. By about 18 months of age, the toddler is able to run, grasp, and manipulate objects, feed himself or herself, play with toys, and communicate with others.
- Toddlers may have erratic eating patterns as compared to infants and older children.
- Toddlers are curious, and with their improved mobility they have no sense of danger, therefore making them vulnerable to serious injury.
- Cognitively, a toddlers' thinking is concrete, and they interpret words literally. They have an increased ability to problem solve through trial and error.
- Toddlers are able to communicate verbally. Their negativism and insistence express an increasing need for autonomy.[34]
- They strive for independence and are strong willed, with their favorite word being "NO."
- Common fears include separation from the caregiver and loss of control. They delight in the ability to control themselves and others. The toddler tends to cling to a caregiver when apprehensive.
- A major task of toddlerhood is toilet training. Physiologic and psychologic readiness (such as sphincter tone and interpretation of urge, respectively) usually occur between 18 to 24 months.[34]
- Toddlers' experiences are still strongly sensory based: Seeing is believing.
- Imitates health behaviors of primary caregivers.

Anatomic and Physiologic Characteristics

- 50th percentile weight is 10 to 12 kg.
- A Babinski reflex is normally present until the toddler starts walking. After 2 years of age the child should have a plantar reflex.
- The toddler continues to use abdominal muscles for breathing.
- The toddler has improved thermoregulatory ability but may still develop cold stress when critically ill or injured and exposed for extended periods of time.
- The head is larger than the rest of the body, making it more vulnerable to injury until approximately 6 to 8 years of age.

Approaching Toddlers

- Approach the toddler gradually. Keep physical contact minimal until the toddler is acquainted with you. Use a quiet, soothing voice.
- Incorporate play while assessing the toddler (e.g., "Show me your bellybutton"). If the child becomes upset or apprehensive, complete the assessment as expeditiously as possible.
- Encourage caregivers to hold and comfort their child during assessments and interventions.
- Introduce and use equipment gradually. Allow the child to handle minor equipment such as a stethoscope.
- Provide the toddler with limited choices such as, "Do you want me to measure your muscle in your right arm or left arm?" This provides the toddler with a sense of control.
- Prepare the child immediately before a procedure, using simple, concrete age-appropriate terms. Throughout the procedure, provide reassurance.
- Tell the child when the assessment or procedure is completed.
- Provide the toddler with positive reinforcement following procedures and praise their assistance, regardless of the child's reaction.

Anticipatory Guidance and Health Promotion for Toddlers

- The toddler has become more mobile, requiring closer supervision. Minimize home hazards for injury, such as placing household products and medications in secure locations, keeping handles from cooking utensils pointed away from the edge of the stove, and eliminating clutter around stairways to lessen risk for stairway falls.
- Child safety restraint devices in motor vehicles are required. Best practice indicates that the safest position for the toddler's car seat is forward facing in the rear seat. References for caregivers include car manual, car seat packaging information, and local car seat

experts (including The National Safe Kids Campaign®, police, and emergency medical services). Review information regarding risk of injury with air bag deployment and inappropriate installation of child safety seats.

- Parents should practice toy safety by choosing toys according to the child's age and development, not according to the child's desires.
- Injury prevention: Children of this age are extremely malleable and observant, and their health behaviors reflect those of their primary caregivers.

Preschoolers (3 to 5 years of age)

Psychosocial Development

- Preschoolers are magical and illogical thinkers. They often confuse coincidence with causation, have difficulty distinguishing fantasy from reality, and have many misconceptions about illness, injury, and body functions (e.g., if they have a cut, their "insides" will leak out).
- Preschoolers' thinking has been described as magical;[35] they often have imaginary playmates.
- Preschoolers often take words and phrases literally. **Table 3-4** reviews words and phrases that are often confusing to this age child.

Table 3-4 Are they hearing what you are saying?

Considerations when communicating with children[1,21,34,35]

Words that have more than one meaning are especially confusing to children, especially the older toddler and preschool-age child. At that age the child is unable to interpret the abstract meaning of words and interprets them literally. If the use of medical terminology is unavoidable, it is imperative to explain these words at the age-appropriate level to the child. It is ideal to hold discussions with parents out of the hearing range of the child to avoid the child misinterpreting words or phases.

Words or Terms to AVOID	Suggested Substitutions
Take ... as in I'm going to take your temperature. May be interpreted as taking something away.	I'm going to measure your temperature.
Dressing change. Interpretation: Why are they going to undress me? I don't want to change my clothes.	I'm going to put a clean bandage on you.
Urine. Interpretation: You're in. You're in what?	Use child's familiar term such as "pee," "your water," or "number one."
Stool. Interpretation: taking a chair away. Why are you taking all the chairs away?	Use child's familiar terms such as "BM," "poop," "do dee," "ca-ca," or "number two."
CT Scan (CAT Scan). Interpretation: Can my cat do it? I'm allergic to cats. I'm afraid of cats.	We're going to take you to get a special picture of your insides.
Shot (also avoid use of the word beesting). Interpretation: With a gun? Are you going to hurt me?	I am going to give you some medicine with a little needle (a little pinch, a little owie) or medicine under the skin.
IV. Interpretation: Ivy? I don't like plants. Are you going to plant me in the yard?	Describe in simple terms. Show if possible and allow touching.
Move you to the floor. Interpretation: Why are you going to take my bed away?	Move you to a new bed.
ICU. Interpretation: Was I invisible before?	Move you to a special room.
I'm going to stick you. Interpretation: With what? I got poked with a stick before.	I'm going to make a little pinch in your arm so we can give you some medicine.
Dye. Interpretation: Am I gonna die?	Use a special medicine.
Put to sleep. Interpretations: They put my dog to sleep. Mommy said my fish was sleeping and she flushed him.	Give you some medicine to give you special sleep, and when you wake up...
We're going to fix your cut. Interpretation: With scissors? Will it hurt?	We're going to make your boo-boo better.
A stretcher's coming to get you. Interpretation: A monster? A machine that will stretch my body?	A special bed on wheels.
We are going to give you some tests. Interpretation: What if I fail? I don't like tests; I'm not good at them.	We are going to find out why you are feeling sick.

- Preschoolers ask a lot of questions and are more independent.
- Common fears include body mutilation, especially genitalia, loss of control, death, darkness, and being left alone; therefore, the preschooler needs a lot of reassurance and simple explanations.
- Health practices are seen as tasks that must be mastered, such as brushing teeth. They have no concept of cause and effect; illness is often seen as punishment.

Anatomic and Physiologic Characteristics
- 50th percentile weight is 14 to 18 kg.
- Normal urinary output is 1 ml/kg/hr.
- The preschooler continues to use abdominal muscles for breathing.

Approaching the Preschooler
- Allow the child to handle equipment (or similar play equipment) such as a stethoscope.
- Immediately before the procedure, prepare the child by using simple concrete terms. Explain in terms of the sensory experience (i.e., hearing, feeling, and seeing). Delays in proceeding with the procedure following preparation can lead to increased anxiety and increased imagination of fearful things. The time lag should be less than 2 minutes.[3]
- Set limits on behavior, but offer choices whenever possible to enhance feelings of control.
- Enlist the child's help (e.g., tell the children to hold still, but give them permission to cry). Do not link "good" behavior with stoic behavior. Avoid the use of the word bad because children tend to link it with themselves being bad.
- Assess the child's level of understanding and correct erroneous or unclear ideas since adult vocabulary may be misleading.
- Consider age-related language in explaining procedures to children.
- Use games to gain cooperation.
- Use dressings freely to promote preschoolers' feelings of body integrity.

Anticipatory Guidance and Health Promotion for Preschoolers
- Motor vehicle safety restraint devices are still required for most children in this age group. Be aware of laws affecting child restraint in your state or country. Many child restraint devices are designed for children up to 80 pounds (36 kg).
- Children of this age are extremely malleable and observant. By this age, children are able to understand the need for injury prevention and the reason

for it. Preschoolers learn through example and will begin noticing if caregivers are not using safety restraints themselves.
- Riding toys are beginning to be used. Remind caregivers that safety helmets must be correctly fitted and worn.
- Instruct caregivers to place beds away from windows because this age group is at risk of falls from windows.
- Provide safety information on stranger danger.

School-Age Children (5 to 11 years of age)

Psychosocial Development
- School-age children are developing a sense of accomplishment and mastery of new skills. Successes contribute to positive self-esteem and a sense of control.
- Although the ability for logical thought processes is beginning, misinterpretation of words and phrases is common. Avoid using technical words and phrases.
- Their concept of time is improved; awareness of possible long-term consequences of illness is present.
- Provide specific instructions to the child about their behavior (e.g., "It's okay to cry as long as you hold your arm still"). Setting limits provides the child with a sense of control and a sense of accomplishment once the procedure is completed.
- By the age of 9, children can understand simple explanations about their anatomy and body functions. They believe that people can be part healthy and part unhealthy.
- Older school-age children tend to hide their thoughts and feelings.
- Common fears include separation from friends, loss of control, and physical disability. Risk-taking behavior is emerging and is most concerning if present by the age of 6.
- School-age children develop a general knowledge of medical intervention often based on media reports, television shows, and nightmarish fantasies.
- They are more likely to want to participate in their care.

Anatomic and Physiologic Characteristics
- 50th percentile weight is 20 to 32 kg.
- By about 8 years of age, the child's respiratory anatomy and physiology approximates that of an adult. The child's circulatory blood volume is 80 ml/kg.

Approaching School-Age Children

Approaching School-Age Children
- Provide the older school-aged child the choice of having the caregiver present during assessment.

- Allow them to participate in their care. Examples of this include opening a bandage, removing a blood pressure cuff, and carrying their chart or papers.
- Explain procedures simply and allow time for questions. The school-age child may be reluctant to ask questions or to admit not knowing something that the child perceives he or she is expected to know.
- Provide privacy. Privacy needs are changing, and some children may not want caregivers in the room when they undress.[36] They are really modest.
- Be honest, explain procedures, and describe how the child can be involved in his or her own care.
- Provide reassuring comments with positive reinforcement following procedures, and praise their assistance regardless of the child's reaction.
- Reassure the child that he or she did nothing wrong. The procedure, illness, or injury discomfort is not punishment and is unrelated to his or her actions.

Anticipatory Guidance and Health Promotion for School-Age Children

- Due to their desire for social acceptance, school-age children may exhibit risk-taking behaviors to prove themselves worthy of acceptance. Because they have limited understanding of casual relationships between events, they may not think through the consequences of their actions.[36]
- Remind the caregivers and the child that bicycle helmets must be worn. Helmets must be replaced every 3 years or sooner, depending on the child's head growth, if cracks or chips develop in the helmet material, or if damage is sustained following a significant crash.
- Remind the caregiver and the child that safety pads for knees, elbows, and wrists must also be worn when in-line skating or skateboarding.
- Caregivers need to ensure safe transportation of children in motor vehicles through appropriate use of car safety restraints (including car seats and seat belts). The safest place in a motor vehicle for all children under 12 years of age is in the rear seat. Provide information regarding injury risks associated with air bag deployment.
- Provide safety information on the avoidance of strangers and "saying no" to the use of alcohol and drugs.

Adolescents (11 to 18 years of age)

Psychosocial Development

- Adolescence is a period of experimentation and risk-taking activity. They have little common sense.
- Adolescents are acutely aware of their body appearance. Anything that differentiates them from their peers is perceived as a major tragedy.
- Psychosomatic complaints are common.
- The adolescent's quest for independence from his or her family often leads to family dissension.
- Peer relationships are the most important relationships and provide psychological support and social development. Sexual interests are common.
- Adolescents may experience mood swings, depression, eating disorders, and violent behavior. These behaviors should be further evaluated as an emerging/developing mental health concern versus normal adolescent behavior.
- Common fears include changes in appearance, dependency, and loss of control.
- Beliefs may be influenced by the peer group in terms of acceptance and rejection.
- To seek comfort, adolescents may regress to earlier stages of development when stressed, ill, or in pain.[21]
- Adolescents progress from concrete to formal operational cognitive development but still lack the conceptual thinking skills of the adult. They need concrete explanations.[23]
- Health is perceived as feeling good and in control.

Anatomic and Physiologic Characteristics

- Weights range from 36 kg to adult weight. This weight range is out of the range for length-based resuscitation tapes.
- Adolescence is characterized by rapid growth and heightened emotions usually associated with hormonal changes.[29]
- Puberty begins between 8 and 14 years of age in females (median age of menarche is 12.5 years[29]) and between 9 and 16 years of age in males.

Approaching Adolescents

- Provide adolescents with concrete information about their illness or injury, normal body functions, and plan of care, treatments, and diagnostic tests.
- Treat the adolescent as an adult. They expect it, but give them a lot of reassurance.
- When talking with adolescents, avoid interruptions and distractions. Encourage the adolescent to ask questions and participate in their own health care. Address his or her concerns first, and then those of the parents.[5]
- Be attentive to nonverbal cues.
- Respect privacy and confidentiality unless the information divulged is harmful to the adolescent or others (such as suicidal ideation or threat of harm of others).

- Issues such as sexual activity, sexually transmitted diseases, and pregnancy must be communicated in a private setting without the presence of the primary caregiver. In many states, testing for any of these issues or concerns can be done without parental consent; however, it is not commonly the initial reason for seeking emergency care.

- Be honest and nonjudgmental. Avoid talking down to the adolescent, and avoid the use of slang terms. Use terms the adolescent can understand.

- Provide feedback about the adolescent's health status. When appropriate, emphasize the normalcy of physical findings.

- Clearly explain how their body will be affected by the illness or procedure.

- Offer the opportunity for the adolescent to choose a support person during assessments and interventions, thus allowing them autonomy and decision making.

- Include a screening for health risk behaviors when obtaining the history. The HEADSS mnemonic (**Box 3-4**) facilitates covering common risk areas for the adolescent.[21,24]

- The rate of suicide and substance abuse is high.

Anticipatory Guidance and Health Promotion for Adolescents

- Promote recreational safety and the use of safety equipment including helmets and other safety equipment.
- Promote proper seat belt use and motor vehicle safety.
- Provide counseling related to reducing the risk of sexually transmitted diseases, use of birth control, safe sexual practices, and responsible sexual behavior.[37]

- Provide injury awareness and prevention literature about driving safely, hazards of driving under the influence of drugs and alcohol, and sexually transmitted diseases. Use resources available through agencies such as the AAP and ENA.

- Promote and provide health guidance information regarding[37]
  - Parenting
  - Development
  - Diet and physical activity
  - Health lifestyles (including sexual behavior and substance use)
  - Injury prevention

- Promote annual preventative services visit with the PCP for the adolescent.[11] The preventative services visit facilitates early recognition of potential and actual health problems and the early establishment of health promotion practices.

Role of Play

Through play, children learn about themselves and the world in which they live. Play functions to develop sensorimotor, intellectual, and socializations skills as well as to foster self-awareness, creativity, and values. Play reflects the child's development and awareness of their environment,[14,16] as outlined in **Table 3-5**. Patterns of play begin with the most simple and become increasingly complex, reflecting the child's stage of development. Play allows children to practice the skills they have already attained and to continually learn and gain new skills.[1] It also helps them cope with stressful situations.

Spontaneous play is child initiated. Therapeutic play is provider initiated and often used to reduce stress related to illness, injury, or medical procedures and to explore relationships with significant members of the child's life.[16]

In any setting, including the ED, play is a useful assessment tool in children. For example, the assessment of a 5-year-old asthmatic following an aerosol treatment reveals a child pale in color with intercostal retractions sitting cross-legged actively engaged in coloring a picture. Reassessment of the child 30 minutes later reveals a child pale in color with intercostal retractions leaning back against the bed holding a crayon but no longer coloring. In this example, the differences in play activity may be subtle indications of the changes in the child's status and the dynamic process of the child's illness or injury.

Box 3-4 HEADSS mnemonic[21,24]

H = Home: Who lives at home? How does everyone get along?

E = Education: What school do you attend and what grade? How are your grades? Do you have an after-school job?

E = Eating: Review eating behaviors, meal frequency, and content.

A = Activities: What activities are you involved in at school? What activities are you involved in after school and on weekends?

A = Affect: What is the adolescent's affect? Is there evidence of depression or anxiety?

D = Drugs: Ask about substance use including illegal drugs, inhalants, alcohol, and smoking. Are peers involved in substance use?

S = Suicidal ideations and attempts: Has the adolescent ever thought about suicide? Have there been any attempts? Are there any suicidal ideations currently?

S = Sexual activity: What is the sexual history including gender of partners, number of partners, use of protection, and date of last sexual activity? Any history of sexually transmitted diseases, treatment received? Any previous pregnancies and outcome? Is there any history of sexual abuse?

General Safety in the Emergency Environment

The health care setting may not always be a safe environment for the child. This is particularly true of the ED setting, with high volume and rapid turnover of patients, transportation of patients and equipment to other areas via wheelchair and stretchers, multiple routes of access and egress, and the "normal" risks for children related to injury. Children must always be supervised; therefore, ED staff should instruct caregivers to keep side rails in the up and locked position, to avoid leaving their child unattended, and to discourage children from running in the hallways. Consider child safety and injury prevention when purchasing furniture, room decorations, and toys for waiting areas, play stations, and patient rooms.

After the Case

Following care of the pediatric patient, take the opportunity for all staff members to learn from the case. Make every effort to

- Discuss and review difficult cases with the team members involved. Discuss alternative treatments and procedures that may have been easier to accomplish and may have resulted in the same or better outcome. If any staff member is unfamiliar with the treatment or procedure, review this information with the individual staff and arrange for an in-service for all staff.
- If the case did not go as well as anticipated, systematically review where the difficulties occurred. For example, identify if the problems occurred with the patient, the equipment, the staff, or the system.

Summary

Providing health care to children requires an understanding of the characteristics of growth and development. It is essential to utilize these facts during your assessment and interventions to obtain accurate information and the most effective treatment possible.

- The child exists within the context of a family. Even the child who has been neglected or maltreated refers to their parents or primary caregivers for support.
- Crying is an infant's and young child's way of communication. Instead of crying being perceived as noise, consider crying as an assessment component to indicate adequate strength and possibly improving status. However, a cry that cannot be alleviated needs further assessment. Different-pitched cries and tones have different meanings—encourage the parents or caregivers to help understand the source.

Table 3-5 Developmental Relationships of Play [7, 14, 16, 32–37]

Stage of development	Play exhibited	Activities
Infancy	Infants seek pleasure through social play by exhibiting social behaviors (i.e., smiling) which elicit positive attention from caregivers. They may be attracted (and distracted) with lights and moving brightly colored objects. In this exploratory stage, they explore their world through the touch of objects.	Speak to the infant in a soft, singsong rhythm. Allow them to hold and touch items you are using (such as stethoscope or tape roll). Use distraction such as flashlight, room light, bubbles, singing, playing peek-a-boo, and clapping.
Toddler	Toddlers participate in parallel play; they play alongside, not with, others. Less complex pretend play often imitates parental roles (i.e., mowing the yard or pushing a grocery cart). They enjoy push-pull toys, blocks, and large balls.	Provide toys that are lifelike (such as telephones and tools). Allow them to keep and hold any item they might bring (i.e., stuffed animal, dolls, or cars).
Early childhood (Preschooler)	Cooperative play with sharing can be seen in the preschooler. Imaginary friends develop with pretend play. Through pretend play children act out the activities of daily life (i.e., acting like a teacher, policeman, or postman).	Provide coloring books, books, videos, and toys and games that encourage imagination.
School-age	Play becomes more competitive and complex. Interest in games, hobbies, and sports. Rules and rituals are important aspects of games and play.	Provide playing cards, puzzles, books, crafts, board and video games.
Adolescent	Competition serves as a motivation for play.	Facilitate private space. Provide radio or other music device, video or computer games. Provide telephone.

- Play is their work. Use it as a part of assessment–a child who is able to stay engaged in play has a relatively intact mental status, whereas, a child who is no longer interested in play has a changing or decreasing mental status.

- Always consider the developmental stage of the child before entering a room to perform an intervention or assessment.

- There are more similarities than differences between adults and children. Approach the parents and family as you do the child—with the same caring and concern.

- An organized approach will help ensure confidence and consistent patient care.

- Anticipatory guidance is the best preventive measure when dealing with children and families. Every interaction with a child and family should include appropriate teaching to deal with a situation before it becomes a problem. In the ED setting, the most beneficial anticipatory guidance involves injury prevention and home safety.

References

1. Hockenberry, M. J., Winkelstein, M. L., Wilson, D., & Kline, N. E. (Eds.). (2003). Family influences on health promotion. In *Wong's nursing care of infants and children* (7th ed., pp. 64–102). St. Louis, MO: Mosby.

2. Horowitz, L., Kassam-Adams, N., & Bergstein, J. (2001). Mental health aspects of emergency medical services for children: Summary of a consensus conference. *Academic Emergency Medicine, 8*(12), 1187–1196.

3. Conway, A. E. (2003). Developmental and psychosocial considerations. In D. O. Thomas, L. M. Bernardo, & B. Herman (Eds.), *Core curriculum for pediatric emergency nursing* (pp. 35–48). Boston: Jones and Bartlett.

4. Muscari, M. E. (2001). Infants. In *Advanced pediatric clinical assessment: Skills and procedures* (pp. 8–16). Philadelphia: Lippincott.

5. Dieckmann, R., Brownstein, D. & Gausche-Hill, M. (Eds.). (2000). Using a developmental approach. In American Academy of Pediatrics (Ed.), *Pediatric education for prehospital professionals* (pp. 16–29). Boston: Jones and Bartlett.

6. McKenzie, I. M. (1997). Developmental physiology and psychology. In I. M. McKenzie, P. B. Gaukroger, P. G. Ragg, & T. C. Brown (Eds.), *Manual of acute pain management in children* (pp. 7–10). New York: Churchill.

7. Muscari, M. E. (2001). Developmental assessment. In *Advanced pediatric clinical assessment: Skills and procedures* (pp. 3–7). Philadelphia: Lippincott.

8. Bove, M. A. (1993). Positioning and securing children for procedures. In L. M. Bernardo & M. A. Bove (Eds.), *Pediatric emergency nursing procedures* (pp. 29–34). Boston: Jones and Bartlett.

9. Bernardo, L. M., & Conway, A. E. (1998). Pain assessment and management. In T. E. Soud & J. S. Rogers (Eds.), *Manual of pediatric emergency nursing* (pp. 686–711). St. Louis, MO: Mosby-Year Book

10. Emergency Nurses Association. (2001). *Family presence at the bedside during invasive procedures and resuscitation* (Position statement). Des Plaines, IL: Author.

11. Boudreaux, E. D., Francis, J. L., & Layacano, T. (2002). Family presence during invasive procedures and resuscitations in the emergency department: A critical review and suggestions for future research. *Annals of Emergency Medicine, 40*(2), 193–205.

12. Eichhorn, D. J., Meyers, T. A., Guzzetta, C. E., Clark, A. P., Klein, J. D., Taliaferro, E., & Calvin, A. O. (2001). During invasive procedures and resuscitation: Hearing the voice of the patient. *American Journal of Nursing, 101*(5), 48–55.

13. Williams, J. M. (2002). Family presence during resuscitation: To see or not to see? *Nursing Clinics of North America, 37*(1), 211–220.

14. Velasco-Whetsell, M., Coffin, D. A., Lizardo, L. M., Lizardo, M. L., MacDougall, B. J., Madayag, T. M., et al. (Eds.). (2000). Growth and development. In *Pediatric nursing* (pp. 66–96). New York: McGraw-Hill.

15. Hockenberry, M. J., Winkelstein, M. L., Wilson, D., & Kline, N. E. (Eds.). (2003). Physical and developmental assessment of the child. In *Wong's nursing care of infants and children* (7th ed., pp. 170–239). St. Louis, MO: Mosby.

16. Hockenberry, M. J., Winkelstein, M. L., Wilson, D., & Kline, N. E. (Eds.). (2003). Family-centered care of the child during illness and hospitalization. In *Wong's nursing care of infants and children* (7th ed., pp. 1031–1100). St. Louis, MO: Mosby.

17. American Heart Association. (2002). Recognition of respiratory failure and shock. In *PALS provider manual* (pp. 23–42). Dallas, TX: American Heart Association.

18. Callahan, J. M. (1997). Pharmacologic agents. In R. A. Dieckman, D. H. Fiser, & S. M. Selbst (Eds.), *Illustrated textbook of pediatric emergency and critical care procedures* (pp. 53–67). St. Louis, MO: Mosby-Year Book. .

19. American Academy of Pediatrics. Committee on Injury Prevention and Poison Prevention. (2001). Injuries associated with infant walkers. *Pediatrics, 108*(3), 790–792.

20. Frose, N., & Constarino, A. J. (1997). Sedation and pain relief: Other agents. In R. A. Dieckmann, D. H. Fiser, & S. M. Selbst (Eds.), *Illustrated textbook of pediatric emergency and critical care procedures* (pp. 68–71). St. Louis, MO: Mosby-Year Book.

21. Deering, C. G., & Cody, D. J. (2002). Communicating with children and adolescents: "Children are all foreigners," Ralph Waldo Emerson said; but it need not always be the case. Here are some specific, age-appropriate tips for understanding the language of children. *American Journal of Nursing, 102*(3), 34–41.

22. Ashburn, M. A., Gauthier, M., Love, G., Basta, S., Gaylord, B., & Kessler, K. (1997). Iontophoretic administration of 2% lidocaine HCL and 1:10,000 epinephrine in humans. *Clinical Journal of Pain, 13*(1), 22–26.

23. American Academy of Pediatrics committee on drugs. (1992). Guidelines for monitoring and management of pediatric patients during and after sedation for diagnostic and therapeutic procedures. (1992). *Pediatrics, 89*(6, Pt 1), 1110–1115.

24. Cohen, E., Mackenzie, R. G., & Yates, G. L. (1991). HEADSS, a psychosocial risk assessment instrument: Implications foe designing effective intervention programs for runaway youth. *Journal of Adolescent Health, 12*(7), 539–544.

25. Bernardo, L. M., & Schenkel, K. (2003). Pediatric trauma. In L. Newberry (Ed.), *Sheehy's emergency nursing: Principles and practice* (5th ed., pp. 379–400). St. Louis, MO: Mosby.

26. Dunn, A. M. (2002). Culture competence and the primary provider. *Journal of Pediatric Health, 16*(3), 105–111.

27. O'Brien, M. M., Creamer, K. M., Hill, E. E., & Welham, J. (2002). Tolerance of family presence during pediatric cardiopulmonary resuscitation: A snapshot of military and civilian pediatricians, nurses, and residents. *Pediatric Emergency Care, 18*(6), 409–413.

28. Jarvis, A. S. (1998). Parental presence during resuscitation: Attitudes of staff on a paediatric intensive care unit. *Intensive Critical Care Nurse, 14,* 3–7.

29. Chumlea, W. C., Schubert, C. M., Roche, A. F., Kulin, H. E., Lee, P. A., Himes, J. H., et al. (2003). Age at menarche and racial comparison in U.S. girls. *Pediatrics, 111*(1), 110–113.

30. Denke, N. J. (2003). End of life in the emergency department. In L. Newberry (Ed.), *Sheehy's emergency nursing: Principles and practice* (5th ed., pp. 183–188). St. Louis, MO: Mosby.

31. MacLean, S. L., Guzzetta, C. E., White, C., Fontaine, D., Eichhorn, D. J., Meyers, T. A., et al. (2003). Family presence during cardiopulmonary resuscitation and invasive procedures: Practice of critical care and emergency nurses. *Journal of Emergency Nursing, 29*(3), 208–221.

32. Hockenberry, M. J., Winkelstein, M. L., Wilson, D., & Kline, N. E. (Eds.). (2003). Health promotion of the newborn and family. In *Wong's nursing care of infants and children* (7th ed., pp. 240–294). St. Louis, MO: Mosby.

33. Hockenberry, M. J., Winkelstein, M. L., Wilson, D., & Kline, N. E. (Eds.). (2003). Health promotion of the infant and family. In *Wong's nursing care of infants and children* (7th ed., pp. 493–553). St. Louis, MO: Mosby.

34. Hockenberry, M. J., Winkelstein, M. L., Wilson, D., & Kline, N. E. (Eds.). (2003). Health promotion of the toddler and family. In *Wong's nursing care of infants and children* (7th ed., pp. 600–627). St. Louis, MO: Mosby.

35. Hockenberry, M. J., Winkelstein, M. L., Wilson, D., & Kline, N. E. (Eds.). (2003). Health promotion of the preschooler and family. In *Wong's nursing care of infants and children* (7th ed., pp. 628–648). St. Louis, MO: Mosby.

36. Hockenberry, M. J., Winkelstein, M. L., Wilson, D., & Kline, N. E. (Eds.). (2003). Health promotion of the school-age child and family. In *Wong's nursing care of infants and children* (7th ed., pp. 698–738). St. Louis, MO: Mosby.

37. Hockenberry, M. J., Winkelstein, M. L., Wilson, D., & Kline, N. E. (Eds.). (2003). Health promotion of the adolescent and family. In *Wong's nursing care of infants and children* (7th ed., pp. 64–102). St. Louis, MO: Mosby.

Web Site Resources

U.S. Consumer Product Safety Commission http://www.cpsc.gov

National Safe Kids Organization http://www.safekids.org/

American College of Emergency Physicians http://www.acep.org

American Academy of Pediatrics http://www.aap.org

Centers for Disease Control http://www.cdc.gov

National Emergency Medical Services for Children
http://www.ems-c.org

National Association of Children's Hospital and Related Institutions
http://www.childrenshospitals.net/nachri

Appendix 3-A

Recommended Childhood and Adolescent Immunization Schedule -- United States, 2003

Vaccine ▼ / Age ▶	Birth	1 mo	2 mos	4 mos	6 mos	12 mos	15 mos	18 mos	24 mos	4-6 yrs	11-12 yrs	13-18 yrs
						range of recommended ages	catch-up vaccination			preadolescent assessment		
Hepatitis B[1]	HepB #1	only if mother HBsAg (-)									HepB series	
			HepB #2			HepB #3						
Diphtheria, Tetanus, Pertussis[2]			DTaP	DTaP	DTaP		DTaP			DTaP	Td	
Haemophilus influenzae Type b[3]			Hib	Hib	Hib	Hib						
Inactivated Polio			IPV	IPV		IPV				IPV		
Measles, Mumps, Rubella[4]						MMR #1				MMR #2	MMR #2	
Varicella[5]						Varicella				Varicella		
Pneumococcal[6]			PCV	PCV	PCV	PCV				PCV	PPV	
Hepatitis A[7]										Hepatitis A series		
Influenza[8]						Influenza (yearly)						

Vaccines below this line are for selected populations

This schedule indicates the recommended ages for routine administration of currently licensed childhood vaccines, as of December 1, 2002, for children through age 18 years. Any dose not given at the recommended age should be given at any subsequent visit when indicated and feasible. ▨ Indicates age groups that warrant special effort to administer those vaccines not previously given. Additional vaccines may be licensed and recommended during the year. Licensed combination vaccines may be used whenever any components of the combination are indicated and the vaccine's other components are not contraindicated. Providers should consult the manufacturers' package inserts for detailed recommendations.

1. Hepatitis B vaccine (HepB). All infants should receive the first dose of hepatitis B vaccine soon after birth and before hospital discharge; the first dose may also be given by age 2 months if the infant's mother is HBsAg-negative. Only monovalent HepB can be used for the birth dose. Monovalent or combination vaccine containing HepB may be used to complete the series. Four doses of vaccine may be administered when a birth dose is given. The second dose should be given at least 4 weeks after the first dose, except for combination vaccines, which cannot be administered before age 6 weeks. The third dose should be given at least 16 weeks after the first dose and at least 8 weeks after the second dose. The last dose in the vaccination series (third or fourth dose) should not be administered before age 6 months. Infants born to HBsAg-positive mothers should receive HepB and 0.5 mL Hepatitis B Immune Globulin (HBIG) within 12 hours of birth at separate sites. The second dose is recommended at age 1–2 months. The last dose in the vaccination series should not be administered before age 6 months. These infants should be tested for HBsAg and anti-HBs at 9–15 months of age. Infants born to mothers whose HBsAg status is unknown should receive the first dose of the HepB series within 12 hours of birth. Maternal blood should be drawn as soon as possible to determine the mother's HBsAg status; if the HBsAg test is positive, the infant should receive HBIG as soon as possible (no later than age 1 week). The second dose is recommended at age 1–2 months. The last dose in the vaccination series should not be administered before age 6 months.

2. Diphtheria and tetanus toxoids and acellular pertussis vaccine (DTaP). The fourth dose of DTaP may be administered as early as age 12 months, provided 6 months have elapsed since the third dose and the child is unlikely to return at age 15–18 months. Tetanus and diphtheria toxoids (Td) is recommended at age 11–12 years if at least 5 years have elapsed since the last dose of tetanus and diphtheria toxoid-containing vaccine. Subsequent routine Td boosters are recommended every 10 years.

3. Haemophilus influenza type b (Hib) conjugate vaccine. Three Hib conjugate vaccines are licensed for infant use. If PRP-OMP (PedvaxHIB® or ComVax® [Merck]) is administered at ages 2 and 4 months, a dose at age 6 months is not required. DTaP/Hib combination products should not be used for primary immunization in infants at ages 2, 4, or 6 months, but can be used as boosters following any Hib vaccine.

4. Measles, mumps, and rubella vaccine (MMR). The second dose of MMR is recommended routinely at age 4–6 years, but may be administered during any visit, provided at least 4 weeks have elapsed since the first dose and that both doses are administered beginning at or after age 12 months. Those who have not previously received the second dose should complete the schedule by the 11- to 12-year-old visit.

5. Varicella vaccine. Varicella vaccine is recommended at any visit at or after age 12 months for susceptible children (i.e., those who lack a reliable history of chickenpox). Susceptible persons aged = 13 years should receive two doses, given at least 4 weeks apart.

6. Pneumococcal vaccine. The heptavalent pneumococcal conjugate vaccine (PCV) is recommended for all children age

2–23 months. It is also recommended for certain children age 24–59 months. Pneumococcal polysaccharide vaccine (PPV) is recommended in addition to PCV for certain high-risk groups. See MMWR2000;49(RR-9);1-38.

7. Hepatitis A vaccine. Hepatitis A vaccine is recommended for children and adolescents in selected states and regions and for certain high-risk groups; consult your local public health authority. Children and adolescents in these states, regions, and high-risk groups who have not been immunized against hepatitis A can begin the hepatitis A vaccination series during any visit. The two doses in the series should be administered at least 6 months apart. See MMWR1999;48(RR-12);1-37.

8. Influenza vaccine. Influenza vaccine is recommended annually for children age = 6 months with certain risk factors (including but not limited to asthma, cardiac disease, sickle cell disease, HIV, diabetes, and household members of persons in groups at high risk; see MMWR 2002;51(RR-3);1-31) and can be administered to all others wishing to obtain immunity. In addition, healthy children age 6–23 months are encouraged to receive influenza vaccine if feasible because children in this age group are at substantially increased risk for influenza-related hospitalizations. Children aged = 12 years should receive vaccine in a dosage appropriate for their age (0.25 mL if age 6–35months or 0.5 mL if aged = 3 years). Children aged = 8 years who are receiving influenza vaccine for the first time should receive two doses separated by at least 4 weeks.

For additional information about vaccines, including precautions and contraindications for immunization and vaccine shortages, please visit the National Immunization Program Web site at www.cdc.gov/nip or call the National Immunization Information Hotline at 800-232-2522 (English) or 800-232-0233 (Spanish).

Approved by the Advisory Committee on Immunization Practices (www.cdc.gov/nip/acip), the American Academy of Pediatrics (www.aap.org), and the American Academy of Family Physicians (www.aafp.org)

Appendix 3-B *Childhood Development (Infant to Adolescent)*

Physical and Motor Development	Intellectual/ Psychosocial Development	Language Development	Pain	Death
Infant Development (1 Month to 1 Year)				
GROWTH • Period of most rapid growth • Infant weight gain—1 oz/day • Weight doubles by age 6 months; triples by 1 year	Trust versus Mistrust (Erikson) • When physical needs are consistently met, infants learn to trust self and environment Common Fears (after 6 months) • Separation • Strangers	Sensorimotor Period (Piaget) • Infants learn by the use of their senses and activities	• Infants do experience pain • Degree of pain perceived is unknown	• Infants do not understand the meaning of death • The developing sense of separation serves as a basis for a beginning understanding of the meaning of death
Toddler Development (1 to 2 Years)				
GROWTH • Rate significantly slows down, accompanied by a tremendous decrease in appetite GENERAL APPEARANCE • Potbellied • Exaggerated lumbar curve • Wide-based gait INCREASED MOBILITY • Hallmark of physical development in the toddler	Autonomy versus Shame and Doubt (Erikson) • Increasing independence and self-care activities • Expanding the world with which the toddler interacts • Need to experience joy of exploring and exerting some control over body functions and activity, while maintaining support of "anchor" (i.e., primary caregiver) Common Fears • Separation • Loss of control • Altered rituals • Pain	Sensorimotor Period (Piaget) • Cognition and language not yet sophisticated enough for children to learn through thought processes and communication	• No formal concept of pain, related to immature thought process and poorly developed body image • React as intensely to painless procedures as to ones that hurt, especially when restrained • Intrusive procedures, such as taking temperatures, are very distressing • React to pain with physical resistance, aggression, negativism, and regression • Rare for toddlers to fake pain • Verbal responses concerning pain are unreliable	• Understanding of death still very limited • Belief that loss of significant others is temporary; reinforced by: - Developing sense of object permanence (i.e., objects continue to exist even if cannot be seen) - Repeated experiences of separations and reunions - Magical thinking - TV shows (e.g., cartoon characters)

Childhood Development (Infant to Adolescent)

Physical and Motor Development	Psychosocial Development	Intellectual/ Lanugage Development	Pain	Death
Preschool Development (3 to 5 Years)				
GROWTH • Weight gain—2 kg/year • Height gain—6 to 8 cm/year • Usually are half adult height by 2 years of age GENERAL APPEARANCE • "Baby fat" and protuberant abdomen disappear	Initiative versus Guilt (Erikson) • Greater autonomy and independence • Still intense need for caregivers when under stress • Initiate activities, rather than just imitating others • Age of discovery, curiosity, and developing social behavior • Sense of self as individual Common Fears • Mutilation • Loss of control • Death • Dark • Ghosts	Preoperational (Piaget) • Time of trial/error learning • Egocentric—view experiences from own perspective • Understand explanations only in terms of real events or what their senses tell them • No logical or abstract thought; coincidence confused with causation • Magical thinking continues • Difficulty distinguishing between reality and fantasy • May see illness or injury as punishment for "bad" thoughts or behavior • Imaginary friends; fascination with superheros and monsters	• Pain perceived as punishment for bad thoughts or behavior • Difficulty understanding that painful procedures help them get well • Cannot differentiate between "good" pain (as a result of treatment) and "bad" pain (resulting from injury or illness) • React to painful procedures with aggression and verbal reprimands (e.g., "I hate you"; "You're mean")	• Incomplete understanding of death fosters anxiety because of fear of death • Death is seen as an altered state of consciousness in which a person cannot perform normal activities, such as eating or walking • Perceive immobility, sleep, and other alterations in consciousness as death like states; associate words and phrases (e.g., "put to sleep") with death • Death is seen as reversible; reinforced by TV and cartoons • Unable to perceive inevitability of death due to limited time concept • View death as punishment
School-Aged Children (6 to 10 Years)				
GROWTH • Relatively latent period	Industry versus Inferiority (Erikson) • Age of accomplishment, increasing competence, and mastery of new skills • Successes contribute to positive self-esteem and a sense of control • Need parental support in times of stress; may be unwilling or unable to ask Common Fears • Separation from friends • Loss of control • Physical disability	Concrete Operations (Piaget) • Beginning of logical thought • Deductive reasoning develops • Improved concept of time; awareness of possible long-term consequences of illness • More sophisticated understanding of causality • Still interpret phrases and idioms at face value	• Reaction to pain affected by past experiences, parental response, and the meaning attached to it. • Better able to localize and describe pain accurately • Pain can be exaggerated because of heightened fears of bodily injury, pain, and death.	• Concept of death more logically based • Understand death as the irreversible cessation of life • View death as a tragedy that happens to others, not themselves • When death is actual threat, may feel responsible for death and experience guilt

Childhood Development (Infant to Adolescent)

Physical and Motor Development	Psychosocial Development	Intellectual/ Lanugage Development	Pain	Death
Adolescent Development (11 to 18 Years)				
GROWTH • Females—growth spurt begins at age 9 1/2 years • Males—growth spurt begins at age 10 1/2 years PUBERTY • Secondary sex characteristics begin to develop between the ages of 8 and 13 years for females; 10 and 14 years for males	• Identity versus Role Confusion (Erikson) • Transition from childhood to adulthood • Quest for independence often leads to family dissension • Major concerns: establishing identity and developing mature sexual orientation • Risk-taking behaviors— feel that nothing bad can happen to them Common Fears • Changes in appearance or functioning • Dependency • Loss of control	• Concrete to Formal Operations (Piaget) • Memory fully developed • Concept of time well understood • Adolescents can project to the future and imagine potential consequences of actions and illnesses • Some adolescents do not achieve formal operations	• Can locate and quantify pain accurately and thoroughly • Often hyperresponsive to pain; reacts to fear of changes in appearance or function • In general, highly controlled in responding to pain and painful procedures	• Understanding of death similar to that of adults • Intellectually believe that death can happen to them, but avoid realistic thoughts of death • Many adolescents defy the possibility of death through reckless behavior, substance abuse, or daring sports activities

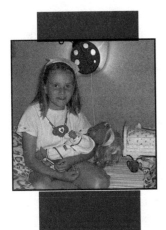

chapter 4

INITIAL ASSESSMENT

Introduction

A systematic process for the initial assessment of every ill and injured pediatric patient is necessary for recognizing life-threatening conditions, identifying indicators of illness and injury, and determining priorities of care based on the assessment findings.[1] Although the majority of children present with non-emergent illness or injury, it is essential to remember that cardiopulmonary failure in children is rarely a sudden event. Rather, arrest is the end result of a progressively deteriorating respiratory or circulatory function.[2]

Emergency care providers should be prepared to identify signs and symptoms of a life-threatening illness or injury and be able to rapidly provide the child with the appropriate interventions, stabilization, and evaluation.[3] Utilizing an organized, systematic approach when approaching each child helps ensure that signs of physiologic compromise will not be missed. The initial assessment is divided into two phases, the primary and secondary assessments. Both phases can be completed within minutes unless resuscitative measures are required.

A Guide to Initial Assessment

The following mnemonic describes the components of the initial assessment of the pediatric patient. The materials presented in this chapter represent comprehensive primary and secondary assessments.

Primary assessment

- A = Airway with simultaneous cervical spine stabilization for any injured child whose mechanism of injury,

symptoms, or physical findings suggest spinal trauma
- B = Breathing
- C = Circulation
- D = Disability or neurologic status
- E = Exposure and environmental control to prevent heat loss

Secondary assessment

- F = Full set of vital signs, including weight, and family presence
- G = Give comfort measures
- H = Head-to-toe assessment and history
- I = Inspect posterior surfaces

Primary Assessment

The primary assessment consists of assessment of the airway with cervical spine stabilization or maintenance of spinal stabilization when trauma is suspected, breathing, circulation, disability or neurologic status, and exposure with environmental control. Interventions to correct any life-threatening conditions must be performed before further assessment is continued. The interventions are listed in order of priority.

Airway

Assessment

Inspect the pediatric patient's airway. Assess for the following.

- Vocalization: Can the pediatric patient talk or cry?
- Tongue obstruction in an unresponsive pediatric patient
- Loose teeth or foreign objects, such as gum or small toys, in the oropharynx or hypopharynx

Objectives

On completion of this chapter, the learner should be able to:

1. Discuss the components of a pediatric primary assessment.
2. Correlate life-threatening conditions with the specific component of the primary assessment.
3. Describe interventions needed to manage life-threatening conditions found during the mary assessment.
4. Identify the components of a pediatric secondary assessment.
5. Evaluate the effectiveness of nursing interventions as related to desired patient outcomes.

- Vomitus, bleeding, or other secretions in the mouth
- Edema of the lips and/or tissues of the mouth
- Preferred posture (e.g., the tripod position is characterized by the pediatric patient sitting up, leaning forward, with the neck extended and head tilted up in an effort to maximize the airway)
- Drooling (in children other than teething infants)
- Dysphagia (difficulty swallowing)
- Abnormal airway sounds such as stridor, snoring, or gurgling. (Inspiratory sounds are characteristic of extrathoracic or upper airway causes of obstruction. Expiratory sounds are characteristic of intrathoracic or lower respiratory tract causes of obstruction.)

Interventions

Airway patent

- For any pediatric patient whose mechanism of injury, symptoms, or physical findings suggest a possible cervical spine injury, manually stabilize the cervical spine or maintain spinal stabilization if completed in the prehospital environment. All airway maneuvers for these children must be performed with the cervical spine in a neutral position to prevent secondary injury to the spinal cord/column.
- If a child is awake and breathing, he or she may have assumed a position that maximizes their ability to maintain a spontaneous airway. Allow the child to maintain this position or a position of comfort.

Airway partially or totally obstructed

- If the pediatric patient is unresponsive and/or unable to maintain a spontaneous airway, position the pediatric patient (sniffing position) and manually open the airway. Techniques to open or clear an obstructed airway during the primary assessment include
  - Jaw thrust
  - Head tilt-chin lift (difficult to do in the younger child). **Do not** use this technique if trauma is suspected.
    - Infants and young children have a large occiput; positioning them supine on a bed or backboard may cause their cervical vertebrae to flex anteriorly. Flexion may contribute to airway compromise or decrease the effectiveness of the jaw thrust or chin lift maneuvers.
    - To provide neutral alignment of the cervical spine and a neutral position for the child's airway, place padding under the younger child's shoulders to bring the shoulders into horizontal alignment with the external auditory meatus.
    - Suction the oropharynx with a rigid tonsil suction to remove debris. Vomitus or secretions

should be removed immediately by suctioning the patient to prevent aspiration. Suctioning or other interventions must be done in a manner to prevent stimulation of the child's gag reflex, which may cause subsequent vomiting or aspiration, as well as bradycardia.

- Suction the nose of the young infant with nasal secretions.
- Follow pediatric basic life support guidelines to relieve foreign body airway obstructions.[4]

If the pediatric patient is unable to maintain a patent airway after proper positioning:

- Insert an appropriate size nasopharyngeal airway if the pediatric patient is conscious and there is no evidence of facial trauma or skull fracture.
- Insert an oropharyngeal airway if the pediatric patient is unconscious or does not have a gag reflex. Proper positioning of the head and jaw must be maintained even in the presence of a patent airway.
- Prepare for endotracheal intubation.

Breathing

Once a patent airway has been established, assess for the following.

Assessment

- Level of consciousness
- Spontaneous respirations
- Rate and depth of respirations
- Symmetric chest rise and fall
- Skin color (cyanosis, first noted in mucous membranes of the mouth, is a late sign of respiratory compromise)
- Presence and quality of bilateral breath sounds
  - Auscultate bilaterally over the axilla. The chest wall of infants and young children is thin: breath sounds may be transmitted from one side to the opposite side, leading to "equal breath sounds," even in the presence of a pneumothorax.
- Presence of indicators of increased work of breathing:
  - Nasal flaring
  - Substernal, subcostal, intercostal, supraclavicular, or suprasternal retractions
  - Head bobbing
  - Expiratory grunting
  - Accessory muscle use
- Jugular vein distention (difficult to assess in infants and young children) and tracheal position
- Paradoxical respirations due to a flail segment

- Soft tissue and bony chest wall integrity
- Measurement of oxygen saturation by a pulse oximeter, if readily available
  - < 95 % at sea level is indicative of respiratory compromise; exceptions include children with uncorrected congenital heart defects

Interventions

Breathing present and effective

- Position the pediatric patient to facilitate respiratory effectiveness and comfort; respiratory mechanics are better with the pediatric patient in an upright position.
- In the spontaneously breathing pediatric patient, deliver supplemental oxygen, as indicated by the pediatric patient's clinical condition.
  - All seriously ill or injured patients should have oxygen administered at the highest concentration in a manner the pediatric patient will tolerate.
  - Consider using a nonrebreather mask at a flow rate sufficient to keep the reservoir bag inflated during inspiration; usually requires 12 to 15 liters/minute..

Breathing ineffective

- Assist ventilation with 100 % oxygen via a bag-mask device for apnea or hypoventilation
  - Assess effectiveness of assisted ventilation by observing chest rise and fall and auscultating for the presence of breath sounds.
- Prepare for endotracheal intubation.
  - Indications for intubation include[4]
    - Inadequate central nervous system control of ventilation resulting in apnea or inadequate respiratory effort (e.g., severe head injury with decreasing level of consciousness or Pediatric Coma Scale score or Glasgow Coma Scale [GCS] score ≤ 8).
    - Loss of protective airway reflexes
    - Functional or anatomic airway obstruction
    - Excessive work of breathing leading to fatigue
    - Need for high peak inspiratory pressures or positive end-expiratory pressures to maintain effective alveolar gas exchange
    - Permitting paralysis or sedation for diagnostic studies while ensuring protection of the airway and control of ventilation
  - Assemble equipment.
    - Suction device: tonsil-tipped or large-bore catheter and suction catheter to fit into endotracheal tube
    - Bag-mask with oxygen source
    - Stylet, laryngoscope blade, and handle

- Endotracheal tubes: three endotracheal tubes (one tube of the estimated required size and tubes 0.5 mm smaller and 0.5 mm larger). Tube size can be estimated using various strategies (see **Table 4-1**).
- Tape or endotracheal tube holder
- Exhaled CO_2 detector (as available)
- Confirm endotracheal tube placement at the time of insertion and each time the child is moved.
  - Initial (primary) confirmation[4]
    - Observe chest rise and fall.
    - Listen for breath sounds bilaterally in the axilla. Listen over the stomach. In infants and small children, referred sounds may be heard over the stomach. Any sounds heard over the stomach should always be fainter than those heard in the axillary areas.
    - Look for water vapor in the tube during expiration.
  - Secondary confirmation involves evaluation of exhaled CO_2 and oxygenation including[4]
    - Assessment of exhaled CO_2 by colorimetric device or continuous capnography (as available)
      - In a child with a perfusing rhythm, exhaled CO_2 detection is the best method for verification of tube placement.[5]
    - Assessment of oxygen saturation by pulse oximeter
    - Assessment of changes or improvement of skin and mucous membrane color
- Secure the tube, maintaining the child's head in a neutral position.
- Document endotracheal tube size, cuffed versus uncuffed tube, and depth by assessing location of tube at the lip, gum, or tooth line.
  - Appropriate depth of insertion can be estimated by one of the following formulas.[5]

Depth of insertion (cm) = internal tube diameter (in mm) x 3

Or in children > 2 years of age:

$$\text{Depth of insertion (cm)} = \frac{\text{Age in years} + 12}{2}$$

Table 4-1 Estimating Tracheal Tube Size

- Tube size (mm) = $\dfrac{\text{Age in years} + 16}{4}$
- Select a tube that matches the diameter of the child's fifth finger
- Use a length-based resuscitation tape such as the Broselow™ tape

Reproduced with permission from Bernardo, L. M. & Lees, W. E. (2001). Infants and children. In K. S. Oman, J. Koziol-McLain, & L. J. Sheetz (Eds.), *Emergency nursing secrets* (pp. 227-231). Philadelphia, PA: Hanley & Belfus, Inc.

- Obtain chest radiograph.
- Insert a gastric tube to decompress the stomach and minimize the risk of aspiration. Gastric distention may impede adequate ventilation by limiting the downward movement of the diaphragm.
- Administer medications to facilitate intubation procedure as ordered.
- If neuromuscular blocking agents are used, a sedative must also be given.
- Resuscitation equipment must be available at the bedside prior to administration of neuromuscular blocking agents.
- Decompress tension pneumothorax via needle thoracentesis, as needed. This may be indicated if the patient is in severe respiratory distress or is intubated and not improving with other interventions.

Circulation

Once adequate breathing is established, assess for the following.

Assessment

- Central and peripheral pulse rate and quality (volume/strength)
  - Palpate a brachial pulse as the central pulse in the infant; palpate a carotid pulse in children > 1 year of age.[6] The femoral pulse may also be used as a central pulse in any patient, regardless of age.
  - The presence of central pulses with absent or weak peripheral pulses is a sign of poor tissue perfusion.
- Skin color (pale, mottled, dusky, cyanotic), temperature, and moisture
- Capillary refill. Blanch the nailbed with sustained pressure for a few seconds and then release pressure. The time it takes for the nail to return to its original color is the capillary refill time.[7] Normal capillary refill is 2 seconds or less in a warm ambient environment. Factors that may affect capillary refill, not related to an alteration in general tissue perfusion, include a cool ambient temperature and injury with vascular compromise.
- Uncontrolled external bleeding

Interventions

Circulation: Ineffective

- Control any uncontrolled external bleeding by applying direct pressure over the bleeding site(s).
- Obtain vascular access by inserting the largest bore catheter that the vessel can accommodate and initiating an intravenous infusion as indicated by the pediatric patient's illness or injury.

- In the unconscious pediatric patient of any age, if peripheral access cannot be rapidly achieved, intraosseous access should be immediately considered.[5]
- Administer a 20 ml/kg fluid bolus of a warmed crystalloid solution (i.e., 0.9% normal saline or lactated Ringer's solution), as indicated by the pediatric patient's perfusion status.
  - In the pediatric patient with a severe volume deficit, the bolus should be infused within 5 to 10 minutes; in the less severely fluid depleted pediatric patient the bolus should be infused over 5 to 20 minutes.[4]
- Repeat the bolus if reassessment findings indicate inadequate tissue perfusion. Boluses should be repeated until systemic perfusion improves.[4] If symptoms of shock persist, the pediatric patient may need blood (hemorrhagic losses), colloid solutions (septic shock), or vasopressors (neurogenic shock).
- Initiate drug therapy as indicated by the illness or injury and perfusion status.
- Initiate synchronized cardioversion, as indicated by dysrhythmias.
- Initiate cardiac compressions if the pulse rate is less than 60 beats/minute and perfusion is ineffective (cardiac output = heart rate x stroke volume)

Disability—Brief Neurologic Assessment

After the assessment of airway, breathing, and circulation, conduct a brief neurologic evaluation to determine the degree of disability, as measured by the pediatric patient's level of consciousness. The findings must be based on the pediatric patient's age and developmental level.

Assessment

- Determine the pediatric patient's level of consciousness by assessing the pediatric patient's response to verbal and/or painful stimuli using the AVPU mnemonic:
  - A = Awake and alert
  - V = Responsive only to verbal stimuli
  - P = Responsive only to painful stimuli
  - U = Completely unresponsive
- In children with chronic neurologic impairment, assess responsiveness in relation to their normal or baseline status; ask the caregiver what the typical level of responsiveness for their child would be.
- Assess pupil size, shape, equality, and reactivity to light.

Interventions

- If the assessment indicates a decreased level of consciousness, conduct further investigation during the secondary assessment to identify the cause.

- Initiate pharmacologic therapy as prescribed.
- Consider the need for endotracheal intubation to maintain airway patency and/or ensure adequate ventilation and oxygenation.

Exposure and Environmental Control

Assessment

Undress the pediatric patient to examine and identify any underlying injury or additional signs of illness. Infants and children have a larger body surface area to body weight ratio and are at a greater risk to rapidly lose body heat when left exposed. Initiate methods to maintain a normothermic state or warm the patient, if hypothermic. Cold stress in critically ill or injured infants can increase metabolic demands, exacerbate the effects of hypoxia and hypoglycemia, and affect responses to resuscitative efforts.

Interventions

- Provide measures to maintain normal body temperature or to warm the patient.
  - Warm blankets
  - Overhead warming lights or other warming device
  - Warm, ambient environment, increasing the room temperature as needed
  - Warm intravenous fluids via fluid warmer when bolus volumes of intravenous fluids are administered. A variety of commercially available fluid warmers are specifically designed to warm intravenous fluids.
- For pediatric patients with fevers, provide measures to cool the patient (metabolic demand increases 10% to 13% for every degree Celsius elevation of temperature above normal; 8% increase for each degree Fahrenheit).[4] Avoid shivering as shivering not only increases metabolic and oxygen demand but also increases the temperature.
  - Remove excessive clothing or blankets.
  - Administer antipyretics per protocol.
  - In the febrile pediatric patient, consider administering intravenous fluids at normal body temperature.

Secondary Assessment

Full Set of Vital Signs

Assessment

Vital signs may be obtained prior to the secondary assessment phase, especially when a team of providers is simultaneously involved in providing care to a seriously ill or injured pediatric patient. If a complete set of vital signs has not yet been obtained, it should be done now. Recognizing subtle and significant alterations in vital signs is an important part of analyzing the assessment data. The following vital signs should be assessed in all pediatric patients.

- Respirations: Assess the rate, rhythm, and depth of respirations.
- Pulse or heart rate: Auscultate an apical pulse as a baseline rate in infants and younger children and in any critically ill or injured infant, child, or adolescent.
  - Compare central and peripheral pulses bilaterally for strength and equality.
  - When evaluating central and peripheral perfusion, palpate the peripheral pulse on an uninjured extremity.
- Blood pressure: Measure the blood pressure by auscultation, palpation, ultrasonic flow meter, or noninvasive blood pressure monitor.
  - Blood pressure cuff size can affect the accuracy of readings. An appropriately sized blood pressure cuff bladder covers one half to two thirds of the pediatric patient's upper arm.
  - Auscultate the initial blood pressure in infants, children, and adolescents with signs of poor perfusion.
    - Noninvasive, automated blood pressure monitors should be used with caution on critically ill or injured pediatric patients. Some models are not accurate for extremely high or low blood pressures. Abnormal readings or significant changes in readings should be validated by auscultation or another manual method.
  - The blood pressure in a pediatric patient may be within normal limits for the pediatric patient's age despite significant fluid/blood loss; pediatric patients can compensate for greater than a 25% volume loss before systolic blood pressure drops.
  - Typical systolic pressure in children 2 years of age or older is[4]
    Normal Systolic BP (mm Hg) = 90 + (2 x age in years)
    - The lowest acceptable limit of systolic pressure in children 2 years of age or older is[4]
      Lower limit of Normal Systolic BP (mm Hg) = 70 + (2 x age in years)
    - Diastolic blood pressure is 2/3 of the systolic pressure.
  - Temperature: Obtain temperature via an appropriate route (e.g., oral, rectal, axillary), considering the child's age and condition. Avoid rectal temperatures in immunocompromised patients. Appendix A provides a conversion table of Celsius and Fahrenheit temperatures.

- Normal pediatric vital signs are listed in **Table 4-2**.
- Apply continuous cardiac, cardiorespiratory, or pulse oximeter monitors, as appropriate, based on the pediatric patient's condition
- Weight in kilograms. The pediatric patient's weight in kilograms is needed for calculating medication doses and intravenous fluid amounts.
  - Obtain a measured weight whenever possible.
  - If circumstances do not permit a measured weight, the weight may be estimated; **Table 4-3** lists strategies for estimating pediatric weights.

Abnormal Vital Signs

- Factors affecting heart rate and respiratory rate are listed in **Table 4-4**.
- Serial blood pressure measurements are useful in identifying subtle changes. A widening pulse pressure (systolic pressure - diastolic pressure) can occur secondary to increased intracranial pressure and early septic shock; a narrowing pulse pressure is seen in early hypovolemic shock.
  - Hypotension is defined by age and can occur secondary to significant fluid or blood losses, sepsis, and certain medications. Hypotension is a late sign of shock in the pediatric patient.
  - Hypertension is defined as blood pressure at or above the 95th percentile for age.
- Temperature variations that may indicate a serious condition include:
  - Rectal temperature $\geq 38°C$ (100.4°F) in infants younger than 2 or 3 months of age
  - Rectal temperature $\geq 40°C$ (104°F) in infants 3 months to 2 years of age with no localized sign of infection
  - Rectal temperature $\leq 36°C$ (96.8°F)

Table 4-2 Vital Signs by Age

Age	Respiratory Rate/ Minute	Heart Rate/ Minute	Blood Pressure Systolic (mm Hg)
Preterm newborn	55-65	120-180	40-60
Term newborn	40-60	90-170	52-92
1 month	30-50	110-180	60-104
6 months	25-35	110-180	65-125
1 year	20-30	80-160	70-118
2 years	20-30	80-130	73-117
4 years	20-30	80-120	65-117
6 years	18-24	75-115	76-116
8 years	18-22	70-110	76-119
10 years	16-20	70-110	82-122
12 years	16-20	60-110	84-128
14 years	16-20	60-105	85-136

Adapted from Proehl, J. A. (1999). Secondary survey. In J. A. Proehl (Ed.), *Emergency nursing procedures* (2nd ed., pp. 4-6). Philadelphia, PA: WB Saunders.

Table 4-3 Strategies For Estimating Pediatric Weights

- Ask the caregiver the child's last measured weight; older children may know their own weight.
- Use a length-based resuscitation tape, such as the Broselow® tape, to estimate the child's weight if 35 kg or less.
- For the child > 1 year of age: Weight in kg = (2 x age in years) + 10
- For the child < 1 year of age: Weight in kg = $\frac{\text{Age in months}}{2}$ + 4

Table 4-4 Factors Affecting Heart Rate and Respiratory Rate

Increased Heart Rate and Respiratory Rate	Decreased Respiratory Rate	Decreased Heart Rate
Fear, anxiety, agitation	Hypoxia (late)	Vagal stimulation
Pain	Hypothermia (late)	Hypoxia (late)
Crying	Increased intracranial pressure	Hypothermia (late)
Fever	Respiratory muscle fatigue	Cardiac pathology
Hypoxia (early)	Medications	Shock (late)
Hypovolemia		Increased intracranial pressure
Hypothermia (early)		Medications
Shock (early)		
Medications		

Family Presence

The family is the pediatric patient's primary support system. The ENA recognizes the role of the family in the health and well-being of the patient and supports allowing families the option of being present for invasive and resuscitative procedures.[8]

- Assign a staff member to provide family support and to provide explanations about procedures.
- Assess the needs of the family—taking into consideration cultural variances.
- Facilitate and support the family's involvement in the pediatric patient's care.

Give Comfort Measures

Initiate comfort measures based on the pediatric patient's chief complaint and obvious injury. Examples are listed in **Table 4-5**.

Head-to-Toe Assessment

Information from the head-to-toe assessment is collected through inspection, palpation, and auscultation. The order and type of information collected in the secondary assessment will vary based on the pediatric patient's developmental level, chief complaint, and clinical appearance.

General Appearance

The general appearance of the pediatric patient can assist the nurse in discerning problems that need further investigation. The pediatric patient's activity level, interaction with the environment, outward appearance (cleanliness, appropriateness of clothing for the season, general nutritional status), and reactions to caregivers are important factors in the overall assessment of the child. Body position and alignment, guarding or self-protective movements, muscle tone, and unusual odors, such as gasoline, chemicals, urine, and feces, may be identified during the secondary assessment.

Head/Face/Neck

During the secondary assessment a more complete neurologic assessment is performed.

- A Pediatric Coma Scale score or GCS may be determined at this time (see **Table 4-6**).
- Determine orientation to person, place, and time in older children or the ability to recognize caregivers in preverbal and young children.

Inspect

- Lacerations, abrasions, ecchymosis, rashes, asymmetry, or edema

- Petechiae, subconjunctival hemorrhage
- Loose teeth or material in the mouth
- Bony deformities or angulation
- Symmetry of facial expressions
- Jugular vein distention

Palpate

- Anterior and posterior fontanels in infants for fullness, bulging, or depression. To provide meaningful information, fontanels should be palpated while the child is upright and calm[10] and not over obvious trauma or bony injury.
- Tracheal position
- Bony depressions/crepitus

Eyes/Ears/Nose

Inspect

- Eye and eyelid position, ear position
  - Color of sclera and conjunctiva. Observe for subconjunctival hemorrhage.
  - Hyphema
  - Ptosis
- Drainage or bleeding
- Lacerations, abrasions, or edema
- Ecchymosis or bruising
  - Periorbital ecchymosis or raccoon's eyes (suggestive of anterior basilar skull fracture)
  - Post auricular ecchymosis or Battle's sign, which is bleeding into the tissue behind the ears (suggestive of posterior basilar skull fracture)
- Eyeglasses or contact lenses
- Pupils, including size, shape, equality, reactivity to light, and opacity
- Extraocular eye movements
  - Observe the child's ability to follow your finger in all six directions.

Table 4-5 Comfort Measures

- Evaluate presence and level of pain. Pain can be assessed using self-report, behavioral observation, or physiologic measures, depending on the age of the child and his or her communication capabilities.[9]
- Stabilize suspected fractures
- Apply cold to injury sites
- Dress open wounds
- Provide a wheelchair or stretcher as indicated by pediatric patient's condition and chief complaint
- Consider nonpharmacologic developmentally-appropriate techniques to reduce pain

- Observe the infant or toddler's tracking of an object in all six directions.

Palpate

- Periorbital tenderness or pain
- Auricle tenderness or pain
- Nasal tenderness or pain

Chest

Inspect

- Respiratory rate, depth, work of breathing, use of accessory muscles, abdominal muscles, paradoxical chest wall movement
- Symmetry of chest wall movements
- Lacerations, abrasions, contusions, lesions/rashes, puncture wounds, impaled objects, ecchymosis, swelling, scars, or presence of central venous access devices
- Scars from healed chest tube sites, central lines, surgical incisions, or penetrating wounds

Auscultate

- Equality of breath sounds (listening over lateral, anterior, and if possible, posterior lung fields)
- Adventitious sounds such as wheezes, crackles, and friction rubs
- Heart sounds for rate, rhythm, and adventitious sounds such as murmurs, gallops, and friction rub

Palpate

- Chest wall tenderness

*Table 4-6 Pediatric Coma Scale**

Eye Opening		
Score	**> 1 year**	**< 1 year**
4	Spontaneously	Spontaneously
3	To verbal command	To shout
2	To pain	To pain
1	No response	No response
Best Motor Response		
Score	**> 1 year**	**< 1 year**
6	Obeys	Spontaneous
5	Localizes pain	Localizes pain
4	Flexion-withdrawal	Flexion-withdrawal
3	Flexion-abnormal (decorticate rigidity)	Flexion-abnormal (decorticate rigidity)
2	Extension (decerebrate rigidity)	Extension (decerebrate rigidity)
1	No response	No response

Best Verbal Response		
Score	**> 5 years**	**2 to 5 years**	**0 to 23 months**
5	Oriented and converses	Appropriate words/phrases	Smiles and coos appropriately
4	Disoriented and converses	Inappropriate words	Cries and is consolable
3	Inappropriate words	Persistent cries and/or screams	Persistent, inappropriate crying and/or screaming
2	Incomprehensible sounds	Grunts	Grunts, agitated, and restless
1	No response	No response	No response

TOTAL = 3 to 15

* Score is the sum of the individual scores from eye opening, best verbal response, and best motor response, using age-specific criteria. GCS score of 13-15 indicates mild head injury, GCS score of 9-12 indicates moderate head injury, and GCS score of ≤ 8 indicates severe head injury.

Reprinted with permission from Pons, P. T. (1999). Head trauma. In R. M. Barkin & P. Rosen (Eds.), *Emergency pediatrics: A guide to ambulatory care* (5th ed., pp. 412-425). St. Louis, MO: Mosby.

- Crepitus
- Subcutaneous emphysema
- Bony deformities

Abdomen

Inspect

- Use of abdominal muscles for breathing
- Lacerations, abrasions, contusions, rashes, impaled objects, or ecchymosis
- Observe for seat belt marks in children involved in motor vehicle crashes.
- Distention
- Feeding tubes or buttons
- Penetrating wounds or scars from healed surgical incisions

Auscultate

- Bowel sounds in all quadrants

Palpate

- All four quadrants for rigidity, tenderness, and guarding. In the infant or young child who is crying, evaluation for firmness or rigidity is more difficult. Palpating the abdomen on inspiration allows for palpation when the abdominal muscles are more relaxed.

Pelvis and Genitalia

Inspect

- Lacerations, abrasions, rashes, or edema
- Drainage from the meatus or vagina
- Scrotal bleeding or edema
- Priapism (indicative of pathologies such as sickle cell crisis or spinal cord injury)

Palpate

- Pelvic stability
- Anal sphincter tone
- Femoral pulses

Extremities

Inspect

- Angulation, deformity, open wounds with evidence of protruding bone fragments, puncture wounds, edema, ecchymosis, rashes, purpura, or petechiae
- Color (with injuries, compare injured extremity to uninjured limb)
- Abnormal movement
- Position
- Scars or venous access devices
- Signs of congenital anomalies such as a club foot, length discrepancies, or clubbing of digits

Palpate

- Skin temperature (with injuries, compare injured extremity to uninjured limb)
- Symmetry and quality of distal pulses. Compare bilateral peripheral pulses for strength and equality.
- Bony crepitus
- Muscle strength and range of motion
- Sensation

Inspect Posterior Surfaces

Inspect

- Bleeding, abrasions, wounds, hematomas, or ecchymosis
- Rashes, petechiae, edema, or purpura
- Patterned injuries or injuries in various stages of healing (suggestive of child maltreatment)

Palpate

- Tenderness and deformity of the spine
- Costovertebral angle tenderness

History

The history is obtained from the caregiver of the infant or young child or from both the caregiver and the older child or adolescent. The history is an important piece of the initial data that assists the health care provider in analyzing assessment findings. The MIVT mnemonic (i.e., mechanism of injury, injuries sustained, vital signs, and treatment) can be used to elicit a history from prehospital providers for children who have sustained trauma. Additional information related to MIVT is provided in Chapter 11, *Pediatric Trauma*. The SAMPLE and CIAMPEDS mnemonics may also be used to elicit the history. **Table 4-7** outlines the components of SAMPLE, and **Table 4-8** describes the components of CIAMPEDS. The ENA recommends following the CIAMPEDS mnemonic.

Additional information, including social and family histories, may also be needed.

Diagnostic Procedures

- The necessity of laboratory and radiographic studies is determined by the pediatric patient's clinical presentation, pattern of injury, history, and specific institutional protocols.
- The infant and toddler with serious illness or injury should have a blood glucose measured (bedside glucose test, serum glucose) because of their risk of hypoglycemia when physiologically stressed.

Table 4-7 SAMPLE

S	Signs and Symptoms	Determination of the onset and nature of the child's symptoms, including pain or fever.
A	Allergies	Evaluation of the child's previous allergic or hypersensitivity reactions: • Document reactions to medications, foods, products (e.g., latex) and environmental allergens. The type of reaction must also be documented.
M	Medications	Evaluation of the child's current medication regimen including prescription medications, over-the-counter medications, and herbal and dietary supplements: • Dose administered • Time of last dose • Duration of use

P	Past Medical History	A review of the child's health status, including prior illnesses, injuries, hospitalizations, surgeries, and chronic physical and psychiatric illnesses. Use of alcohol, tobacco, drugs, or other substances of abuse should be evaluated, as appropriate:
		• The past medical history of the neonate should include the prenatal and birth history:
		  - Maternal complications during pregnancy or delivery
		  - Infant's gestational age and birth weight
		  - Number of days infant remained in hospital post-birth
		• The past medical history of the menarche female should include the date and description of her last menstrual period.
		• The past medical history for sexually active patients should include:
		  - Type of birth control used
		  - Barrier protection
		  - Prior treatment for sexually transmitted diseases
		  - Gravida (pregnancies) and para (births, miscarriages, abortions, living children)

	Parent's/ Caregiver's Impression of the Child's Condition	Evaluation of the caregiver's concerns and observations of the child's condition. • Especially significant in evaluating the special needs child • Consider cultural differences that may affect the caregiver's impressions
L	Last meal	Assessment of the child's recent oral intake and changes in eating patterns related to the illness or injury: • Time of last meal and last fluid intake • Changes in eating patterns or fluid intake • Usual diet: Breast milk, type of formula, solid foods, diet for age and developmental level, cultural differences • Special diet or diet restrictions

E	Events Surrounding the Illness or Injury	Evaluation of the onset of the illness or circumstances and mechanism of injury:
		• Illness:
		  - Length of illness, including date and day of onset and sequence of symptoms
		  - Treatment provided prior to ED visit
		• Injury:
		  - Time and date injury occurred
		  - M: Mechanism of injury, including the use of protective devices (seat belts, helmets)
		  - I: Injuries suspected
		  - V: Vital signs in prehospital environment
		  - T: Treatment by prehospital providers
		  - Description of circumstances leading to injury
		  - Witnessed or unwitnessed

- The need for continuous physiologic monitoring is determined by the pediatric patient's condition, risk for deterioration, or the need to evaluate physiologic responses to treatment. A combination of cardiac, pulse oximeter, and noninvasive blood pressure monitoring may be indicated. Invasive blood pressure and exhaled CO_2 monitoring are valuable adjuncts for the care of the critically ill or injured child.

Planning and Implementation

Interventions for life-threatening conditions are performed as soon as the condition is recognized. Corresponding interventions have been listed with each component of the primary assessment. Additional interventions may be identified during or following the secondary assessment. These interventions may include the following.

Table 4-8 CIAMPEDS

C	Chief Complaint	Reason for the child's ED visit and duration of complaint (e.g., fever for past 2 days)
I	Immunizations	Evaluation of the child's current immunization status
		• The completion of all scheduled immunizations for the child's age should be evaluated.
		• If the child has not received immunizations due to religious or cultural beliefs, document this information.
	Isolation	Evaluation of the child's exposure to communicable diseases (e.g., meningitis, chickenpox, shingles, whooping cough, tuberculosis)
		• A child with active disease or who is potentially infectious must be placed in respiratory isolation on arrival to the ED.
		• Other exposures that may be evaluated include exposure to meningitis and scabies.
A	Allergies	Evaluation of the child's previous allergic or hypersensitivity reactions
		• Document reactions to medications, foods, products (e.g., latex) and environmental allergens. The type of reaction must also be documented.
M	Medications	Evaluation of the child's current medication regimen including prescription and over-the-counter medications, herbal and dietary supplements
		• Dose administered
		• Time of last dose
		• Duration of use
P	Past Medical History	A review of the child's health status, including prior illnesses, injuries, hospitalizations, surgeries, and chronic physical and psychiatric illnesses. Use of alcohol, tobacco, drugs, or other substances of abuse should be evaluated, as appropriate.
		• The past medical history of the neonate should include the prenatal and birth history
		- Maternal complications during pregnancy or delivery
		- Infant's gestational age and birth weight
		- Number of days infant remained in hospital post-birth
		• The past medical history of the menarche female should include the date and description of her last menstrual period
		• The past medical history for sexually active patients should include
		- Type of birth control used
		- Barrier protection
		- Prior treatment for sexually transmitted diseases
		- Gravida (pregnancies) and para (births, miscarriages, abortions, living children)
	Parent's/Caregiver's Impression of the Child's Condition	• Identify the child's primary caregiver
		• Consider cultural differences that may affect the caregiver's impressions
		• Evaluation of the caregiver's concerns and observations of the child's condition
		- Especially significant in evaluating the special needs child

Table 4-8 cont. CIAMPEDS

E	Events Surrounding The Illness or Injury	Evaluation of the onset of the illness or circumstances and mechanism of injury
		• Illness
		- Length of illness, including date and day of onset and sequence of symptoms
		- Treatment provided prior to ED visit
		• Injury
		- Time and date injury occurred
		- M: Mechanism of injury, including the use of protective devices (seat belts, helmets)
		- I: Injuries suspected
		- V: Vital signs in prehospital environment
		- T: Treatment by prehospital providers
		- Description of circumstances leading to injury
		- Witnessed or unwitnessed
D	Diet	Assessment of the child's recent oral intake and changes in eating patterns related to the illness or injury
		• Changes in eating patterns or fluid intake
		• Time of last meal and last fluid intake
		• Usual diet: Breast milk, type of formula, solid foods, diet for age and developmental level, cultural differences
		• Special diet or diet restrictions
	Diapers	Assessment of the child's urine and stool output
		• Frequency of urination over last 24 hours, changes in frequency
		• Time of last void
		• Changes in odor or color of urine
		• Last bowel movement; color and consistency of stool
		• Change in frequency of bowel movements
S	Symptoms Associated with the Illness or Injury	Identification of symptoms and progression of symptoms since the time of onset of the illness or injury event

- Prepare for admission or transfer to a pediatric tertiary care center, as indicated by the pediatric patient's clinical condition.

- Obtain vascular access for the administration of maintenance fluids or medication(s).

  - The administration of maintenance intravenous fluids may be required to replace insensible losses (skin, respiratory tract) and ongoing losses (vomiting, diarrhea). The rate and type of fluid is tailored to the specific needs of the pediatric patient. The appropriate fluid is based on the child's glucose, sodium, and potassium needs. Solutions commonly used include 5% dextrose/0.2% saline or 0.45% normal saline (U.S.); 4% dextrose in ¼ or 1/5 normal saline (Australia).

    - Fluid requirements are calculated based on the child's weight (see **Table 4-9**).

    - In some circumstances, maintenance fluids may be restricted (i.e., patients with increased intracranial pressure, pulmonary contusion). Restricted rates are calculated by the following method.

Maintenance volume/hour x desired degree of restriction

- For a 15-kg patient who is placed on two-thirds maintenance, the hourly rate is: 50 ml/hour (maintenance) x 2/3 (restricted) = 33 ml/hour.

- Insert a gastric tube to decompress the stomach as indicated. Consult a chart or length-based resuscitation tape to determine the correct tube size. See Appendix B for a list of tube sizes based on age.

- Determine the need to keep the pediatric patient without food or drink.

- Monitor the pediatric patient's intake and output, as indicated by condition.

- Insert an indwelling urinary catheter, as indicated by pediatric patient's condition, unless urethral injury is suspected. In infants and young children, the decision may be made to weigh diapers rather than insert a urinary catheter:

1 gram increase in diaper weight = 1 ml of urine
- Consult a chart or length-based resuscitation tape to determine the correct tube size. See Appendix B for a list of tube sizes based on age.
- Normal hourly urine output varies with the size and age of the child (see **Table 4-10**).

- Administer medications (e.g., antibiotics, vaccines, pain medication) as prescribed.
- Initiate appropriate isolation measures.
- Facilitate family presence in the treatment area, as guided by the assessment of family needs and institutional protocols.
  - Provide timely and clear explanations of procedures and treatment plans.
  - Assign a health care professional to provide ongoing explanation and support.
- Provide psychosocial support to help the pediatric patient cope with fear of treatment procedures.
- Evaluate for indicators of child maltreatment (see Chapter 13, *Child Maltreatment*)

Evaluation and Ongoing Assessment

The evaluation phase of the nursing process occurs when the nurse evaluates the patient's responses to the interventions and the continued effects of the illness or injury event. The achievement of expected outcomes is evaluated, and the treatment or intervention plan is adjusted as needed to attain unmet outcomes. If the pediatric patient's condition deteriorates, the primary assessment must be repeated. General evaluation of the pediatric patient's progress includes ongoing assessment of the following.

- Airway patency
- Breathing effectiveness
- Level of consciousness, activity level
- Skin temperature and color, color of mucous membranes
- Pulse rate and quality
- Intake and output
- Vital signs and pulse oximeter.
- Pain
- Body systems, as appropriate, based on assessment findings and desired outcomes

Summary

The initial assessment of ill or injured pediatric patients requires a systematic process that recognizes life-threatening conditions, identifies injuries, and determines priorities of care based on the assessment. Recognition of life-threatening conditions requires knowledge of normal growth and development, as well as the anatomic and physiologic characteristics unique to infants, children, and adolescents. The key to a successful outcome is early recognition of the prearrest state with the goal to prevent arrest with appropriate treatment. The nurse must strive to be proactive when providing care for the pediatric patient.

Table 4-9 Calculating Maintenance Fluid Requirements

4 ml/kg/hour for the first 10 kg of body weight
+ 2 ml/kg/hour for the second 10 kg of body weight
+ 1 ml/kg/hour for each additional kg over 20 kg

Ex: The hourly maintenance fluid needed for a 15-kg child would be:

4 ml x 10 kg = 40 ml/hour
+ 2 ml x 5 kg = 10 ml/hour
15 kg = 50 ml/hour

Ex: The hourly maintenance fluid needed for a 25-kg child would be:

4 ml x 10 kg = 40 ml/hour
+ 2 ml x 10 kg = 20 ml/hour
+ 1 ml x 5 kg = 5 ml/hour
25 kg = 65 ml/hour

Adapted from American Heart Association. (2002). Postarrest stabilization and transport. In *Pediatric advanced life support* (pp. 229-247). Dallas, TX: Author.

Table 4-10 Normal Urine Output By Age

Infant	2 ml/kg/hour
Child	1 to 2 ml/kg/hour
Adolescent	0.5 to 1 ml/kg/hour

References

1. Twedell, D. M. (2000). Nursing process: Assessment and priority setting. In K. S. Jordan (Ed.), *Emergency nursing core curriculum* (5th ed., pp. 1-25). Philadelphia: Saunders.

2. Young, K. D., & Seidel, J. S. (1999). Pediatric cardiopulmonary resuscitation: A collective review. *Annals of Emergency Medicine, 33*(2), 195–205.

3. Emergency Nurses Association. (2001). *Educational recommendations for nurses providing pediatric emergency care* [Position statement]. Des Plaines, IL: Author.

4. American Heart Association.(2002). *Pediatric advanced life support provider manual*. Dallas, TX: Author.

5. American Heart Association (AHA) in collaboration with the International Liaison Committee on Resuscitation. (2000). Guidelines 2000 for cardiopulmonary resuscitation and emergency cardiovascular care. Part 10: Pediatric advanced life support. *Circulation, 102*(8 suppl.), I291–I342.

6. American Heart Association (AHA) in collaboration with the International Liaison Committee on Resuscitation. (2000). Guidelines 2000 for cardiopulmonary resuscitation and emergency cardiovascular care. Part 9: Pediatric basic life support. *Circulation, 102*(8 suppl.), I253–I290.

7. Hockenberry, M. J., Wilson, D., Winkelstein, M. L., & Kline, N. E. (Eds.). (2003). Physical and developmental assessment of the child. In *Wong's nursing care of infants and children* (7th ed., pp. 170–239). St. Louis, MO: Mosby.

8. Emergency Nurses Association. (2001). *Family presence at the bedside during invasive procedures and resuscitation* [Position statement]. Des Plaines, IL: Author.

9. The assessment and management of acute pain in infants, children, and adolescents. (2001). *Pediatrics, 108*(3), 793–797.

10. Benjamin, V. L. (1998). Pediatric history and physical examination. In T. E. Soud & J. S. Rugers (Eds.), *Manual of pediatric emergency nursing* (pp. 70–88). St. Louis, MO: Mosby-Year Book.

11. Bernardo, L. M., & Lees, W. E. (2001). Infants and children. In K. S. Oman, J. Koziol-McLain, & L. J. Sheetz (Eds.), *Emergency nursing secrets* (pp. 227–231). Philadelphia: Hanley & Belfus.

Appendix 4-A

Temperature Conversion

To convert Celsius to Fahrenheit: (9/5 x temperature) + 32 OR (temperature x 1.8) + 32

To convert Fahrenheit to Celsius: (temperature - 32) x 5/9 OR (temperature - 32) ÷ 1.8

Celsius	Fahrenheit	Celsius	Fahrenheit
34.2	93.6	38.6	101.4
34.6	94.3	39.0	102.2
35.0	95.0	39.4	102.9
35.4	95.7	39.8	103.6
35.8	96.4	40.2	104.3
36.2	97.1	40.6	105.1
36.6	97.8	41.0	105.8
37.0	98.6	41.4	106.5
37.4	99.3	41.8	107.2
37.8	100.0	42.2	108.0
38.2	100.7	42.6	108.7

Appendix 4-B

*Sizes for Selected Pediatric Equipment**

Device	Neonate (3-4 kg)	Infant (4-10 kg)	1-3 yr (10-15 kg)	3-9 yr (15-30 kg)	9-14 yr (30-50 kg)
Endotracheal tube (mm)	3.0-3.5	3.5-4.5	4-5	4.5-6.5	6.5-7.0
Gastric tube (F)	5	8	8-10	10-12	12-16
Urinary catheter (F)	5	8	8-10	10-12	12-16
Chest tube (F)	10-14	14-20	14-24	16-32	28-38
Suction catheter (F)	6	6-8	8	8-10	10-12
Blood pressure cuff	Newborn	Infant	Infant-child	Child	Child-adult

*Suggested sizes only. Consider individual child's size and clinical condition when selecting equipment.

Reprinted with permission from Andreoni, C. P. and Klinkhammer, B. (2000). *Quick reference for pediatric emergency nursing* (p.23). Philadelphia, PA: W. B. Saunders.

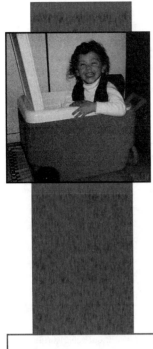

chapter 5

TRIAGING THE PEDIATRIC PATIENT

Case Scenario A

A 6-year-old child arrives to the emergency department (ED) walking with her mother. The Pediatric Assessment Triangle (PAT) reveals that the child is interactive, her color is pink, and she has mild intercostal retractions with nasal flaring.

Case Scenario B

An 18-month-old arrives to the ED carried by his mother. The PAT reveals that the child is pale with unlabored respirations and reacts minimally to strangers.

Case Scenario C

A 1-year-old arrives to the ED in a stroller pushed by her father. She is crying but consolable, her skin appears pale, and she has unlabored respirations.

Which of the preceding patients, according to the PAT, requires the most immediate intervention?

See answers at the end of the chapter.

Objectives

On completion of this chapter, the learner should be able to:

1. Identify the components of the pediatric triage process.

2. Compare and contrast the differences between triage of pediatric and adult patients.

3. Discuss the differences between the three-level, four-level and five-level triage classification systems.

4. Demonstrate understanding of the triage process for pediatric patients through case scenario presentations.

5. Review the red flags of pediatric triage assessment.

The process of triage occurs primarily in the ED, but also in a variety of other locations where patients are received. This includes inpatient receiving units, pre- and postprocedure areas, freestanding urgent care settings, clinic settings, schools, and field settings, such as emergency medical services (EMS), interfacility transport, disaster management, search and rescue, and the armed services.

The systematic process of triage begins when the patient comes into view of the nurse or health care provider performing the triage process. Triage, from the French word trier, meaning to sort, is a process that originated during wartime. Injured soldiers were often sorted to enable the less-injured soldiers to receive medical attention before the more seriously injured soldiers. This allowed the less-injured soldiers to return to the front line more quickly. The process of triage continues today. However, patients are now sorted according to their urgency of need for emergency care.

In the ED, triage is the first place that a patient or family makes contact when seeking emergency care.[1] Like the evolution of health care in the past decade, the triage process has also evolved to acknowledge the increasing volume of patients presenting for care, the definition of customer satisfaction, and the dwindling market of limited resources.[2] The overall goals of triage are the same for both adults and children—to rapidly assess the patients presenting for emergency care and to determine the severity of illness or injury and the corresponding need for emergency care. The challenge in assessing a pediatric patient and assigning triage acuity is to understand the effects of developmental and physiological characteristics of children and compare that against the assessment findings.[3]

An effective triage system serves to make certain that all patients receive health care in a timely manner according to their level of urgency based on a triage assessment. The initiation of emergency care essentially depends on the assessment and acuity assigned by the triage nurse. The triage nurse serves as the gatekeeper for the ED to promote patient flow and the efficient use of resources (including staffing, rooms, and equipment) by appropriate assignment of acuity.[4]

The Emergency Nurses Association's Standard of Practice for Triage describes the comprehensive triage process to include the evaluation and prioritization of patients presenting to the ED, the initiation of interventions based on patient need, the ordering of diagnostic and procedural interventions (based on standing triage protocols), and the performance of ongoing reassessments for patients pending room placement and definitive emergency care.[5, 6, 7]

The Triage Process for Children

There are four components to pediatric triage. These components include the Pediatric Assessment Triangle (PAT), the physical assessment (objective information), the history using CIAMPEDS (subjective information), and the triage decision. Although the PAT is most commonly the initial component and the assignment of triage acuity is last, it is recognized that the four components to pediatric triage are often done simultaneously.

Different than the triage of adult patients, the triage of pediatric patients generally involves additional assessment and history taking to arrive at the triage decision. The rationale for additional assessment includes

- The significance of the developmental stage of each child, their current behavior as compared to their norm
- The awareness of illnesses and injuries that are common with different developmental stages
- The identification of risk factors for child maltreatment
- The extent of the compensatory mechanisms of children that may mask serious illness or injury
- The risk for rapid deterioration once compensatory mechanisms fail

Similarly, the rationale for additional history taking includes

- The communication with the family or primary caregiver about parental concerns and perceptions
- The consideration for the absence of mature communication skills in most children
- The portability of children with caregivers who often ignore the use of EMS and delay definitive care
- The identification of risk factors for child maltreatment
- Any treatments provided prior to arrival, including the use of cultural and home treatments and their effects
- The lack of primary health care and preventive care by many children and families

The Pediatric Assessment Triangle (PAT)

Children often have an exaggerated response to the approach of strangers, and health care providers may provoke this response. Children may express apprehension and fear in the health care setting as a result of previous experiences or as a new unknown experience. This apprehension and fear may be demonstrated physiologically as agitation, inconsolability, combativeness, withdrawal, tachycardia, or tachypnea. These same symptoms can also indicate significant illness or injury. Due to this exaggerated response, the most accurate assessment will occur as you approach the child from across the room.[10,11] **Table 5-1** describes general tips when triaging children and their families.

Table 5-1 Pediatric Triage Tips[8,9]

- Approach the child slowly and calmly.
- If possible, allow the child to remain with the caregiver or in the stroller.
- Avoid standing over the child—position yourself at eye level with the child.
- Avoid direct eye contact with young children, especially toddlers, as they may feel threatened.
- Always observe before touching.
- If age appropriate, allow the child to touch equipment (i.e., stethoscope).
- Use distraction while doing assessment. Make the beeping or moving equipment into a game (i.e., a car race, a song, a video machine, a TV).
- Be sure to involve the child while the assessment is occurring. Speak directly to them by calling their name and enlist their help (i.e., press the button, remove the blood pressure cuff).
- Explain the expected course of treatment to the parents, including the triage findings and concerns.
- Reassure the caregivers that their child is doing okay—this will help calm the parents and indirectly calm the child. If the child is not doing well, find at least one thing that is good (i.e., he is breathing on his own).
- With vital signs, do least invasive first.
- ALWAYS look under a cover. This includes blankets or wound dressings.
- Call the child by the name their parents call them, not necessarily their given name.
- Talk and look at the child, even though you may be asking the parent a question.
- Allow parents to help—give directions if needed and invite them to participate (within reason). Remember that most parents often feel a loss of control with the situation.
- Reassure, reassure, reassure.

The Pediatric Assessment Triangle provides a physiological assessment of three areas to rapidly identify how sick the pediatric patient is and to determine how quickly treatment is required.[10,12] As the child and family enter triage (or the area in which you are working), quickly assess the following parameters using visual and auditory observation assessment skills only: (1) the child's activity level (interest in play, interest in environment, and body position), (2) airway (abnormal airway sounds, drooling), (3) breathing (respiratory rate and effort), and (4) circulation (skin color). Primary caregivers and parents can assist with distracting the pediatric patient, changing positions to facilitate better visualization, and removing or lifting clothing.

As the "across-the-room assessment," the PAT precedes the initial assessment and vital signs components of triage assessment. Outside the triage area, the PAT can be used to provide a quick ongoing evaluation of the pediatric patient to identify changes in condition and response to interventions. It allows for a rapid assessment of the pediatric patient's overall physiological stability and the development of an overall general impression—looks good versus looks bad.[10, 13]

To more effectively utilize the PAT, the nurse can seek the answers to the following questions.

- *General Impression:* Does the child look ill? Does the child look well? Is the child playful? Does the child seem aware of his or her surroundings? Is the child running, walking, requiring assistance to ambulate, or being held by the caregiver? Is the child alert, crying continuously, sleepy, or unresponsive? What is the child's interaction with the environment and caregiver?
- *Work of Breathing:* What is the position of comfort to facilitate air entry—sniffing or tripod? Are there audible airway sounds such as stridor, grunting, or wheezing? Is the child coughing? Is the child drooling? How is the child breathing—rapid, labored, or shallow? Is the respiratory rate slow, normal for age, or rapid? Is there nasal flaring? Are there signs of accessory muscle use?
- *Circulation to skin:* Is the child's skin color pale, dusky, cyanotic, mottled, or flushed? Is there any obvious bleeding? Is the child diaphoretic?

The three components of the PAT help to quickly identify a pediatric patient in need of rapid intervention and treatment. General appearance points to neurological function and how well the body is compensating; work of breathing and circulation point to the vital functions that are sensitive in the pediatric patient. **Table 5-2** offers interpretations of the PAT that will assist the triage nurse in formulating a clinical impression.

Pediatric patients with a good general appearance (vital functions intact, no respiratory distress or peripheral vasoconstriction) are stable enough to warrant comprehensive triage and designation of a low-acuity triage classification. Pediatric patients with poor general appearance (compromise with respirations, shock, or altered level of consciousness) require high-acuity triage classification with rapid interventions initiated.[10]

Physical Assessment

Following the PAT, the initial primary and secondary assessment begins. For the pediatric patient who does not have a patent airway, is not breathing adequately, does not have adequate perfusion, or has a decreased level of consciousness or is unresponsive, the triage process is interrupted, and appropriate interventions are initiated. For the pediatric patient who appears to be stable and compensating, the triage process progresses to a more thorough primary and secondary assessment.

Table 5-2 Interpretation of the Pediatric Assessment Triangle

General Appearance	Work of breathing	Circulation to skin	Systems involved	Compensated	Ill
Good	Normal	Normal	No active compromise to vital functions	Yes	No
Good	Increased	Normal	Respiratory distress (varying degrees)	Yes	No
Poor	Increased —poor effort	Normal	Respiratory failure	No	Yes
Good	Normal	Abnormal	Peripheral vasoconstriction (medications, fever, hypothermia)	Yes	Probably not
Poor	Normal to mildly increased	Abnormal	Shock	No	Yes
Poor	Normal	Normal	CNS dysfunction (postictal, head injury, drugs)	No	Yes
Poor	Poor effort	Abnormal	Cardiopulmonary failure	No	Yes
Poor	None	None	Cardiopulmonary arrest	No	Yes

Reprinted with permission from Romig, L. E. (2001). PREP: Patient physiology, rescuer responses, equipment, protocols. Size-up & approach tips for pediatric calls. *Journal of Emergency Medical Services, 26*(5), 24–33.

The systematic approach will follow the A to I mnemonic as described in Chapter 4, *Initial Assessment.* Nurses who are accustomed to triaging pediatric patients may complete the primary assessment more quickly and modify their secondary assessment to a more problem-focused or system-focused secondary assessment. For example, in a child who presents with a laceration to the leg, the airway and breathing portions of the primary assessment would be completed rapidly—the child is awake, alert, and talking without difficulty; while a more focused assessment would be completed of the circulatory status, extremity including neurovascular status, and comfort level. Emergency nurses who are more accustomed to triaging adults and less-experienced pediatric nurses should follow the systematic triage process to avoid missing any subtle cues or red flags (see **Table 5-3**).

The measurement of vital signs is a central component of the physical assessment of pediatric patients because they often provide subtle information regarding the child's status. However, vital signs are not the first priority when triaging a child. Vulnerable populations may benefit from having all or part of the vital signs obtained in triage because it may affect the triage decision. These children include infants less than 3 months of age, children with chronic illnesses, and children returning within 24 hours.

Considerations for obtaining vital signs in children in the triage area include the following.
- The ability to provide privacy
- The availability of adequate space to accommodate the parent(s) and child
- The length of time required to obtain vital signs in children
- The acuity of ill or injured child
- The ability to console and comfort family with the information obtained

Normal ranges of vital signs vary with age and size of the pediatric patient. Resources should be available in the triage area to quickly identify vital signs that are out of range or abnormal.[11,12] Vital signs that are within normal range may mean that they are normal or that the pediatric patient is compensating well for the illness or injury. Vital signs should be interpreted in conjunction with the context of the clinical assessment and observation of the pediatric patient. In one study, 25% of patients less than 15 years of age had their triage decision changed as a result of the vital signs obtained.[16]

When possible, vital signs, including heart rate, respiratory rate, temperature, blood pressure, and weight, should be obtained in triage to establish a baseline on arrival and offer the opportunity to trend vital signs on an ongoing basis. Keep in mind that a kilogram weight is needed to calculate any fluids or medications needed. Changes in vital signs (increasing or decreasing) may suggest a loss of compensatory mechanisms, worsening hypoxia, shock, or improvement after treatment.[10,12] It must be acknowledged that apprehensive or crying children, especially those less than 3 years of age, will have altered vital signs not necessarily indicative of their illness or injury.[12] Ideally, interventions to calm the child and reduce anxiety should be instituted before vital signs are obtained. If interventions fail and vital signs are obtained under these conditions, it should be documented in the triage note.

Table 5-3 Red Flags of Pediatric Triage[3,8,10,12,14,15]

Airway	Apnea
	Choking
	Drooling
	Audible airway sounds
	Positioning
Breathing	Grunting
	Sternal retractions, increased work of breathing
	Irregular respiratory patterns
	RR > 60 breaths/minute
	RR < 20 breaths/minute for children less than 6 years of age
	RR < 15 breaths/minute for children less than 15 years of age
	Absence of breath sounds
	Cyanosis
Circulation	Cool or clammy skin
	Tachycardia, bradycardia
	HR > 200 beats/minute
	HR < 60 beats/minute
	Hypotension
	Diminished or absent peripheral pulses
	Decreased tearing, sunken eyes
Disability	Altered level of consciousness
	Inconsolability
	Sunken or bulging fontanel
Exposure	Petechia
	Purpura
	Signs and symptoms of abuse
Full set of vital signs	Hypothermia
	Fever in an infant less than three months > 38°C (100.4°F)
	Temperature > 40.0°C to 40.6°C (104°F to 105°F) at any age
Give comfort	Severe pain
History	History of a chronic illness
	History of a family crisis
	Return visit to ED within 24 hours

Rectal temperatures are the most dependable means of obtaining a temperature when an accurate temperature is needed to make a triage decision.[29] However, avoid obtaining rectal temperatures in children with any potential or actual immunocompromise (including neonates) or with a chronic illness such as sickle cell anemia, because it may allow for the entrance of bacteria through an abraised rectal mucosal wall. Rectal temperatures should also not be taken in any child who has had rectal surgery or who currently has diarrhea.[31]

The Crying Child

One of the most challenging aspects of caring for children in the ED is dealing with a child (usually less than 2 years of age) who presents with nonspecific symptoms such as crying and irritability. Due to the child's inability to communicate and to localize complaints, these symptoms can indicate a wide range of nonurgent and emergent problems, such as colic and meningitis. Be sure to assess for the following.

- Signs of an infectious process including fever, bulging fontanel, ear pain, nuchal rigidity, vomiting, and diarrhea
- Signs of pain including ear pain (otitis media), eye pain (corneal abrasion), joint and bone pain (toxic synovitis, nurse maid's elbow, or fracture), testicular pain, teething or aphthous stomatitis, hair tourniquets of toes and genitalia, or abdominal pain (intussusception or constipation).

Crying and irritability are vague symptoms. The overall appearance and stability of the child should guide the triage process. In most children presenting with crying and irritability, the general appearance and ability of the child to be consoled may be the best indication of the child's status.

Case Scenario D

An 8-year-old is brought to triage with the chief complaint of vomiting for the past 3 hours. The child was carried in by his father and is now quietly sitting in a chair, appears pale, and has nonlabored respirations. Initial assessment reveals a child with a patent airway. There are no abnormal airway sounds or signs of increased work of breathing. He is pale in color and has abrasions to the right side of his body and head. He speaks slowly when responding to questions but answers appropriately; pupils are unequal—right larger than left. Respiratory rate 24 breaths/minute, heart rate 120 beats/minute, capillary refill 3 seconds, and blood pressure 96/60 mm Hg.

1. Based on the PAT and initial assessment, how rapidly should this child be treated?

2. Which components of the CIAMPEDS history would further assist you in identifying the urgency of need for emergency care for this child?

3. What is your impression of the vital signs?

See answers at the end of the chapter.

The Triage History

The triage history is completed through a verbal exchange of information between the triage nurse, the parent (or caregiver), and the pediatric patient (as age appropriate). If there is a language or communication barrier, the exactness of the history will be diminished and may affect the accuracy of the triage decision. Consideration should be made to identify the language barrier based on appropriate verbal responses (other than yes or no) rather than nonverbal responses (such as nodding).

Translators should be obtained as quickly as possible from resources within the facility or by using a service such as the AT&T Language Line. Although staff at your facility should be familiar with confidentiality when translating, friends and family members may not. When using friends and family members to translate, consider the information you are requesting them to ask, discuss confidentiality, and request the confidentiality discussion be translated to the caregiver and child. Caution should be used when using nonprofessional translators (including nurses, social workers, family, friends and siblings) because more errors are likely to occur than with professional translators.[30] In one study of the errors that occurred, 68% had potential clinical implications, with omission of information being the most common type of error (52%).[30] **Box 5-1** identifies specific tips to be used with a translator.

Box 5-1 Tips When Using a Translator[28]

- Meet with translator and explain purpose of the interview.
- Encourage translator to avoid inserting his or her own ideas and from omitting information.
- Avoid using medical jargon. Speak in simple terms using short sentences.
- Avoid requesting too much information at one time. Break down a question into small sections.
- Encourage the translator to interpret the information in the patient's own words.
- Restate and seek clarification as needed.
- Speak directly to the caregivers and child, not to the translator.
- Observe nonverbal communication.

Communication barriers (such as hearing impaired or verbally impaired) must also be identified implementing the most appropriate method of communication (as identified by the patient or family). Alternative communication methods include writing, signing, or using a Teletype machine (TTY) or computer.[9, 17]

Obtaining the history is part of the secondary assessment. Information may be obtained from a variety of sources including prehospital providers, the caregiver, and the child. The goal in obtaining a history is to elicit accurate information regarding the problem or chief complaint and specific information regarding the illness or injury to help determine the urgency of need for emergency care.

Specific factors place children at risk for certain patterns of illness and injury and these should be considered during the history. These factors include (1) biological factors such as age and gender, (2) behavioral factors such as poor nutritional intake or substance use, (3) sociocultural factors such as cultural health practices, (4) environmental factors such as seasonal changes or inner-city living, and (5) developmental factors such as prematurity or developmental delay.[20]

There are a variety of formats used to elicit information in the emergency setting such as CIAMPEDS (Table 4-7) or SAMPLE (Table 4-8) which were described in Chapter 4, *Initial Assessment*.

Triage Decision

The triage decision is made based on the PAT, physical assessment findings, and subjective information obtained from the history. According to assessment findings on severity of illness and potential for deterioration, the patient is classified into an acuity level based on the triage classification system being utilized. There are a number of triage classification systems including the three-level, four-level, and five-level systems.[3,8]

In the United States, many EDs use a three-level triage classification system, which prioritizes patients into emergent, urgent, and nonurgent levels (see **Table 5-4**).[21] The three-level system has many gray areas in which assessment findings challenge triage level classification because they do not match a classification level. As a result, a higher number of patients are overtriaged or undertriaged. An overtriage, or incorrect emergent classification, misuses resources and needlessly impedes other patients' care. Inversely, an incorrect nonurgent triage classification potentially results in poor patient outcomes, extended waiting times, and patient dissatisfaction.[1,19] Reliability and interrater agreement with this classification system is poor,[21] ranging from 11% to 63%.[22]

Table 5-5 reviews the four-level triage classification that is used by a small number of facilities in the United States.[5,8] This system takes the Urgent category of the three-level system and further clarifies distinctions in patient criteria creating the four levels. This system also

Table 5-4 Three-Level Triage Classification[3]

	Description	Time to Definitive Care	Example
Emergent	Pediatric patients with life- or limb-threatening conditions who require resuscitation or immediate intervention to avoid loss of life or permanent disability. Also includes patients who are at risk for deterioration and require immediate intervention.	Less than 20 minutes	• Moderate to severe respiratory distress • Multisystem injury • Shock • Suicide attempt • Extremity injury with neurovascular compromise • Altered neurologic status
Urgent	Pediatric patients with illness, injury, or mental health conditions requiring prompt but not immediate care. Reassessment of these patients must occur to assess for any deterioration during the delay.	Less than 2 hours	• Mild wheezes with minimal respiratory distress • Mild to moderate dehydration • Fracture of the forearm • Single-system trauma without associated symptoms
Nonurgent	Pediatric patients with minor, stable illness or injury. Reassessment of these patients must occur to assess for any deterioration during the delay	Less than 4 hours	• Ear discomfort • Minor wounds without active bleeding • Isolated soft tissue injury • Sore throat • Fever

fails to provide reliability and reproducibility between raters when assigning a triage level.[22]

Compared to the three-level and four-level systems, five-level triage classification systems have consistently demonstrated reliability.[4,22] The five-level classification system is used internationally and is the primary or only triage classification system used in Australia, Canada, New Zealand, and the United Kingdom. The National Triage Scale (NTS), later revised to the Australian Triage Scale (ATS), was implemented in Australia in 1994 and was the first five-level triage classification system that continuously demonstrated reliability.[4,18,19] The Canadian Triage and Acuity Scale (CTAS), based on the NTS and developed in 1995, became the official policy of Ontario in 1997 and is also used in some U.S. emergency departments.[21,22] The CTAS has also been tested to demonstrate reliability. In England a five-level classification system, adapted from the NTS, was developed between the Royal College of Nursing Accident and Emergency Association and the British Association for Accident and Emergency Medicine and revised into the Manchester Triage System.[22] The Emergency Severity Index is a five-level classification system that is used in the United States, and also demonstrates reliability.[1,18,24,25] **Table 5-6** provides a review of the five-level triage classification systems.

Recently, the Emergency Nurses Association (ENA) and the American College of Emergency Physicians (ACEP) jointly approved a policy statement stating that "quality of patient care would benefit from implementing a standardized ED triage scale and acuity categorization process. Based on expert consensus of currently available evidence ACEP and ENA support the adoption of a reliable, valid five-level triage scale." The joint task force indicated that further research was needed in order to recommend one scale over another (personal communication, July 2003). Use of a standard five-level system in the United States would improve triage accuracy and patient outcomes and would promote standardized education and triage competency.[8,18] Currently momentum is building for the development of an international triage system incorporating the five-level classification system.[26]

From time to time, the triage nurse may feel uncomfortable about a patient's clinical appearance or subtle assessment findings. This feeling, intuition, or "sixth sense" is frequently accurate and should not be ignored. Also, the intuition of the parent as indicated by statements such as "I don't know what's wrong, he's just not acting right" should flag this pediatric patient for a more in-depth triage assessment or more frequent reassessments while awaiting room placement. In gen-

Table 5-5 *Four-level Triage Classification*[5,8]

	Description	Time to Definitive Treatment	Example
Critical	Delay may be harmful to patient; condition threatens life or function	Immediate	• Cardiac or respiratory arrest • Severe respiratory distress • Alteration in level of consciousness • Shock
Acute	High risk for patient deterioration if not provided care	15 to 30 minutes	• Infant < 28 days with fever • Moderate respiratory distress • Hemophiliac with bleeding • Severe abdominal pain
Urgent	Does not require immediate attention	30 to 60 minutes	• Fever in infant < 3 months • Laceration without active bleeding • Eye injury without visual disturbance • Mild respiratory distress
Nonurgent	Minor health condition; patient is stable	1 to 2 hours	• History of coughing without cyanosis • Fever > 38°C to 40.9°C (100.4°F to 105.6°F) in children > 12 weeks of age • Ear pain • Upper respiratory symptoms

eral, it may be preferable to place the potentially ill or injured patient in a higher triage category to prevent the possibility of delays in treatment. If, during any part of the triage assessment, the nurse determines that the child has an emergent condition, the triage process should be interrupted and appropriate interventions initiated. Pediatric patients waiting in the ED must be frequently monitored. Serial, timely reassessment is essential to identify the deterioration of children awaiting room placement.

Interventions performed in triage should be implemented through standardized triage-initiated policies or protocols and should be based on specific patient criteria. These interventions may be diagnostic or therapeutic in nature; however, the goal of triage-initiated interventions is not to provide a diagnosis in triage. Interventions initiated by triage nurses for patients waiting to receive definitive care often expedite care and improve patient outcomes.[19,27] The most common triage interventions performed include splinting an injured extremity, obtaining a urinalysis, obtaining blood glu-

cose and other blood specimens, initiating pulse oximetry, administering antipyretic to a febrile child, application of and interpretation of cardiac and pulse oximetry monitoring, initiation of oral rehydration therapy, administering nebulized medications, and initiating intravenous access.[19,27]

Legal Implications of Emergency Care and Triage in the United States[8, 28]

Nurses practicing in the ED must be aware of the legal issues affecting practice and patient care. In the United States, the 1986 Emergency Medical Treatment and Active Labor Act (EMTALA), part of the Consolidated Omnibus Budget and Reconciliation Act (COBRA), specifically affects health care workers providing care in Medicare-participating hospitals with EDs. Also known as the antidumping law, EMTALA was designed to protect patient rights and prevent inappropriate transfers of

Table 5-6 Five-level Triage Classification[1,4,19,23,24,25]

	Description	Time to Definitive Treatment	Example
Resuscitation	Unstable vital functions with maximum resource utilization	Immediate	• Cardiac and respiratory arrest • Unconscious • Active seizure • Major trauma
Emergent	Threatened vital functions with potential threat to life or limb; high resource utilization	Within 10 minutes	• Altered level of consciousness • Chest pain • Moderate to severe respiratory distress • Fever in infant < 6 weeks of age
Urgent	Stable vital functions; not likely to threaten life; medium resource utilization	Within 30 to 60 minutes	• Abdominal pain • Dehydration • Nonpenetrating eye injury • Moderate pain
Semiurgent	Stable vital functions with low need for resources	Within 1 to 2 hours	• Simple laceration • Extremity trauma • Head trauma without symptoms • Fever in child 3 months to 3 years
Nonurgent	Stable vital functions without need of resources	Within 2 to 3 hours	• Sore throat • Earache • Mild gastroenteritis • Fever in child > 36 months

patients regardless of ability to pay for treatment. Additionally, the Health Insurance Portability and Accountability Act (HIPAA) of 1996 is a multifaceted legislation with many health care implications.

The EMTALA statute is triggered when patients present seeking emergency care. Once this occurs, a medical screening exam (MSE) must be performed to determine if the individual seeking care has an emergency medical condition. If one exists, the patient must be stabilized within the capabilities of the hospital. Should further stabilization be required, the patient must be transferred to a hospital with specialized capabilities, and the receiving hospital must accept the patient if it has the space and personnel available. Hospital policies and procedures must identify who may perform the MSE; however, it must be realized that triage does not satisfy the MSE requirement of EMTALA. EMTALA compliance dilemmas may exist when there is missing triage documentation of patients, particularly for those patients who left without being seen.[3] If triage staff becomes aware that a patient is planning on leaving without being seen, the patient should be reassured that emergency care will be provided and be informed of the risks of leaving. These efforts should be documented on the triage note.

HIPAA covers three areas, including insurance portability (ability to change insurance without losing coverage), fraud enforcement (accountability), and administrative simplification of all patients' health information. For ED staff, the last area has the most impact. HIPAA requirements affect all patient-identifiable health-related information, whether it is oral, written, or electronic. Communication of patient health-related information should be limited to those who need to know the information to provide treatment, payment, and health care administration.

Summary

The triage process for ill or injured pediatric patients involves a systematic process that recognizes life-threatening conditions, identifies injuries, and determines priorities of care. The nurse's responsibility in triaging pediatric patients is first to be able to differentiate between the well child and those with illness or injury requiring more acute care. The systematic approach of triage consists of four components—the Pediatric Assessment Triangle, physical assessment, history, and the triage decision. Identifying the abnormal assessment findings and the subtle cues communicated by the pediatric patient will enable the triage nurse to accurately and effectively designate triage decisions.

Answers to Case Scenarios A, B, C

Of these three children, Case B is the most ill and requires the most rapid intervention. This toddler has a poor general appearance as evidenced by the altered level of consciousness (reacts minimally to strangers) and abnormal circulation to skin (pale skin color). She is no longer able to compensate for her illness or injury. There is a high suspicion of shock or central nervous system dysfunction. History revealed that the child had ingested an unknown amount of her mother's nerve pills 30 minutes prior to arrival.

The school-age child from Case A has an increased work of breathing (nasal flaring and mild intercostals retractions) with normal skin color and normal general appearance (interactive and walking). She appears to be compensating for her illness or injury and seems to be adequately ventilating and oxygenating herself. History revealed that the child has hyperactive airway disease (asthma) and started wheezing after she developed an upper respiratory infection. She was given a nebulizer treatment 30 minutes prior to arrival.

The toddler from Case C has a good general appearance (the child is crying but is consolable by father) with normal work of breathing, but has abnormal circulation to skin (pale skin color). Although she appears ill, she is compensating well. History reveals that she started vomiting during the night and diarrhea started this morning. The father states that she starts crying just before she vomits.

Answers to Case Scenario D

Based on the PAT, this child is concerning and should receive a more in-depth triage evaluation. His general appearance is abnormal, and his circulation to skin color is abnormal (pale), possibly indicating that he has neurological or circulatory problem. Additional findings include unequal pupils R > L, which further point toward a closed head injury.

2. CIAMPEDS History

Past medical history/parent perception:

Q: Does he have any past medical history?
Answer = No.

Q: Is he acting normally?
Answer = He's a little quieter than usual.

Q: Is he speaking normally?
Answer = Yes, his cerebral palsy sometimes makes him talk that way.

Q: What does the parent think?
Answer = Parent concerned about the vomiting.

Events surrounding:

Q: What happened before he started vomiting?
Answer = Nothing.

Q: What caused the abrasions?
Answer = He fell off his bicycle this morning going over a curb.

Q: Did he lose consciousness after falling?
Answer = No

Diet/diapers:

Q: How many times has he vomited?
Answer = 4 times in the past hour

Q: Any diarrhea?
Answer = No

3. Vital sign interpretation:

RR—high end of normal, HR—tachycardia due to blood or fluid loss, fear, pain, CR—slightly delayed (what is body temperature?), BP—WNL

References

1. Wuerz, R.C., Milne, L. W., Eitel, D. R., Travers, D., & Gilboy, N. G. (2000). Reliability and validity of a new five-level triage instrument. *Academic Emergency Medicine, 7*(3), 236–242.

2. Fry, M., & Burr, G. (2001). Current triage practice and influences affecting clinical decision-making in emergency departments in NSW, Australia. *Accident and Emergency Nursing, 9*(4), 227–234.

3. Holleran, R. S. (2003). Triage. In D. O. Thomas, L. M. Bernardo, & B. Herman (Eds.), *Core curriculum for pediatric emergency nursing* (pp. 89–95). Boston, MA: Jones and Bartlett.

4. Considine, J., Ung, L., & Thomas, S. (2000). Triage nurses' decisions using the national triage scale for Australian emergency departments. *Accident & Emergency Nursing, 8*(4), 201–209.

5. Murphy, K. S. (Ed.). (1997). *Pediatric triage guidelines.* St. Louis, MO: Mosby-Year Book.

6. Considine, J., Ung, L., & Thomas, S. (2001). Clinical decisions using the national triage scale: How important is postgraduate education? *Accident and Emergency Nursing, 9*(2), 101–108.

7. Emergency Nurses Association. (1999). *Standards of emergency nursing practice* (4th ed.). Des Plaines, IL: Author.

8. Thomas, D. O. (2002). Special considerations for pediatric triage in the emergency department. *Nursing Clinics of North America, 37*(1), 145–159.

9. Handysides, G. (1996). *Triage in emergency practice.* St. Louis, MO: Mosby.

10. Romig, L. E. (2001). PREP for peds—patient physiology, rescuer responses, equipment, protocols. Size-up & approach tips for pediatric calls. *Journal of Emergency Medical Services, 26*(5), 24–33.

11. Velasco-Whetsell, M., Coffin, D., Hamilton, O., Hartley, J., Hunt, C., Lizardo, L., et al. (Eds.). (2000). *Pediatric nursing.* New York: McGraw-Hill.

12. American Academy of Pediatrics. (Eds.). (2000). *Pediatric education for prehospital professionals.* Boston, MA: Jones and Bartlett.

13. Bernardo, L. M., & Lees, W. E. (2001). Infants and children. In K. S. Oman, J. K. Koziol-McLain, & L. J. Scheetz (Eds.), *Emergency nursing secrets* (pp. 227–231). Philadelphia: Hanley & Belfus.

14. American Heart Association. (2002). *PALS provider manual.* Dallas, TX: Author.

15. Andreoni, C. P., & Klinkhammer, B. (2000). *Quick reference for pediatric emergency nursing.* Philadelphia: Saunders.

16. Cooper, R. J., Schriger, D. L., Flaherty, H. L., Lin, E. J., & Hubbell, K. A. (2002). Effect of vital signs on triage decisions. *Annals of Emergency Medicine, 39*(3), 223–232.

17. Zimmermann, P. G. (2002). Guiding principles at triage: Advice for new triage nurses. *Journal of Emergency Nursing, 28*(1), 24–33.

18. Travers, D. A., Waller, A. E., Bowling, J. M., Flowers, D., & Tintinalli, J. (2002). Five-level triage system more effective than three-level in a tertiary emergency department. *Journal of Emergency Nursing, 28*(5), 395–400.

19. Gerdtz, M. & Bucknall, T. (2000). Australian triage nurse's decision-making and scope of practice. *Australian Journal of Advanced Nursing, 18*(1), 24–33.

20. Muscari, M. E. (2001). *Advanced pediatric clinical assessment: Skills and procedures.* Philadelphia: Lippincott Williams & Wilkins.

21. Wuerz, R., Fernandes, C. M., & Alarcon, J. (1998). Inconsistency of emergency department triage. *Annals of Emergency Medicine, 32*(4), 431–435.

22. Zimmermann, P. G. (2001). The case for a universal, valid, reliable, 5-tier triage acuity scale for US emergency departments. *Journal of Emergency Nursing, 27*(3), 246–254.

23. Beveridge, R., Ducharme, J., Janes, L., Beaulieu, S., & Walter, S. (1999). Reliability of the Canadian emergency department triage and acuity scale: Interrater agreement. *Annals of Emergency Medicine, 34*(2), 155–159.

24. National Triage Task Force. (2001). Canadian paediatric triage and acuity scale: Implementation guidelines for emergency departments. *Canadian Journal of Emergency Medicine, 3*(4 Supplement), S1–S27.

25. Wuerz, R. C., Travers, D., Gilboy, N., Eitel, D. R., Rosenau, A., & Yazhari, R. (2001). Implementation and refinement of the emergency severity index. *Academic Emergency Medicine, 8*(2), 170–176.

26. Jelinek, G. A. (2001). Towards an international triage scale. *European Journal of Emergency Medicine, 8*(1), 3–7.

27. Cheung, W. W., Heeney, L., & Pound, J. L. (2002). An advance triage system. *Accident and Emergency Nursing, 10*(1), 10–16.

28. Mitchiner, J. C. & Yeh, C. S. (2002). The emergency medical treatment and active labor act: What emergency nurses need to know. *Nursing Clinics of North America, 37*(1), 19–34.

29. Casky, Courtney. (2003). Pediatric emergencies. In L. Newberry (Ed.), *Sheehy's emergency nursing: Priniciples and practice* (5th ed., pp. 719–743). St. Louis, MO: Mosby.

30. Flores, G., Laws, M. B., Mayo, S. J., Zuckerman, B., Abreu, M., Medina, L., & Hardt, E. J. (2003). Errors in medical interpretation and their potential clinical conse-quences in pediatric encounters. *Pediatrics, 111*(1), 6–14.

31. Hockenberry, M. J., Wilson, D., Winkelstein, M. L., & Kline, N. E. (Eds.). (2003). Physical and developmental assessment of the child. In *Wong's nursing care of infants and children* (7th ed., pp. 170–239). St. Louis, MO: Mosby.

Internet Resources

Emtala.com
www.emtala.com

American College of Emergency Physicians
www.acep.org

Centers for Disease Control and Prevention
www.cdc.gov

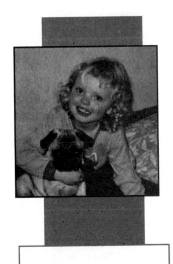

chapter 6

RESPIRATORY DISTRESS AND FAILURE

Objectives

On completion of this chapter, the learner should be able to:

1. Identify the anatomic and physiologic characteristics of the respiratory system that contribute to the signs and symptoms of respiratory distress or failure.

2. Identify the most frequent causes of respiratory distress and failure in children.

3. Delineate the specific interventions needed to manage the pediatric patient with respiratory distress or failure.

4. Evaluate the effectiveness of nursing interventions related to patient outcomes.

5. Identify health promotion strategies related to respiratory distress and failure.

Introduction

Respiratory disorders are a major cause of illness and hospitalization in the pediatric population.[1] Children are unique in their responses to respiratory problems because of their anatomic, physiologic, and developmental characteristics. Respiratory compromise in children can be caused by upper and lower respiratory tract infections, sedative medications, central nervous system disorders, musculoskeletal deformities, or congenital anomalies and disorders.

Respiratory distress is part of a continuum that, if left untreated, results in respiratory failure, which is the most common pathway to cardiopulmonary arrest in children. The outcomes for children following cardiopulmonary arrest are dismal; thus early recognition and treatment of the child in respiratory distress is critical.[2]

Anatomic, Physiologic, and Developmental Characteristics as a Basis for Signs and Symptoms

Central Control of Respiration

The respiratory center is located in the brainstem and controls the rate of ventilation by responding to changes in arterial carbon dioxide ($PaCO_2$) and hydrogen ion concentrations (H^+). An excess of either substance causes a direct excitatory effect on the respiratory center, resulting in an increased rate of ventilation.

↑ $PaCO_2$ or ↑ H^+ = ↑ Respiratory Rate

Oxygen (O_2) does not have a significant effect on the respiratory center, but instead acts on chemical receptors (chemoreceptors) located in the carotid and aortic bodies. Chemoreceptors indirectly control the rate of ventilation by sending signals to the respiratory center through afferent nerves. Though chemoreceptors are sensitive to $PaCO_2$ and H^+ levels, they are most strongly stimulated when arterial PaO_2 decreases below 60 mm Hg.[3]

↓ PaO_2 = ↑ Respiratory Rate (early sign) and ↓ Respiratory Rate (late sign)

In the infant, the central nervous system and peripheral nerves are not well developed, and there are fewer peripheral chemoreceptors. Although healthy infants and children will compensate for hypercarbia, hypoxia, and acidosis with hyperventilation, younger infants are less able to compensate for these stressors. Premature infants, rather than responding with hyperventilation, may initially respond with tachypnea followed by bradypnea and apnea.[4]

The child's ventilatory system is in a constant state of growth and development until approximately 7 to 8 years of age, when it is similar to that of the adult. **Table 6-1** summarizes key anatomic characteristics and their clinical significance to respiratory distress and failure.

Definition of Respiratory Distress and Failure

Respiratory distress is a clinical state characterized by signs of increased work of breathing, including tachypnea, hyperpnea, nasal flaring, use of accesso-

Table 6-1 Key Anatomic Characteristics

CHARACTERISTICS	CLINICAL SIGNIFICANCE
Nares have little support cartilage.	Nasal flaring is an early sign of distress.
Infants younger than 4 months of age are obligate nasal breathers.	Nasopharyngeal secretions or nasogastric tubes can cause airway obstruction.
Head is large in proportion to body with weak supporting musculature and occipital prominence.	Flexion of airway when the pediatric patient is supine; head bobbing occurs when he or she is distressed.
Tongue is large in proportion to oropharynx.	Tongue can easily occlude airway when supine.
Epiglottis is U-shaped, higher, and more anterior to the airway.	Epiglottis is more prone to infection and trauma.
Larynx is positioned more anteriorly and cephalad.	Position of larynx increases risk of aspiration.
Cricoid cartilage is narrowest part of the airway and the trachea is funnel shaped.	Provides an anatomic cuff for endotracheal tubes and a frequent site of foreign-body obstruction.
Airway diameter in the infant and child is smaller and shorter than an adult's.[5] The infant's tracheal diameter approximates the diameter of the little finger.	Airway obstruction can quickly develop in infants and small children. A small amount of edema or secretions can markedly increase airway resistance and result in partial or complete airway obstruction.
Tracheal length is proportional to the child's size. The length for an infant is approximately 7 cm.	Correct depth of tracheal tube insertion varies with size of child. Right mainstem intubation occurs when tracheal tube is inserted beyond tracheal length.
Tracheal and bronchial cartilaginous support rings are "C" rather than "O" shaped.	Allows airway collapse than can be exacerbated during illness or when the neck is hyperextended or flexed.
Alveoli increase in number until middle childhood to 9 times as many as were present at birth.[6] Alveoli have less elastic recoil and less supportive elastic tissue.	Less alveolar surface is available for gas exchange in infants and small children. A child requires faster respiratory rates for normal function; respiratory rate increases with distress. Alveoli are more prone to collapse at the end of expiration.
Lung (tidal) volume is approximately 10 ml/kg (e.g., 100 ml in a 10-kg child) as compared to that in the adult, which is 500 ml.	Results in low residual capacity and oxygen reserve. Variation in tidal volume must be considered when bag-mask ventilation is performed to avoid overinflation or underinflation.
Metabolic rate is twice that of adults with twice the oxygen consumption.	Hypoxia occurs more rapidly when the child is in respiratory distress. Other factors that increase metabolic rate (e.g., fever) contribute to respiratory demands.
Rib orientation is more horizontal than vertical.	Chest diameter is maximally expanded at baseline and cannot be increased with distress (barrel chested).
Ribs are cartilaginous and intercostal muscles are immature.	Allows chest wall collapse rather than expansion during distress causing retractions.
Chest wall is thin; thorax is small with organs in close proximity.	Allows transmitted breath sounds. Breath sounds from one area are heard in other areas of the chest and not easily differentiated.
Diaphragm is the major muscle of breathing.	Ventilation is directly affected when diaphragmatic excursion is impeded by pressure from above, such as with the hyperexpansion seen in asthma or from below, as with abdominal distension from gastric insufflation. Abdominal breathing is common.
Hemoglobin concentrations vary by age. A low value of 9.5 grams/100 ml occurs at 3 months and volume increases until adult values are reached at puberty.[7]	Cyanosis develops when 5 gm of hemoglobin are desaturated or when as much as 50% of the child's blood is deoxygenated. Therefore, cyanosis is a late sign of distress.

ry muscles, and inspiratory retractions.[5] Respiratory failure is characterized by inadequate oxygenation, ventilation, or both.[5] Therefore, respiratory distress and failure represent the two ends of a continuum of ventilatory dysfunction. The clinical manifestations of progression in this continuum can be subtle and are often not recognized early.

Respiratory failure is frequently described in the physiologic terms of the concentration of partial pressure of oxygen (PaO_2) or carbon dioxide ($PaCO_2$). Unfortunately, arterial blood gas (ABG) values alone may be easily subject to misinterpretation and are not always available when intervention is required. Respiratory failure occurs when the pediatric patient can no longer compensate to maintain adequate gas exchange. Fatigue from excessive work of breathing is often a precipitating factor. Work of breathing and an evaluation of ventilatory effectiveness may be more helpful in determining the child's potential for respiratory failure than ABG results alone. Ventilatory assistance must never be delayed while awaiting ABG results because rapid deterioration and respiratory arrest may occur.

Causes of Respiratory Distress and Failure

In the pediatric patient, the most common causes of respiratory distress and failure are upper or lower airway

Table 6-2 Causes of Respiratory Distress and Failure

Upper Airway	Lower Airway
Bacterial tracheitis	Acute respiratory distress syndrome
Croup	Aspiration
Epiglottitis	Asthma
Foreign-body aspiration	Atelectasis
Retropharyngeal abscess	Bronchiolitis
Smoke inhalation	Bronchomalacia
Subglottic stenosis	Foreign bodies
Tracheomalacia	Pertussis
Trauma	Pleural effusions
	Pneumo/hemothorax
	Pneumonia
	Pulmonary contusion
	Pulmonary edema
	Smoke inhalation
	Trauma
	Vascular rings

obstructive disorders (**Table 6-2**). Other causes of respiratory failure include central nervous system depression, musculoskeletal disorders, and thoracic disorders. It is not always necessary to identify the cause of the distress immediately. It is more important to recognize that respiratory distress exists and to initiate the proper interventions to prevent the deterioration to respiratory failure or arrest.

Nursing Care of the Pediatric Patient with Respiratory Distress or Failure

The pediatric patient who is in respiratory distress or failure requires simultaneous assessment and the initiation of critical interventions. Refer to Chapter 4, *Initial Assessment*, for a review of a comprehensive primary and secondary assessment. Additional or specific history data important to the evaluation of respiratory distress are listed following. Assessment findings that may indicate respiratory distress or failure are listed in the signs and symptoms section.

Additional History

- Time of onset
- Characteristic of onset (rapid or gradual)
- Previous episodes of respiratory distress

Signs and Symptoms

- Altered level of consciousness. Any alteration in the level of consciousness must be considered a result of cerebral hypoxia until proven otherwise.
  - Inability to recognize caregivers
  - Decreased interaction with environment
  - Restlessness
  - Anxiety
  - Confusion
  - Inability to be consoled
- Increased work of breathing
  - Nasal flaring
  - Retractions (see **Figure 6-1**)
  - Head bobbing
  - Grunting. Created by premature closure of the glottis in an attempt to increase the physiologic positive end expiratory pressure. It is a compensatory mechanism to relieve collapsing alveoli.
- Tripod position. Leaning forward while sitting up allows the tongue to remain forward and open the airway.

- Paradoxical respirations. Often called "seesaw" breathing and represents increased dependence on diaphragm to breathe.
- Pallor
- Cyanosis. Late sign; represents significant hypoxia.
- Unusual drooling. Inability to swallow may indicate pharyngeal obstruction.
- Decreased gag reflex. May be from decreased level of consciousness or muscle tone.
- Altered respiratory rate
  - Tachypnea
  - Bradypnea or a sudden decrease in respiratory rate. Late sign; represents fatigue and impending arrest.
  - Apnea. Apnea is usually considered pauses in breathing of more than 15 to 20 seconds. Periodic breathing that occurs in neonates is irregular breathing with pauses of less than 15 seconds.
- Altered heart rate
  - Tachycardia
  - Bradycardia. Late sign; represents impending arrest.
- Snoring. Represents partial obstruction of nasopharyngeal space.
- Stridor. Inspiratory sound representing partial obstruction or collapse of the trachea.
- Adventitious breath sounds. Wheezing and crackles are common in reactive airway disease, asthma, bronchiolitis, pneumonia, and pulmonary edema.

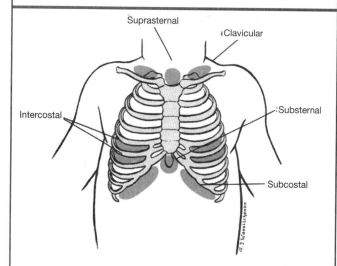

Figure 6-1 Location of Retractions

Suprasternal
Clavicular
Intercostal
Substernal
Subcostal

Reprinted with permission from Hockenberry, M. J., Wilson, D., Winkelstein, M. L., & Kline, N. E. (Eds.). (2003). The child with disturbance of oxygen and carbon dioxide exchange. In *Wong's nursing care of infants and children* (7th ed., pp. 1303–1342). St. Louis, MO: Mosby.

- Decreased, absent, or unequal breath sounds. Physical examination findings may vary over time due to secretions, bronchoconstriction, fluid shifts, or airway collapse.

Diagnostic Procedures

A variety of radiographic, imaging, and laboratory studies may be performed based on the suspected etiology of the pediatric patient's condition. Definitive diagnostic testing is completed while the resuscitation effort is in progress or after the pediatric patient has been stabilized.

Monitors
- Pulse oximetry
  - Poor perfusion may impede the monitor's ability to obtain an accurate reading.
  - A normal reading does not negate the pediatric patient's need for supplemental oxygen.
- Cardiac monitor, as indicted.
- Capnography, as indicated.

Radiographic Studies
- Chest radiograph to determine the presence of enlarged heart, foreign body, pulmonary infection, pulmonary edema, hyperexpansion, or pneumothorax or hemothorax.
- Lateral radiograph of the neck or thorax to evaluate the presence of a foreign body or pleural effusions.
- Other radiographic and imaging studies may be indicated based on the clinical presentation of respiratory compromise.

Laboratory Studies
- Arterial or capillary blood gas may be obtained, depending on the pediatric patient's condition and clinical concern. Capillary blood gas may be used to evaluate pH and CO_2 levels. A decreasing pH indicates a worsening of the cellular oxygen debt which results from the development of metabolic acidosis from anaerobic metabolism and lactic acid production. An elevated $PaCO_2$ indicates respiratory acidosis and impaired ventilation of the alveoli. A low PaO_2 indicates hypoxia.
- Increasing carbon dioxide retention represents hypoventilation. This can be measured with blood gases and monitored or trended with the use of capnography.
- Other laboratory studies including cultures may be indicated based on the pediatric patient's condition and treatment plan.

Planning/Implementation

Refer to Chapter 4, *Initial Assessment*, for a description of the general nursing interventions for the pediatric patient. After a patent airway, breathing, and circulation are assured, the following interventions are initiated, as appropriate for the pediatric patient's condition.

Additional Interventions

- Position the pediatric patient to facilitate respiratory effectiveness and comfort.
  - Raise the head of the bed to the most comfortable angle.
  - Try to avoid invasive procedures or actions that may upset the pediatric patient until the airway is secured (e.g., patients with partial airway obstruction from a foreign body or epiglottitis)
- Suction the infant's nares with a bulb syringe when secretions are present.
- Administer supplemental oxygen by the most appropriate method, delivering the highest concentration of oxygen, as appropriate for the pediatric patient's condition.
- Give nothing by mouth, as appropriate.
  - Pediatric patients with extreme tachypnea, severe respiratory distress, or impending failure must be kept NPO (nothing by mouth) because of the risk of aspiration and potential need for intubation.
  - Feeding may also compound the respiratory problem in infants because it increases metabolic demand and oxygen requirements.
  - For those with mild distress, encourage oral intake because tachypnea can lead to increased insensible fluid losses. If the child is to receive nothing by mouth for a significant period, intravenous fluids are required.
- Relieve any conditions that are impeding diaphragmatic excursion.
  - Insert a gastric tube to reduce gastric distention. Air in the stomach from swallowing air or bag-mask ventilation will result in gastric distention, which can impede ventilatory efforts.
  - If a gastrostomy tube is in place for feeding, decompression via the gastrostomy tube may be needed.
- Prepare and administer medications, per protocol, including antipyretics.
- Anticipate the need and prepare for assisted ventilation, intubation, and other advanced support measures, as appropriate.
  - Assess endotracheal tube placement.
    - Observe for symmetric chest rise.
    - Auscultate for breath sounds bilaterally at the midaxillary areas and over the epigastrium. Compare pitch, intensity, and location of the sounds.
    - Exhaled CO_2 detector and/or an esophageal detection device (EDD) can be used to confirm tube placement. EDDs should not be used in children < 1 year of age.
    - Confirm endotracheal tube positioning with a chest radiograph.
    - Record position of endotracheal tube at level of the gum, lip, or teeth.
- Rapid sequence induction for intubation may be required for the pediatric patient in impending and actual respiratory failure.
- Prepare for alternate airway and breathing support measures, if indicated.
  - A laryngeal mask airway (LMA) may be indicated for the unresponsive pediatric patient.
  - A needle cricothyrotomy is indicated only in cases of complete upper airway obstruction when all other interventions have failed to produce an adequate airway.
  - An emergency tracheostomy is rarely indicated in children and must be performed only by experienced physicians.
- Prepare for needle decompression of tension pneumothorax.

Evaluation and Ongoing Assessment

Pediatric patients with respiratory emergencies require meticulous and frequent reassessment of airway patency, breathing effectiveness, perfusion, and mental status. The etiologies of respiratory distress and failure encompass a broad range of disorders. Initial improvements may not be sustained, and additional interventions may be required. The pediatric patient's response to interventions and trending of the pediatric patient's condition must be closely monitored for achievement of desired outcomes. To evaluate the pediatric patient's respiratory progress, monitor the following.

- Airway patency
- Level of consciousness and interaction with environment
- Work of breathing
- Breath sounds and quality of air exchange
- Peak flow measurements
- Oxygen saturation and exhaled CO_2, as indicated
- Vital signs

Selected Emergencies

Upper Airway

Respiratory distress and failure can result when structures of the upper airway are occluded by edema, secretions, foreign bodies, or anatomic defects. Examples of these include croup, epiglottitis, bacterial tracheitis, foreign-body obstruction, obstructive sleep apnea, and tracheomalacia or vascular rings. Croup, epiglottitis, and foreign-body obstruction are further compared in **Table 6-3**.

Table 6-3 Common Causes of Upper Airway Emergencies

CROUP[8]	EPIGLOTTITIS[8]	FOREIGN-BODY ASPIRATION[8]
Acute viral illness usually causing partial airway obstruction due to tracheal narrowing from edema.	Acute bacterial illness, which usually progresses to complete airway obstruction if untreated because of cellulites of the epiglottis and surrounding soft tissues.	Acute upper or lower airway partial or complete obstruction.
Caused by parainfluenza virus, rhinovirus, influenza A, or respiratory syncytial virus.	Most commonly caused by *Haemophilus influenzae* type B (Hib); incidence has decreased due to Hib immunization. May also be caused by *Streptococcus pneumoniae* and *staphylococcus*.	Most often caused by food items, especially peanuts, but may also be toys, coins, latex balloons, and small disc batteries. Frequently follows history of gagging.
Occurs most commonly in children 6 months to 36 months in age.	Occurs most in underimmunized children and those children too young to have received the vaccine.	Occurs most commonly in children younger than 4 years of age but may occur in any age group.
Presents with gradual onset of cold symptoms, a "barking cough" that is worse at night, hoarse voice, and low-grade fever. Tachypnea, tachycardia, retractions, and inspiratory stridor are common, and expiratory wheezing may be present.	Presents acutely with high fever, sore throat, difficult swallowing, and muffled voice, which leads quickly to respiratory distress. Drooling may be present and may use tripod positioning to maintain airway patency. The pediatric patient may appear anxious and ill.	Presentation varies depending on: (1) when the aspiration occurred and (2) location and degree of obstruction. Signs and symptoms may include drooling, stridor, wheezing or unequal breath sounds, or chest pain.
Neck radiograph may note tracheal narrowing referred to as the "steeple sign."	Lateral neck radiograph may note epiglottic and aryepiglottic swelling referred to as the "thumb sign" and the "posterior triangle." Most blood cultures are positive for the causative agent.	Chest radiograph anterior/posterior, lateral, and decubitus views may reveal radiopaque or obstructing items. Partially obstructing, nonradiopaque items can be very difficult to evaluate by radiograph. Direct visualization by deep laryngoscopy or bronchoscopy may be required for definitive diagnosis.

1. Provide cool mist with supplemental oxygen as tolerated.
2. Monitor oxygen saturation.
3. Encourage fluids.
4. Administer medications as ordered:
  • Nebulized racemic epinephrine 0.25 ml in 3 to 5 ml normal saline. Children should be monitored for 2 to 3 hours, as medication effect may not be sustained (the "rebound effect").
  • Use of steroids (e.g., dexamethasone) may be considered.[9]
	1. Keep in position of comfort and do not separate from caregiver.
	2. No invasive procedures until airway stabilized, including
	  • Throat examination, as it can precipitate gagging and complete obstruction
	  • Rectal temperature
	  • Blood work or intravenous access
	3. Provide blow-by oxygen as tolerated.
	4. Anticipate tracheal intubation in surgery.
	5. Complete intravenous access, radiographs, laboratory work, and antibiotics once the airway is stabilized.
		1. Initiate pediatric basic life support techniques to relieve choking as appropriate.
		2. Keep in position of comfort and do not separate from caregiver.
		3. No invasive procedures until airway stabilized, including
		  • Throat examination
		  • Rectal temperature
		  • Blood work or intravenous access
		4. Provide blow-by oxygen, as needed.
		5. Complete intravenous access and radiographs once airway is stabilized.

Lower Airway

Respiratory distress and failure can also result when edema, bronchoconstriction, secretions, foreign bodies, weak muscle walls, or anatomical defects occlude structures of the lower airway. Examples of these include asthma, bronchiolitis, pneumonia, foreign-body obstruction, bronchomalacia, muscular dystrophy, and scoliosis or kyphosis.

Asthma

Asthma is the most common chronic illness in children, affecting more than 5 million children in the United States alone.[10] Asthma is defined as a chronic inflammatory disorder of the airways.[11] The disease is characterized by hyperreactiveness of the airway, widespread inflammatory changes, bronchospasm, and mucous plugging. Recurrent episodes may include any of the following: wheezing, breathlessness, chest tightness, and coughing. Seasonal and environmental allergies, exercise, infections, medications, irritants, weather changes, smoking, exposure to secondhand smoke, and emotions often precipitate asthmatic exacerbations.

Confirmation of the diagnosis of asthma is usually delayed until the child has had repeated episodes and is older than 1 year of age. Diagnosing asthma in infants is often difficult, and underrecognition and undertreatment are common problems in this age group. Treatment is best directed toward long-term control rather than episodic emergency care.[11]

Additional History
- Frequent coughing, especially at night
- Recurrent wheezing
- Recurrent breathlessness
- Recurrent chest tightness
- Fatigue
- Known triggers or exposure to any of the following prior to this illness
  - Exercise
  - Viral infection
  - Animals with fur or feathers
  - House dust mites
  - Molds or pollen
  - Smoke from tobacco or wood
  - Weather changes
  - Strong emotional expression such as laughing or crying hard
  - Airborne chemicals or dust
  - Medications such as salicylates or nonsteroidal anti-inflammatory drugs

- Atopic dermatitis or eczema
- Previous history of reactive airway disease, asthma, previous wheezing episodes
  - Frequency of symptoms
  - Number of school days missed
  - Present medications including dose, route, and frequency
  - Morning baseline peak flow volumes
  - Number of ED visits per year
  - Number of hospitalizations; date of last hospitalization
  - Number of critical care unit admissions; date of last admission to critical care unit
  - Number of tracheal intubations; date of last intubation
- Management by primary care provider, pulmonologist, or an allergy specialist

Signs and Symptoms
- Wheezing on inspiration or expiration
- Prolonged expiratory phase
- Decreased or unequal breath sounds
- Tachypnea
- Retractions
- Coughing, especially at night and early morning

Diagnostic Procedures
Laboratory Studies

Arterial blood gas for severe exacerbations. A $PaCO_2$ > 42 mm Hg or PaO_2 < 90 mm Hg with signs of muscle fatigue or a declining level of consciousness, despite maximal therapy, may indicate impending respiratory failure and the need for endotracheal intubation.[11]

Additional Interventions
- Deliver supplemental oxygen per protocol. Monitor oxygen saturation until a clear response to bronchodilator therapy has occurred.[11]
- Obtain peak expiratory flow or forced expiratory volume measurement. Record percentage of predicted best.
- Administer medications as ordered (see **Table 6-4** for medications and recommended doses)
  - Short-acting beta-2 agonists. May be delivered as nebulized aerosol or metered dose inhaler.
  - Nebulizers are usually administered every 20 minutes to a total of three treatments or may be administered continuously, depending on patient condition.
  - Anticholinergics may potentiate bronchodilatory effect of beta-2 agonists.

Table 6-4 Dosages of Drugs for Asthma Exacerbations in Emergency Medical Care or Hospital

Medications	Adult Dose	Child Dose	Comments
Inhaled Short-Acting Beta$_2$-Agonists			
Albuterol Nebulizer solution (5mg/mL)	2.5-5 mg every 20 minutes for 3 doses, then 2.5-10 mg every 1-4 hours as needed, or 10-15 mg/hour continuously	0.15 mg/kg (minimum dose 1.5 mg) every 20 minutes for 3 doses, then 0.15-0.3 mg/kg up to 10 mg every 1-4 hours as needed, or 0.5 mg/kg/hour by continuous nebulization.	Only selective beta$_2$-agonists are recommended. For optimal delivery, dilute aerosols to minimum of 4 mL at as flow of 6-8 L/min.
MDI (90 mcg/puff)	4-8 puffs every 20 minutes up to 4 hours, then every 1-4 hours as needed	4-8 puffs every 20 minutes for 3 doses, then every 1-4 hours inhalation maneuver. Use spacer/holding chamber.	As effective as nebulized therapy if patient is able to coordinate
Bitolterol Nebulizer solution (2 mg/mL)	See albuterol dose	See albuterol dose; thought to be half as potent as albuterol on a mg basis.	Has not been studied in severe asthma exacerbations. Do not mix with other drugs.
MDI (370 mcg/puff)	See albuterol dose	See albuterol dose	Has not been studied in severe asthma exacerbations.
Pirbuterol MDI (200 mcg/puff)	See albuterol dose	See albuterol dose; thought to be half as potent as albuterol on a mg basis.	Has not been studied in severe asthma exacerbations.
Systemic (Injected) Beta$_2$-Agonists			
Epinephrine 1:1000 (1 mg/mL)	0.3-0.5 mg every 20 minutes for 3 doses sq	0.01 mg/kg up to 0.3-0.5 mg every 20 minutes for 3 doses sq	No proven advantage of systemic therapy over aerosol.
Terbutaline (1 mg/mL)	0.25 mg every 20 minutes for 3 doses sq	0.01 mg/kg every 20 minutes for 3 doses then every 2-6 hours as needed sq	No proven advantage of systemic therapy over aerosol.
Anticholinergics			
Ipratropium bromide Nebulizer solution (0.25 mg/mL)	0.5 mg every 30 minutes for 3 doses then every 2-4 hours as needed	.25 mg every 10 minutes for 3 doses, then every 2 to 4 hours	May mix in same nebulizer with albuterol. Should not be used as first-line therapy; should be added to beta$_2$-agonist therapy.
MDI (18 mcg/puff)	4-8 puffs as needed	4-8 puffs as needed	Dose delivered from MDI is low and has not been studied in asthma exacerbations.
Corticosteroids			
Prednisone Methylprednisolone Prednisolone	120-180 mg/day in 3 or 4 divided doses for 48 hours, then 60-80 mg/day until PEF reaches 70% of predicted or personal best	1 mg/kg every 6 hours for 48 hours then 1-2 mg/kg/day (maximum = 60 mg/day) in 2 divided doses until PEF 70% of predicted or personal best	For outpatient "burst" use 40-60 mg in single or 2 divided doses for adults (children: 1-2 mg/kg/day, maximum 60 mg/day) for 3-10 days

Note:
* No advantage has been found for higher dose corticosteroids in severe asthma exacerbations, nor is there any advantage for intravenous administration over oral therapy provided gastrointestinal transit time or absorption is not impaired. The usual regimen is to continue the frequent multiple daily dosing until the patient achieves an FEV_1 or PEF of 50 percent of predicted or personal best and then lower the dose to twice daily. This usually occurs within 48 hours. Therapy following a hospitalization or emergency department visit may last from 3 to 10 days. If patients are then started on inhaled corticosteroids, studies indicate there is no need to taper the systemic corticosteroid dose. If the followup systemic corticosteroid therapy is to be given once daily, one study indicates that it may be more clinically effective to give the dose in the afternoon at 3:00 p.m., with no increase in adrenal suppression (Beam et al. 1992).

Table 6-5 Classifying Severity of Asthma Exacerbations

	Mild	Moderate	Severe	Respiratory Arrest Imminent
Symptoms				
Breathlessness	While walking Can lie down	While talking (infant-softer, shorter cry; difficulty feeding) Prefers sitting	While at rest (infant-stops feeding) Sits upright	
Talks in	Sentences	Phrases	Words	
Alertness	May be agitated	Usually agitated	Usually agitated	Drowsy or confused
Signs				
Respiratory rate	Increased	Increased	Often > 30/min	
		Guide to rates of breathing in awake children *Age* *Normal rate* < 2 months < 60/minute 2-12 months < 50/minute 1-5 years < 40/minute 6-8 years < 30 minute		
Use of accessory muscles; suprasternal retractions	Usually not	Commonly	Usually	Paradoxical thoracoabdominal movement
Wheeze	Moderate, often only end expiratory	Loud; throughout exhalation	Usually loud; throughout inhalation and exhalation	Absence of wheeze
Pulse/minute	< 100	100-120	> 120	Bradycardia
		Guide to normal pulse rates in children: *Age* *Normal rate* 1-12 months < 160/minute 1-2 years < 120/minute 2-8 years < 110/minute		
Pulsus paradoxus	Absent < 10 mm Hg	May be present 10-25 mm Hg	Often present > 25 mm Hg (adult) 20-40 mm Hg (child)	Absence suggests respiratory muscle fatigue
Functional Assessment				
PEF % predicted or % personal best	> 80%	Approx. 50-80% or response lasts < 2hrs	< 50% predicted or personal best	
PaO_2 (on air)	Normal (test not usually necessary)	> 60 mm Hg (test not usually necessary)	< 60 mm Hg: possible cyanosis	
and/or				
PCO_2	< 42 mm Hg (test not usually necessary)	< 42 mm Hg (test not usually necessary)	≥ 42 mm Hg: possible respiratory failure (see text)	
SaO_2% (on air) at sea level	> 95% (test not usually necessary)	91-95%	< 91%	
	Hypercapnia (hypoventilation) develops more readily in young children than in adults and adolescents.			

Note:
- The presence of several parameters, but not necessarily all, indicates the general classification of the exacerbation.
- Many of these parameters have not been systematically studied, so they serve only as general guides.

Reprinted with permission from *Guidelines for the diagnosis and management of asthma. National Asthma Education Program, Expert Panel Report 2.* Washington, DC: U.S. Department of Health and Human Services, National Institutes of Health publication 99-4051, July 1997.

- Systemic corticosteroids. Oral administration of prednisone has been shown to have effects equivalent to those of intravenous methylprednisolone sodium succinate.[11]

- Reassess patient after dose of inhaled bronchodilator and at least every 60 minutes thereafter. More frequent assessment may be required for severe exacerbations.

- Classify the severity of the asthma exacerbation. See **Table 6-5**.

- Prepare for admission or transfer if the child's condition does not improve.[11]

- Prepare for discharge if the child's condition has improved and desired outcomes achieved (peak expiratory flow > 70%, response sustained 60 minutes after last treatment, no distress, and normal physical examination).[11,12]

- Review home management of asthma with caregivers including

  - Medications: dose, frequency, and purpose

  - Proper use of the nebulizer or metered dose inhaler and spacer; return demonstration from caregiver

- Review measurement of peak expiratory flow.

  - Have the caregiver demonstrate use of the peak flow meter to assure proper technique and review indications for change in the child's treatment.

  - At home, peak expiratory flow is usually obtained in the morning prior to bronchodilator therapy and is used to guide the home therapy plan.[11,12]

- Discuss trigger avoidance with caregiver.

- Emphasize the need for regular care in an outpatient setting. Refer the patient to a primary care provider.

- Recommend follow-up appointment with primary care provider or asthma specialist.

Bronchiolitis

Bronchiolitis is a lower respiratory infection in infants younger than 1 year of age and is most commonly caused by the respiratory syncytial virus (RSV). The infectious process causes destruction of the lining of the bronchioles, causing bronchoconstriction and mucous plugging. Edema and secretions of the lower respiratory tract cause gradual lower airway obstruction. Extensive mucous plugging may progress to atelectasis and pneumonia. It is more often seen in the winter and early spring. Pediatric patients with a history of prematurity and cardiac and pulmonary diseases are at greater risk for severe life-threatening manifestations of the virus.[8]

Additional History

- Symptoms of upper respiratory infection

- History of vomiting and poor fluid or food intake

- Preexisting conditions such as chronic pulmonary insufficiency, congenital heart disease, or pulmonary hypertension

Signs and Symptoms

- Cough

- Tachypnea

- Retractions

- Wheezing and a prolonged expiratory phase

- Decreased air entry or exchange

- Volume depletion secondary to decreased oral intake

- Apnea spells

- Low-grade fever common in early infection

Additional Interventions

- Place in contact isolation.

- Consider obtaining a nasopharyngeal swab for RSV for viral culture. Rapid RSV tests, ELISA, and direct fluorescent antibody staining have 90% specificity, and results are obtained more quickly than with the viral culture.[13]

- Administer medications as ordered. Although still somewhat controversial, recent studies indicate that the use of bronchodilators and systemic corticosteroids do not shorten the course of illness, alter its severity, or decrease the length of hospital stays.[13–15] When admitted to the hospital, certain infants may be candidates for ribavirin, which is an antiviral aerosol medication: those with complicated congenital heart disease, cystic fibrosis, infants younger than 6 weeks of age, born at less than 37 weeks gestational age, taking immunosuppressive medication, or requiring mechanical ventilation.[16]

Pertussis

Pertussis, commonly referred to as whooping cough, is a highly contagious, acute bacterial infection caused by Bordetella pertussis. Prior to the availability of the pertussis vaccine in the 1940s, more than 200,000 cases were reported annually in the United States. The incidence of pertussis has been gradually increasing since the 1980s, with 7,687 cases reported in 2000.[17] This disease has an incubation period of 7 to 10 days and is characterized by three phases: the catarrhal stage, the paroxysmal stage, and the convalescent stage. An insidious onset of runny nose, low-grade fever, and a mild occasional cough characterizes the catarrhal stage. The cough becomes more severe over 1 to 2 weeks, and the paroxysmal stage begins. This stage of the disease is when pertussis is usually first suspected and is characterized by the following.

- Paroxysms of numerous, rapid coughs secondary to thick mucus in the tracheobronchial tree
- Long inspiratory effort with high-pitched whoop
- Cyanosis may occur during a paroxysm
- Vomiting and fatigue follow each episode
- Occurs more frequently at night

The paroxysmal stage usually lasts 1 to 6 weeks, followed by gradual recovery or the convalescent stage, which occurs over 2 to 3 weeks. Complications associated with pertussis occur most frequently in infants: pneumonia (11.8%) and neurologic complications such as seizures and encephalopathy (0.8% and 0.1%, respectively).[17]

Additional History
- Underimmunized status
- Recent upper respiratory infection symptoms

Signs and Symptoms
- Bursts of coughing averaging 15 attacks in 24 hours
- Ill and distressed appearance when coughing
- Appears normal when not coughing
- Infants less than 6 months of age may not exhibit the whoop, but paroxysms of coughing are present.

Additional Interventions
- Airborne droplet precautions
- Supportive care
- Administer medications as ordered. Erythromycin is the antibiotic of choice and may be given to all close contacts.[17]
- Counsel caregivers on need to obtain a booster or begin immunizations for other children in the home

Pneumonia

Pneumonia is a lower respiratory infection caused by a viral, bacterial, parasitic, or fungal organism.[18] Most pneumonias in children are viral in origin. Pneumonia can occur in any age group and can vary in etiology and severity, depending on the child's age and immune status. It may be a primary condition or result secondary to other respiratory problems, such as asthma or bronchiolitis. It presents as an acute inflammatory reaction in the lung tissue. As fluid and cellular debris accumulate in the areas of infection, compliance and vital capacity decrease and work of breathing increases.

Additional History
- Worsening of symptoms of upper respiratory infection

- Abrupt onset of fever and chills with bacterial pneumonia
- History of vomiting and poor fluid or food intake
- Preexisting conditions such as chronic pulmonary insufficiency, congenital heart disease, or pulmonary hypertension

Signs and Symptoms
- Cough
- Tachypnea
- Grunting
- Unequal breath sounds
- Crackles
- Wheezes
- Retractions
- Chest pain
- Apnea spells
- Fever
- Abdominal pain, which is more common in children with lower lobe pneumonia and may include abdominal distension and tenderness

Additional Interventions
- Administer antimicrobial medications as ordered.

Health Promotion
- Instruct caregivers to protect young children from foods or objects that commonly cause airway obstruction.
- Provide anticipatory guidance on childproofing the environment to avoid aspiration of small objects.
- Encourage caregiver to obtain training in basic pediatric life support techniques.
- Provide caregivers with information on childhood immunizations, especially pertussis and *Haemophilus influenzae* vaccine, and the importance of keeping the pediatric patient up to date. Provide referral and resources for immunizations, as appropriate.
- For children with asthma, provide information regarding precipitating triggers to avoid, such as tobacco smoke, aspirin, dust, pollen, molds, and animal fur or feathers.
- Instruct caregivers to administer medication to their children as ordered by the physician.
- Provide referral or information on obtaining a primary care provider if one is not already established.

Summary

This chapter has outlined the pediatric patient's unique responses to respiratory problems because of specific anatomic, physiologic, and developmental characteristics. Respiratory compromise in children can occur during upper and lower respiratory tract infections, when they receive sedation for procedures, from musculoskeletal deformities, or even from congenital anomalies. Selective respiratory emergencies, including croup, epiglottitis, foreign-body aspiration, asthma, bronchiolitis, pertussis, and pneumonia have been reviewed.

Respiratory distress is part of a continuum that results in respiratory failure if left untreated, and respiratory failure is the most common pathway to cardiopulmonary arrest in children. Further interventions for the pediatric patient with respiratory compromise have been delineated in this chapter. In addition, suggestions for health-promotion strategies directed at altering the adverse outcomes of respiratory distress and failure have been offered. A collaborative, systematic approach to care reduces fragmentation and enhances the opportunity to improve outcome.

References

1. Health Resource and Service Administration's Maternal and Child Health Bureau. (2000). *Child health USA 2000.* Washington, DC: Government Printing Office.

2. Smith, M. F., & Lyons, A. (2001). Resuscitation and transport of infants and children. In M. A. Q. Curley & P. A. Moloney-Harmon (Eds.), *Critical care nursing of infants and children* (2nd ed., pp. 1025-1053). Philadelphia: Saunders.

3. Hansen, M. (1998). Disorders of pulmonary ventilation. In M. Hansen (Ed.), *Pathophysiology: Foundations of disease and clinical intervention* (pp. 444–482). Philadelphia: Saunders.

4. Pillitteri, A. (2003). Nursing care of the high risk infant and family. In *Maternal and child health nursing: Care of the childbearing and childrearing family* (4th ed., pp. 716–766). Philadelphia: Lippincott Williams and Wilkins.

5. American Heart Association. (2002). Recognition of respiratory failure and shock. In *Pediatric advanced life support (Provider manual)* (pp. 23–42). Dallas, TX: Author.

6. Hockenberry, M. J., Wilson, D., Winkelstein, M. L., & Kline, N. E. (Eds.). (2003). The child with disturbance of oxygen and carbon dioxide exchange. In *Wong's nursing care of infants and children* (7th ed., pp. 1303–1342). St. Louis, MO: Mosby.

7. Pillitteri, A. (2003). Nursing care of the child with a hematologic disorder. In *Maternal and child health nursing: Care of the childbearing and childrearing family.* (4th ed., pp. 1329–1358). Philadelphia: Lippincott Williams and Wilkins.

8. Jardine, J. (2003). Respiratory emergencies. In D. Thomas, L. Bernardo, & B. Herman (Eds.), *Core curriculum for pediatric emergency nursing* (pp. 177–189). Sudbury, MA: Jones and Bartlett.

9. Grant, M. J. C., & Curley, M. A. Q. (2001). Pulmonary critical care problems. In M. A. Q. Curley & P. A. Moloney-Harmon (Eds.), *Critical care nursing of infants and children* (2nd ed., pp. 655–694). Philadelphia: Saunders.

10. Centers for Disease Control and Prevention. (2001). *Profile of the nation's health. CDC Fact Book 2000/2001.* Retrieved February 9, 2003 from http://www.cdc.gov/maso/factbook/main.htm.

11. National Institutes of Health: National Heart, Lung, and Blood Institute. (1997). Pharmacologic therapy: Managing exacerbations of asthma. In *Guidelines for the diagnosis and management of asthma. National Asthma Education Program, Expert Panel Report 2* (pp.105–121).Washington, DC: U.S. Department of Health and Human Services, National Institutes of Health publication 99-4051.

12. National Institutes of Health. (2002). *Guidelines for the diagnosis and management of asthma. National Asthma Education and Prevention Program. Expert Panel Report 2-Update on Selected Topics 2002.* Washington, DC: U.S. Department of Health and Human Services, National Institutes of Health.

13. Wright, R. B., Pomerantz, W. J., & Luria, J. W. (2002). New approaches to respiratory infections in children. Bronchiolitis and croup. *Emergency Medicine Clinics of North America, 20*(1), 93–114.

14. Patel, H., Platt, R. W., Pekeles, G. S., & Ducharme, F. M. (2002). A randomized, controlled trial of the effectiveness of nebulized therapy with epinephrine compared with albuterol and saline in infants hospitalized for acute viral bronchiolitis. *Journal of Pediatrics, 141*(6), 818–824.

15. Mallory, M. D., Shay, D. K., Garrett, J., & Bordley, W. C. (2003). Bronchiolitis management preferences and the influence of pulse oximetry and respiratory rate on the decision to admit. *Pediatrics, 111*(1), e45–51.

16. American Academy of Pediatrics Committee on Infectious Diseases. (1996). Reassessment of the indications for ribavirin therapy in respiratory syncytial virus infections. *Pediatrics, 97*(1), 137–140.

17. Centers for Disease Control and Prevention. *Pertussis.* Retrieved December 2, 2002 from http:www.cdc.gov/nip/publications/pink/pert.pdf

18. Hansen, M. (1998). In M. Hansen, (Ed.), *Pathophysiology: Foundations of disease and clinical intervention* (pp. 499–501). Philadelphia: Saunders.

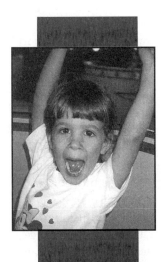

chapter 7

SHOCK

Introduction

In contrast to cardiac arrest in adults, cardiopulmonary arrest in infants and children is rarely a sudden event. Often it does not result from a primary cardiac cause.[1] In the child, the most common causes of cardiopulmonary arrest are conditions that represent a terminal event of progressive shock or respiratory failure. Even though cardiopulmonary arrest in children is not common, the survival rate is dismal following a documented cardiac arrest, less than 7 to 11 %.[1,2]

Causes of shock are heterogenous and vary with age, the child's health status, and the location of the event. Trauma, sudden infant death syndrome, near drowning and sepsis are causes of cardiopulmonary compromise and subsequent shock in children.[1,2]

Anatomic, Physiologic, and Developmental Characteristics as a Basis for Signs and Symptoms

There are specific characteristics in the cardiovascular system of the pediatric patient with important clinical significance. These are summarized in **Table 7-1**.

Definition of Shock

Shock is the manifestation of cellular metabolic insufficiency. There are multiple causes of shock, but the common denominator of shock, no matter what its etiology, is the reduction in the amount of oxygen made available to cells.[3,4] The final common pathway in all types of shock is impairment of cellular metabolism leading to cellular death.

Compensated Shock

The etiology of shock can be dissimilar, but the body's response is uniform, allowing the caregiver to identify signs and symptoms of shock. In early shock, the body will attempt to compensate for the alterations in perfusion that have occurred. Because the child is unable to alter stroke volume (SV) to change cardiac output (CO), the heart rate (HR) will increase, and tachycardia will be an early sign of compensated shock. Remember, CO = SV x HR. Additional signs and symptoms will include tachypnea, mild irritability, and decreased peripheral perfusion.[3,4] The child's body will attempt to compensate during early shock by increasing cardiac output to maintain perfusion to the brain, heart, and kidneys.

Decompensated Shock

As shock progresses and early compensatory mechanisms fail, the body's response becomes more complex and may have lethal consequences. There are systemic as well as cellular responses that are initiated to meet the body's oxygen demands. Decompensated shock is present when signs of shock are associated with systolic hypotension.[3,4,7] The body's responses to decompensated shock and its physiologic complications are summarized in the following table (see **Table 7-2**).

The consequences of decompensated shock include

- Fluid shifts from plasma into the interstitial space are caused by damage to cellular membranes. Generalized edema is found first in dependent areas, then in soft tissues including face, sclera, fingers, and genitalia.

- Disseminated intravascular coagulation and the development of other coagulopathies is caused by stimulation of the coagulation cascade. Petechiae begin to appear under areas of pressure, then become prominent over the trunk and extremities. Bleeding begins at all puncture sites of the skin and in the retina, kidneys, and digestive tract. Urine and feces will test positive for blood (heme +). Eventually hematuria and bloody stools will be present. Petechiae may coalesce into purpuric lesions on the skin, particularly over areas of movement or pressure (joints).

- The continued release of vasoactive and inflammatory mediators allow the inflammatory response to go unchecked. Increased respiratory effort with tachypnea may be difficult to relieve with oxygen administration alone. Airway swelling and closure may also result, requiring rapid endotracheal intubation.

- Pulmonary tissue hypoxia may lead to acute respiratory distress syndrome (ARDS). This noncardiac pulmonary edema causes severe hypoxia. Positive pressure ventilation with expiratory pressure support is necessary to maintain oxygen, carbon dioxide, and pH levels within normal limits.

- Multiple organ dysfunction syndrome and eventually multiple organ failure and death may result if the progress of decompensated shock state cannot be controlled.[3,4] Kidney and liver functions are altered due to decreased perfusion, oxygenation, and microemboli formation. Small bowel and pancreatic function is decreased due to these same conditions. Digestive enzymes and *E. coli* can permeate via diffusion from the small intestine into nearby tissues due to changes in tissue permeability. Bowel necrosis and sepsis can ensue. Fever, abdominal pain with rigidity, hypotension, rising liver function tests, and altered blood glucose levels are signs of this process.

Causes of Shock

Causes or types of shock are described in **Table 7-3**.

Table 7-1

CHARACTERISTICS	CLINICAL SIGNIFICANCE
The myocardium has poor compliance (myocardial fibers are shorter and less elastic), contractile mass is less, stroke volume cannot be increased (1.5 ml/kg/beat/min as compared to 75 to 90 ml/beat/min in an adult).	Heart rate rather than stroke volume increases to maintain cardiac output, which falls precipitously with bradycardia or heart rates exceeding 200 beats/min.
Infants have a higher cardiac output (200 ml/kg/min versus 100 ml/kg/min in the adult).	Cardiac output provides for increased oxygen needs, but leaves little cardiac output in reserve.
The pediatric patient has a high oxygen demand per kilogram of body weight because the child's metabolic rate is high. Oxygen consumption in infants is 6 to 8 ml/kg/min compared to 3 to 4 ml/kg/min in adults.[7]	Any stressors such as hypothermia or sepsis can lead to acute deterioration. Apnea, inadequate alveolar ventilation, hypoxemia, and potential tissue hypoxia can develop more rapidly. A slow or irregular respiratory rate in an acutely ill infant or child is an ominous clinical sign.[7]
A child needs increased circulating blood volume. This is because children have a greater percent of total water body weight. Infant: 90 ml/kg; child: 80 ml/kg; adult: 70 ml/kg.	There is a greater potential for dehydration. Small blood losses can cause circulatory compromise.
A child can maintain adequate cardiac output for long periods due to strong compensatory mechanisms. Rapid deterioration can occur when compensatory mechanisms are exhausted.	Hypotension is a late sign of circulatory decompensation. Children may remain normotensive until 25% of their blood volume is lost. Assess capillary refill as an indicator of peripheral perfusion (capillary refill should be < 2 seconds in a warm ambient environment).

Table 7-2 The Body Systems' Responses to Shock[4]

Cellular level	• Impairment of cellular metabolism • Decreased production of ATP • Failure of the sodium-potassium pump • Development of anaerobic metabolism • Vascular to interstitial compartment fluid shifts • Destruction of cellular membranes due to cellular edema • Impaired glucose delivery and uptake • Lysosomal enzyme release • Sluggish capillary flow • Activation of the clotting cascade
Immune system (Anaphylactic and septic shock)	• Activation of complement cascade system • Phagocytic cells initiate activity (macrophages, monocytes, and neutrophils) • Primary mediator release (cytokines, tumor necrosis factor, interleukin 1, and anaphylatoxin-C5A) • An intense cellular response occurs and releases secondary mediators (cytokines, prostaglandins, tumor necrosis factor, platelet-activating factor, and oxygen-free radicals) • Inflammatory cascade results in continued activation of the above processes leading to cellular destruction
Cardiac system	• Myocardial depressant factor • Decrease in cardiac output and systemic vascular resistance • Development of ischemia and dysrhythmias
Pulmonary system	• Increased permeability (to fluid shift) • Decreased oxygen transport/diffusion • Hypoxia and acidosis
Neurologic system	• Decreased brain perfusion leads to alteration in consciousness • Blood brain barrier and autoregulation may fail
Renal system	• Decrease in glomerular perfusion • Decrease in urinary output • Decrease in detoxification • Activation of the renin-angiotensin 1 to angiotensin 2 feedback loop system for increased vasoconstriction in the periphery
Adrenal system	• Aldosterone is released to stimulate sodium reabsorption in the kidney • Stress hormones are released including epinephrine, norepinephrine and cortisol.
Gastrointestinal system	• Microcirculatory failure • Loss of gut barrier with systemic spread of bacteria
Hepatic system	• Glycogenolysis is activated by epinephrine resulting in breakdown of glycogen to glucose [5] • Glucose stores may be used up rapidly in a child • Hepatic vessels constrict to redirect flow to vital areas[5] • The body shifts from using glucose to protein for energy resulting in increased ammonia production. Ammonia is toxic to cells.[4]
Integumentary system	• Blood is shunted away from skin causing sluggish, delayed capillary refill[7] • The skin will be prone to injury and breakdown • Hypothermia • Bleeding and edema may be difficult to control

Table 7-3 Types of Shock

Hypovolemic shock	• Characterized by an overall decrease in circulating blood or fluid volume. • Hemorrhage or vomiting and diarrhea may cause this low volume shock. Other causes of hypovolemic shock include third spacing, as seen in burns or sepsis, and diabetic ketoacidosis. Fluid shifts outside the vascular bed due to increased tissue permeability. • Hypovolemic shock is the most common cause of shock in children.[7]
Cardiogenic shock	• Characterized by the inability of the myocardium to maintain an adequate cardiac output, usually due to myocardial ischemia or death. The pumping ability of the heart is severely decreased. • In children, cardiogenic shock is rare but may follow open-heart surgery for congenital heart disease, viral myocarditis, drug ingestion, or occur secondary to cardiac dysrhythmia (e.g., asystole, ventricular fibrillation, supraventricular tachycardia).
Distributive shock	• Results from vasodilatation and pooling of blood in the peripheral vasculature • Types of distributive shock include: - Septic shock: One of the most common types of shock in the pediatric patient. It is generally caused by a systemic infectious process. Most common bacteria responsible for sepsis include *E. coli,* streptococcus, *Neisseria meningitis,* and staphylococcus.[6] - Neurogenic shock: Characterized by a loss of sympathetic tone and can be caused by spinal cord trauma, anesthetic agents, or the ingestion of drugs (e.g., barbiturates).
Obstructive shock	• Results from an inadequate circulating volume due to an obstruction in or compression on the great veins, aorta, pulmonary arteries, or the heart. • Obstructive shock may occur from conditions such as pericardial tamponade, tension pneumothorax, mediastinal mass, or congenital abnormality of the great vessels.[5]

Adapted from Hazinski, M. F., & Jenkins, M. E. (2002). Shock, multiple organ dysfunction syndrome, and burns in children. In K. L. McCance & S. E. Huether (Eds.), *Pathophysiology: The biologic basis for disease in adults and children* (4th ed., pp. 1513–1539). St. Louis, MO: Mosby.

Nursing Care of the Pediatric Patient with Shock

Assessment

The pediatric patient who is suffering from shock requires a rapid assessment simultaneous with the initiation of critical interventions.

Additional History

Refer to Chapter 4, *Initial Assessment*, for general questions to obtain a history. Additional or specific history data important in the evaluation of shock include the following.

• Any obvious bleeding sites or history of blood loss
• Vomiting or diarrhea
• Decreased fluid intake
• Any obvious sites of fluid loss such as a burn injury
• Congenital heart disease
• Potential source of infection (e.g., tracheostomy, urinary catheter, G-tube, asplenic, meningitis)
• History of recent trauma
• History of recent surgery

Signs and Symptoms

• Altered level of consciousness (LOC). Although an altered LOC may result from several factors, such as injury to the brain, drugs, or hypoxia, any alteration in LOC should be considered a result of decreased cerebral perfusion until proven otherwise. In a child, an altered LOC may be assessed as
  - Confusion
  - Inability to recognize caregivers
  - Decreased response to environment
  - Anxiety, restlessness, irritability
• Agitation alternating with lethargy[7]
• Tachypnea
• Tachycardia
• Hypotension. In the early stages of shock, the pediatric patient may be normotensive or demonstrate a slightly increased systolic pressure with a widened pulse pressure. Hypotension and bradycardia are late, ominous signs in the pediatric patient in shock.
• Changes in skin color and temperature are caused by the body's compensatory mechanisms that shunt blood away from the skin to vital organs to maintain a blood pressure compatible with life. Vasoconstriction of the skin causes it to appear pale, cool, clammy, ashen, mottled, or cyanotic.

- Changes in the quality of peripheral and central pulses are due to decreased vascular volume. When assessed they will be weak, thready, unequal, or absent.
- Difficulty in obtaining a blood pressure is due to vasoconstriction and decreased cardiac output. It may be difficult to obtain an accurate blood pressure reading by the use of a mechanical noninvasive blood pressure (NIBP) device. Obtain the initial blood pressure manually by auscultation, palpation or ultrasonic Doppler techniques. Correlate NIBP reading with manual measurements.
- Decreased or absent bowel sounds are due to increased sympathetic tone and lowered vascular perfusion.
- Decreased or absent urinary output. The pediatric patient should have urine output of 1 to 2 cc/kg/hr. Decreases are due to severe changes in glomerular filtration rate that result from insufficient perfusion.

Diagnostic Procedures

A variety of radiographic and laboratory studies may be indicated based on the suspected etiology of the pediatric patient's condition. Definitive diagnostic testing is performed as the resuscitation effort is in progress or after the pediatric patient is stabilized. The following procedures and studies may be indicated for the pediatric patient with shock.

Monitors
- Cardiac monitor
- Pulse oximeter. Poor perfusion may impede the monitor's ability to obtain an accurate reading. A normal reading does not negate the pediatric patient's need for supplemental oxygen. Although the saturation reading may be within normal limits, shock results in decreased tissue oxygenation.
- Capnography (in the intubated patient)
- 12-lead ECG

Radiographic Studies
Chest radiograph is completed to determine the presence of an enlarged heart, a pulmonary infection, or a hemothorax or pneumothorax

Other Diagnostic Procedures
- Ultrasound
- Echocardiogram
- Laboratory studies
- Complete blood count and coagulation studies
- Serum or whole blood glucose test
- Electrolytes
- Blood sample for typing
- Arterial pH, PaO_2 and $PaCO_2$. Decreasing pH indicates a worsening of the cellular oxygen debt as metabolic acidosis develops due to anaerobic metabolism and lactic acid production. An elevated $PaCO_2$ may indicate respiratory acidosis and impaired ventilation of the alveoli. A low PaO_2 indicates hypoxia.
- Cultures
  - Blood
  - Body fluids including cerebral spinal fluid
  - Wounds
  - Indwelling devices
- Urinalysis

Planning/Implementation

Refer to Chapter 4, *Initial Assessment*, for a description of the general nursing interventions for the pediatric patient. After ensuring a patent airway and effective ventilation, the following interventions are initiated as appropriate for the pediatric patient's condition.

Additional Interventions

- For absent or ineffective pulse, initiate cardiopulmonary resuscitation utilizing the universal pediatric template when indicated by the pediatric patient's condition (see **Figure 7-1**). Initiate chest compressions in all pediatric patients with heart rates too low to adequately perfuse their vital organs. Chest compressions are initiated if the infant or child's heart rate is less than 60 beats/minute and accompanied by signs of poor systemic perfusion. See Chapter 14, *The Neonate*, for neonatal indicators.
- Effective chest compressions should produce a central pulse. The technique for compressions is based on the age and size of the child. The child less than 1 year of age is considered an infant and chest compressions are performed with two fingers over the sternum just below the nipple line or by using the encircling 2-hand method. This method uses both thumbs to compress the sternum with the fingers placed around the back of the infant. Chest compressions are performed with one hand for the child 1 to 8 years of age. Chest compressions for children over 8 years of age are performed in the same fashion as adults.[8]
- Control any obvious bleeding
- Obtain vascular access according to Pediatric Advanced Life Support (PALS) guidelines.[9]
  - Peripheral venous access can be difficult and time consuming once cardiopulmonary arrest has occurred. Insertion of an intraosseous (IO) line should be used if access is needed emergently and cannot be obtained by conventional means. (See Chapter 10 for information on IO insertion techniques).

- Defibrillate or provide synchronized cardioversion based on cardiac rhythm.
- Initiate volume replacement.
  - Administer a 20 ml/kg bolus of warmed isotonic crystalloid solution. A bolus of fluid is given in its entirety over 5 to 20 minutes based on the child's clinical condition and can be repeated based on the pediatric patient's response. After each bolus reevaluate airway, breathing, and circulation/perfusion, assessing for any changes. Additional crystalloid fluid boluses, blood (for hemorrhagic losses), or colloid solutions may be required for persistent signs of shock.
  - Because approximately one fourth of the crystalloid solution remains in the plasma compartment, infusion of four to five times the fluid lost may be required to restore plasma volume.[1,10]
  - Colloids are more efficient volume expanders than crystalloids because they remain in the intravascular compartment longer than crystalloid solutions. However, colloids may not be as readily available as crystalloid solutions, and they may cause sensitivity

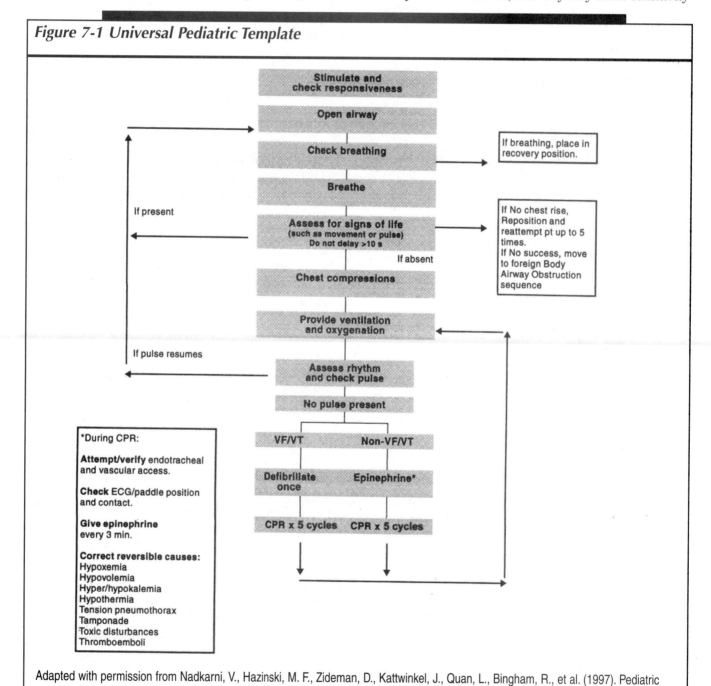

Figure 7-1 Universal Pediatric Template

Adapted with permission from Nadkarni, V., Hazinski, M. F., Zideman, D., Kattwinkel, J., Quan, L., Bingham, R., et al. (1997). Pediatric resuscitation: An advisory statement from the Pediatric Working Group of the International Liaison Committee on Resuscitation. *Circulation, 95*(8), 2185–2195.

reactions. Certain types of shock may respond better to the administration of colloid solutions whereas blood products may be indicated for replacement of blood loss or treatment of coagulopathies.

- Rapid administration of cold blood, blood products, crystalloids, or colloids may contribute to the development of hypothermia. This is of special concern in the pediatric patient who may be experiencing some degree of hypothermia due to environmental exposure. Hypothermia may adversely affect myocardial and metabolic functions.

- Administer medications, such as antipyretics, analgesics, and antibiotics, as indicated.

- Administer 100% oxygen via high-flow delivery.

- Correct hypoglycemia.

  - Infants have limited glycogen stores that are rapidly depleted during periods of stress. A whole blood glucose (bedside glucose test) or serum glucose level is required for any pediatric patient who is critically ill. Glucose monitoring should be performed during resuscitation as well as in the postresuscitation phase. Documented hypoglycemia is treated with intravenous glucose at a dose of 0.5 to 1 g/kg.

  - Administer 2 to 4 ml/kg of 25% glucose solution (D_{25}) slowly via IV or IO. If a prepared D_{25} solution is unavailable, mix equal amounts of D_{50} and sterile water. For example, if 20 ml of D_{25} is ordered, mix 10 ml of D_{50} with 10 cc of sterile water. Administration of D_{25} through small peripheral veins can cause vascular and tissue injury; therefore, further dilution to a 12.5% solution may be necessary in smaller pediatric patients with only peripheral access.

  - In neonates, administer 2 ml/kg of $D_{10}W$ IV over 1 minute for documented and symptomatic hypoglycemia.

  - Reassess serum glucose 15 to 20 minutes after the dextrose bolus and hourly until glucose level is stable.

- Treat the underlying cause of shock.

  - If sepsis is suspected, anticipate the need for antibiotic therapy and lumbar puncture. Early administration of antibiotics is key in the unstable patient in septic shock; however, antibiotic therapy may result in a period of vascular instability due to the endotoxins that are released as some bacteria die. Lumbar puncture may be delayed until the pediatric patient is more stable.

  - If a dysrhythmia has resulted from an electrolyte imbalance or a metabolic derangement, administer medications as prescribed.

- In obstructive shock the goal is to decrease intrathoracic pressure that inhibits cardiac filling or emptying. The causes of this type of shock include pneumothorax, pericardial tamponade, ruptured aorta, or a ruptured diaphragm. Treating these causes is essential in saving the pediatric patient's life. With a pneumothorax, immediate needle decompression with subsequent chest tube insertion is indicated. With pericardial tamponade, pericardiocentesis will assist with removal of blood in the pericardium. When great vessels are injured or when the diaphragm has been ruptured, immediate surgical reconstruction is required. Open thoracotomy may be performed in the emergency room immediately if death is eminent from any of these causes.

- Initiate vasoactive agents as ordered.

  - In the unstable pediatric patient, continuous infusions of vasoactive agents may be used to improve cardiac output and treat postresuscitation myocardial dysfunction.

  - Inotropes, vasopressors, vasodilators, and inodilators are classes of medications that may be used to support circulatory function.

- Correct cardiac dysrhythmias.

  - Because children rarely present to the emergency department with primary cardiac dysrhythmia, antidysrhythmic drugs are seldom used. Epinephrine is the preferred drug in the treatment of bradydysrhythmias or asystole (after initiation of a patent airway, ventilation, and oxygenation) due to the prominent alpha-adrenergic effects in the vascular bed and beta-adrenergic effects on the heart. Atropine is used to diminish vagally mediated bradycardia associated with intubation, symptomatic bradycardia, and atrioventricular block.[1,10]

  - Hypoxia is the most common cause of bradycardia in infants and young children and generally responds to assisted ventilation of 100% oxygen at an age-appropriate rate with adequate tidal volume. Administration of atropine for intubation or preoperatively may mask hypoxia-induced bradycardia; therefore the pediatric patient's oxygen saturation level must be continuously monitored.[1,11]

- Correct electrolyte and acid-base imbalances.

  - Buffers (i.e., sodium bicarbonate) may be administered to the pediatric patient with documented severe acidosis but only after the provision of adequate oxygenation and ventilation because most acidosis is caused by respiratory failure in children.[10]

- In infants less than three months of age a 4.2% solution is used.
- The initial dosage for children in shock is 1mEq/kg of 8.4% solution.
- There is no specific level of acidosis that requires treatment with sodium bicarbonate. The decision to administer sodium bicarbonate is determined by the acuity and severity of the acidosis and the pediatric patient's circulatory state.[1] Sodium bicarbonate is recommended in the treatment of symptomatic patients with hyperkalemia, hypermagnesemia, and poisonings.

- Provide supplemental warmth (i.e., overbed warmers, warm blankets, warm IV fluids, warm humidified oxygen).
  - In children, the combination of body exposure to the environment, high body surface area to volume ratio, and the infusion of large amounts of room temperature intravenous fluids can lead to hypothermia.
  - Hypothermia causes shunting of blood away from the periphery resulting in poor peripheral perfusion and further complicating assessment of the pediatric patient.
  - The pediatric patient who is hypothermic may respond poorly to resuscitative efforts.
  - Additionally, hypothermia depletes compensatory reserves of the already stressed cardiovascular system.
- Continually monitor vital signs and the pediatric patient's response to specific interventions.
- Accurately document the initial assessment, interventions, and the pediatric patient's response to each intervention.
- Promote and support the family's involvement in the pediatric patient's care. Assign a health care professional to provide explanations of procedures and treatment plan to the caregivers. Assign a staff member to provide emotional support and be with the family during the time in the emergency department. Involve the pediatric patient's family as soon as possible in the resuscitation process. The majority of pediatric pulseless arrests have dismal outcomes; therefore decisions may need to be made about the termination of resuscitative efforts and organ donation. Involve the caregivers in this decision-making process.[1,5,12]

Evaluation and Ongoing Assessment

The pediatric patient who is in shock requires meticulous and frequent reassessment of airway patency, breathing effectiveness, perfusion and mental status. The etiologies of shock and cardiovascular compromise encompass a broad range of disorders. Initial improvements may not be sustained and additional interventions may be required. The pediatric patient's response to interventions and trending of the pediatric patient's condition must be closely monitored. To evaluate the pediatric patient's progress, monitor the following:

- Airway patency, including adequacy and patency of airway adjuncts
- Effectiveness of breathing: ventilation and oxygenation
- Perfusion
  - Pulse rate and quality (central vs. peripheral)
  - Skin color and temperature
  - Capillary refill
  - Blood pressure
- Level of consciousness and pupillary reaction
- Urinary output
- Cardiac rhythm
- Oxygen saturation
- Exhaled CO_2, if available (intubated patients)
- Arterial pH, PaO_2, and $PaCO_2$

Health Promotion

Prevention measures and recommendations that have an impact on shock-related morbidity and mortality include

- Educate caregivers about the necessity to schedule infants, children, and adolescents for well-child check-ups with their primary health care providers.
- Identify strategies to educate and encourage caregivers to assure that infants, children, and adolescents receive vaccinations to prevent illness.
- Develop strategies to educate caregivers, children, and their communities about trauma prevention.
- Develop and implement strategies to decrease the risk of infection in children with indwelling devices such as tracheostomies and long-term intravenous access devices.
- Encourage families to attend basic life support classes.

Summary

Evaluation of the pediatric patient in shock requires astute assessment of peripheral perfusion, vital signs, level of consciousness, and urinary output. Shock and respiratory failure are common pathways to cardiovascular collapse and subsequent cardiac arrest in the pediatric patient. The outcome of cardiac arrest in the child is most frequently death or recovery with poor neurological outcome. Early recognition of the signs of shock is critical to the initiation of prompt intervention and the prevention of adverse outcomes. The central piece of the puzzle in the care for the pediatric patient in shock is the interlocking relationship between early recognition of life-threatening illnesses and injuries that cause shock and the initiation of the rapid interventions.

References

1. American Heart Association (AHA) in collaboration with the International Liaison Committee on Resuscitation. (2000). Guidelines 2000 for Cardiopulmonary Resuscitation and Emergency Cardiac Care: International Consensus on Science. Part 10: Pediatric Advanced Life Support. (2000). *Circulation, 102*(suppl I), I-292–296, 305–320.

2. American Heart Association. (2002). The chain of survival and emergency medical services for children. In *Pediatric advanced life support (Provider manual)*(pp. 1–22). Dallas, TX: Author.

3. Guyton, A. C., & Hall, J. E. (2000). Circulatory shock and physiology of its treatment. In A. C. Guyton & J. E. Hall (Eds.), *Textbook of medical physiology* (10th ed., pp. 253–262). Philadelphia: Saunders.

4. Hazinski, M. F., & Jenkins, M. E. (2002). Shock, multiple organ dysfunction syndrome, and burns in children. In K. L. McCance & S. E. Huether (Eds.), *Pathophysiology: The biologic basis for disease in adults and children* (4th ed., pp. 1513–1539). St. Louis, MO: Mosby.

5. Emergency Nurses Association. (2000). Shock. In B. B. Jacobs & K. S. Hoyt (Eds.), *Trauma nursing core course (Provider manual)* (5th ed., pp. 65–83). Des Plaines, IL: Author.

6. Nichols, D. G., Yster, M., Lappe, D. G., & Haller, J. A. (1996). *Golden hour: The handbook of advanced pediatric life support* (2nd ed.). St. Louis, MO: Mosby.

7. American Heart Association. (2002). Recognition of respiratory failure and shock. In *Pediatric advanced life support (Provider manual)* (pp. 23–42). Dallas, TX: Author.

8. American Heart Association. (2002). Basic life support for the PALS healthcare provider. In *Pediatric advanced life support (Provider manual)* (pp. 43–80). Dallas, TX: Author.

9. American Heart Association. (2002). Vascular access. In *Pediatric advanced life support (Provider manual)* (pp. 155–172). Dallas, TX: Author.

10. American Heart Association. (2002). Fluid therapy and medications for shock and cardiac arrest. In *Pediatric advanced life support (Provider manual)* (pp. 127–153). Dallas, TX: Author.

11. American Heart Association. (2002). Airway, ventilation, and management of respiratory distress and failure. In *Pediatric advanced life support (Provider manual)* (pp. 81–126). Dallas, TX: Author.

12. American Heart Association. (2002). Ethical and legal aspects of CPR in children. In *Pediatric advanced life support (Provider manual)* (pp. 409–424). Dallas, TX: Author.

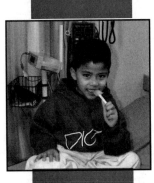

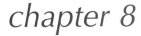 *chapter 8*

VASCULAR ACCESS

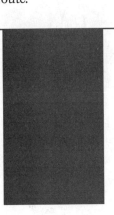

Objectives

On completion of this chapter, the learner should be able to:

1. Identify the indications for each vascular access route.

2. Identify the preferred sites for each vascular access route.

3. Describe the appropriate preparation required for each vascular access route.

4. Describe how to evaluate the patency of each vascular access route.

Introduction

Vascular access is commonly required for children in an emergency care setting for fluid and/or intravenous medication (IV) administration. Access routes include peripheral, intraosseous (IO), and central lines. The technique for rapid fluid bolus administration is discussed in Chapter 10, *Medication Administration*.

Peripheral Vascular Access

- When rapid fluid administration and resuscitation are required, insert the largest catheter that the vessel will accommodate.[1]

- Over-the-needle catheters are preferred because of their stability in the vein. Butterfly needles are rarely used in pediatric patients except in phlebotomy procedures.[1]

- Preparation of the caregiver and pediatric patient prior to the procedure is critical.
  - Use age-appropriate techniques (see Chapter 3, *From the Start—Dealing with Children*)
  - If a treatment room is unavailable prepare equipment prior to the procedure out of sight of the pediatric patient.
  - When time permits, consider the use of dermal anesthetic, iontophoresis, or ice wrapped in a towel.
  - Use distraction and other nonpharmacological interventions.
  - Tell the caregiver and pediatric patient when you are finished.
  - Offer reward stickers and praise any positive behavior.

- IV sites commonly used in infants and children are the scalp (infant), hands, feet, and antecubital fossa.
  - In nonemergent cases attempt distal sites first.
  - For emergent cases the antecubital vein is often the first site.
  - During cardiopulmonary resuscitation (CPR) or in an infant or child with altered level of consciousness the preferred site is the one that is most rapidly accessed without interruption of resuscitation efforts. Most often this will be IO access.[3]
  - Ideally, the sites to avoid for vascular access include an injured extremity or any areas that are edematous or burned.
  - Superficial scalp veins in the infant are frontal, superficial temporal, posterior auricular, supraorbital, occipital, and posterior facial veins (see **Figure 8-1**).
    - A tabbed rubber band can be use as a tourniquet.
    - Shave the area the catheter and tape will cover to avoid pulling hair out from the root when removing the catheter. Save the hair and offer to parents as a "first hair cut" as appropriate. Avoid shaving the head unless you actually see or feel a vein for cannulation.
    - Palpate the vein for absence of a pulse prior to accessing.
    - Insert the needle in either direction.
    - Contraindications to scalp vein insertion include age greater than 9 months, hydrocephalus, ventricular shunt, anencephaly, and skull fracture.

- Upper extremity veins include cephalic, median basilic, and antecubital veins in the upper arm. In the dorsum of the hand, the cephalic and basilic veins may be used.[1]
  - Opt for the nondominant hand if possible.
  - The dorsum of the hand is a good site in chubby infants.
  - It may be helpful to close the child's hand tightly and flex the wrist.
  - In non-Caucasian chubby infants, a povodine solution may make it easier to visualize veins.
  - In small, thin infants a transilluminator or light source under the hand may assist you in finding veins.
- Lower extremity veins include the saphenous vein and veins in the dorsal arch.
  - Avoid lower extremity insertions if the child is ambulatory

Figures 8-2 and **8-3** illustrate IV access sites in upper and lower extremities, respectively.

- Positioning the child appropriately and securing the selected extremity and insertion site are critical steps of the procedure.
- Avoid depending on the caretaker to provide securing the pediatric patient. Use the caretaker for providing comfort measures.
- When inserting a small-gauge catheter, stop once you have pierced the skin to allow for the movement of the extremity as the pediatric patient may jerk when the needle penetrates the skin. Advance the catheter slowly because blood return may be delayed for a few seconds due to the diameter of the needle.

- Visualizing the flashback may be facilitated by inserting the catheter bevel side down in vascular-compromised children.[1,2]

- Avoid shearing the catheter; never reintroduce the stylet into the catheter once it has been withdrawn.

- Blood samples may be drawn prior to initiating fluid therapy. Insert the vacuum adapter directly into the catheter hub or use a T-connector. If a smaller-gauge IV needle is used, the suction from the Vacutainer may collapse the vessel. Consider attaching a syringe

Figure 8-2 Veins of the hand and forearm

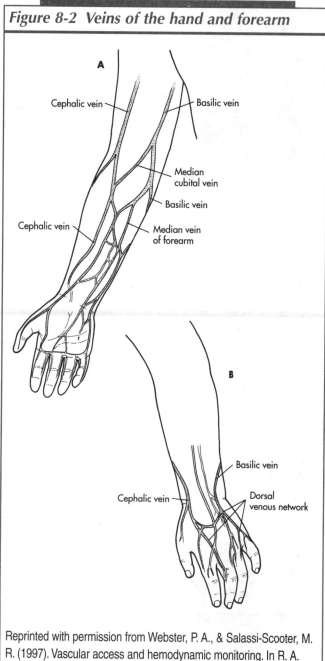

Reprinted with permission from Webster, P. A., & Salassi-Scooter, M. R. (1997). Vascular access and hemodynamic monitoring. In R. A. Dieckmann, D. H. Fiser, & S. M. Selbst (Eds.), *Pediatric emergency and critical care procedures* (pp. 187-195). St. Louis, MO: Mosby.

Figure 8-1 Superficial Scalp Veins

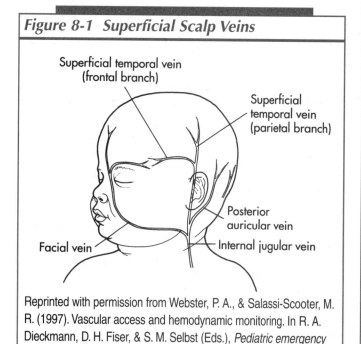

Reprinted with permission from Webster, P. A., & Salassi-Scooter, M. R. (1997). Vascular access and hemodynamic monitoring. In R. A. Dieckmann, D. H. Fiser, & S. M. Selbst (Eds.), *Pediatric emergency and critical care procedures* (pp. 187-195). St. Louis, MO: Mosby.

directly to the hub and gently drawing off the sample. If a T-connector is used, withdraw the blood sample before flushing the T-connector with normal saline.

- Attach a T-connector flushed with normal saline to the hub of the catheter after the stylet is removed. The T-connector provides an access port at the closest point to the site.

- Secure the catheter with tape and gauze or a nonocclusive dressing. **Figure 8-4** illustrates securing of an IV catheter in the hand

  - Tape the catheter securely while maintaining visualization of the site.

  - When taping use caution not to bend the hub of the catheter.

  - Use tape to secure the extremity to an appropriate-sized arm board.

    - Position the pediatric patient's fingers to grasp the arm board rather than remaining outstretched.

    - Use gauze rolls to support the pediatric patient's extremity in a functional position.

  - Loop the IV tubing away from the catheter and secure with tape. Take any tension off the tubing.

  - Label the site and tubing per institution policy.

  - Protect the catheter and IV site. Use a nonrestrictive covering that allows for visualization of the site. Commercially prepared devices are available.

- Evaluate the site per institution policy. Observe for signs of infiltration and whether the dressing is intact, and check any connections.

Intraosseous Access[2]

- IO access is indicated during CPR or the treatment of the critically ill child when immediate vascular access cannot be obtained by conventional means.

- The IO route is a safe and rapid method of accessing the circulatory system and is associated with a low complication rate.

- Obtain IO access by inserting a rigid needle into the medullary cavity of a bone providing access to a non-collapsible venous plexus.[3]

  - The tibia is the preferred site; alternative sites include distal femur, medial malleolus, and anterior superior iliac spine (see **Figure 8-5**). In older children alternate sites include distal tibia, radius and ulna, and anterior superior iliac spine.

  - Check the needle to ensure the bevels of the outer needle and the internal stylet are aligned.

Figure 8-3 Veins of the lower extremity

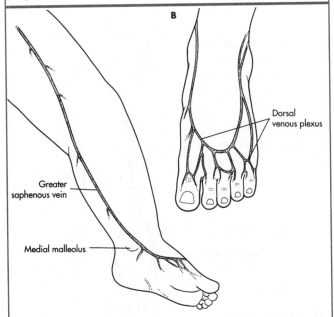

Reprinted with permission from Webster, P. A., & Salassi-Scooter, M. R. (1997). Vascular access and hemodynamic monitoring. In R. A. Dieckmann, D. H. Fiser, & S. M. Selbst (Eds.), *Pediatric emergency and critical care procedures* (pp. 187-195). St. Louis, MO: Mosby.

Figure 8-4 Securing of an IV catheter in the hand

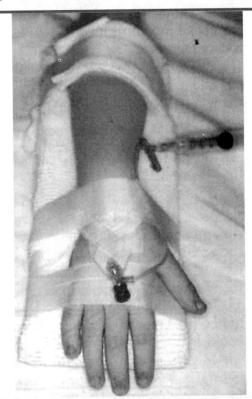

Reprinted with permission from Cunningham, F. J., Engle, W. A., & Rescorla, F. J. (1998). Pediatric vascular access and blood sampling techniques. In J. R. Roberts & J. R. Hedges (Eds.), *Clinical procedures in emergency medicine* (3rd ed., pp. 281-308). Philadelphia: Saunders.

- Support the leg on a rolled blanket or firm surface. Hold the leg without any portion of your hand behind the calf.
- Using sterile technique insert the needle with a twisting motion. In the tibia insert (twist and push simultaneously) 1 to 3 cm below the tibial tuberosity (one finger breath) in the middle of the anteromedial surface of the tibia.
- In other sites make sure you angle slightly away from any growth plates.
- Once you feel a decrease in resistance, stop advancing.
- Unscrew the cap and remove the stylet (if present), attempt to aspirate bone marrow followed by a flush.
- Bone marrow that is aspirated may be placed in lab tubes because many labs are able to process standard tests on the bone marrow. Tests that cannot be processed using bone marrow include a complete blood count, coagulation profiles, and arterial blood gases. Be sure to label the tube appropriately as containing bone marrow. Remember, you may not see any aspirate.

- While flushing make sure to check the tissues around the cannulated bone as well as the dependent area of the extremity for any swelling. This is the definitive method of verifying placement.[1,2]
- Stabilize the needle and connect to fluids. Reassess for signs of infiltration.
- Although the IO needle is typically a larger gauge needle than a pediatric peripheral IV, the actual fluid port tends to be small. In addition, bone marrow is somewhat pressurized, which may prevent fluids from flowing freely by gravity. Therefore, fluids may be given by pushing them manually, by applying a pressure bag, or through an infusion pump.

- When the IO needle is removed apply manual pressure for several minutes; then apply an ointment dressing and label as an IO site.[1]
- Follow medication administration with a 5-ml normal saline flush.
- Complications: fracture, compartment syndrome, skin necrosis, air, fat or bone embolus.
- Contraindications: fracture of the bone selected, cellulitis, osteogenesis imperfecta/osteopetrosis, previous attempts in the same bone.

Figure 8-5 Locations for IO infusion

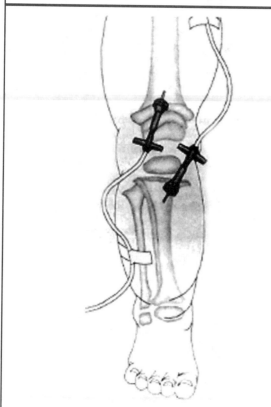

Reprinted with permission from Manley, L., Haley, K., & Dick, M. (1988). Intraosseous infusion: Rapid vascular access for ciritically ill or injured infants and children, *Journal of Emergency Nursing*, 4,63-68.

Figure 8-6 Central Venous Insertion Sites

Internal jugular vein
External jugular vein
Superior vena cava
Right atrium junction
Xiphisternum
Inferior vena cava
Umbilicus
Common iliac vein
Femoral vein
Great saphenous vein

Adapted from Lavelle, J., & Costarino, A. (1997). Central venous access and central venous pressure monitoring. In F. M. Henretig & C. King (Eds.), *Textbook of pediatric emergency procedures* (p. 252). Philadelphia: Lippincott Williams & Wilkins.

Central Venous Access

- Central venous catheters allow for more secure access to the circulation and provide the ability to deliver medications that may otherwise damage tissue if they infiltrate from a peripheral site. In addition, they also allow for central venous pressure to be monitored if needed.
- Infants and children tend to have more complications from central venous catheterization than adults do.[2]
- Central venous access can be obtained in the femoral, internal jugular, or subclavian veins (see **Figure 8-6**). The internal jugular site is difficult to access in children with short necks.
- Central venous access should only be attempted by clinicians experienced with the technique as well as familiar with the unique anatomical features of the pediatric central venous system.
- Long-term central venous access devices are inserted when prolonged or frequent venous access is needed and/or peripheral access is not obtainable. The pediatric patient may present to the emergency department with a long-term device in place.

  - Subcutaneous infusion ports, central venous catheters (Broviac®, Hickman®) and peripherally inserted central catheter (PICC) lines are used in pediatric patients.
  - Confer with the primary caregiver regarding the care of the vascular access device.
  - Follow appropriate procedures to access these devices. Use sterile technique during the access procedure and during line dressing changes.
  - Noncoring needles (Huber® needles) are required to access most subcutaneous infusion ports.
  - Clamping of the catheter is dependent on the type of catheter that is in place. The Hickman and Broviac catheters must be clamped when accessed; the Groshong® catheter should not be clamped because it contains a two-way valve.
  - Following the collection of blood specimens or on completion of an infusion, the device is flushed with heparin solution to maintain patency. The child's weight, the catheter or device size and type, and institution policy will influence the concentration of heparin and saline that is used.

Points to Remember

- Always maintain universal precautions when performing any procedure.
- Explain all procedures to the pediatric patient and family in an age-appropriate and developmentally appropriate manner.
- Use pharmacological and nonpharmacological pain management techniques to decrease pain and stress related to the procedure.
- Reward and comfort the pediatric patient after the procedure. Reinforce positive behaviors.
- In the pediatric patient requiring frequent phlebotomy or IV access attempt to use the pediatric patient's preferred sites.
- Offer choices that you can live up to, such as type of reward, Band-Aid™ or music.
- When attempting peripheral venous access avoid the dominant hand if possible. If the pediatric patient sucks his or her thumb, avoid the favored hand if possible.
- Evaluate all potential IV sites prior to attempting access. Avoid prolonged use of tourniquets and access over bony prominences.
- Obtain assistance with securing and comforting the pediatric patient.
- Avoid using parents to secure the child.
- Obtain assistance if unable to obtain venous access in two or three attempts.
- Monitor IV and IO sites for signs of infiltration at least every hour when administering fluid boluses.

References

1. Infusion Nurses Society. (2000). *Infusion nursing standards of practice*. Retrieved on September 9, 2003 from http://www.ins1.org/philosophy.htm. Standards are: (2) nursing practice, (43) site selection and device placement, and (57) catheter site care.
2. American Heart Association. (2000). Vascular access. In M. F. Hazinski (Ed.), *Pediatric advanced life support* (Provider manual) (pp. 155–172). Dallas, TX: Author.
3. American Academy of Pediatrics. (2000). Using a developmental approach. In R. Dieckmann, D. Brownstein, & M. Gausche-Hill (Eds.), *Pediatric education for prehospital professionals* (pp. 16–29). Sudbury, MA: Jones and Bartlett.

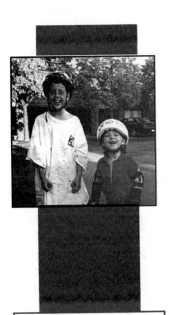

Chapter 9

RHYTHM DISTURBANCES

Objectives

On completion of this chapter, the learner should be able to:

1. Recognize the broad class of dysrhythmias that may occur in the pediatric population.

2. Recognize unstable conditions or dysrhythmias that require immediate intervention.

3. Describe the immediate interventions and/or medications required to stabilize an unstable rhythm.

4. Differentiate supraventricular tachycardia (SVT) from sinus tachycardia (ST).

5. Describe the use of electrical therapy for dysrhythmias.

Introduction

The most common causes of cardiopulmonary arrest in adults are lethal dysrhythmias related to heart disease. In the child, however, the most common causes of cardiopulmonary arrest are conditions that lead to shock and heart failure. Even though cardiopulmonary arrest in children is not common, rates of survival from documented asystole are dismal. This chapter will focus on selected broad categories of dysrhythmias because these are the most common causes of cardiovascular compromise.

Anatomic, Physiologic, and Developmental Characteristics as a Basis for Signs and Symptoms

There are specific characteristics in the cardiovascular system of the pediatric patient with important clinical significance. These are summarized in **Table 9-1**.[1]

Autonomic Nervous System

Cardiac function is regulated by the hypothalamus, which stimulates the cardiovascular control centers located in the medulla oblongata and the pons. These centers receive impulses from the heart and, by means of a reflex loop, send signals to target organs through the sympathetic and parasympathetic systems.

During the first few weeks of life there are numerous changes in the autonomic nervous system and the cardiac conduction system. Sympathetic innervation of the heart is incomplete; therefore, the newborn is particularly sensitive to the effects of parasympathetic stimulation. Stimulation of the parasympathetic pathway (vagal stimulation such as suctioning or defecating) is a common cause of transient bradycardia in the newborn.[2] As the child matures, sympathetic innervation increases; however, older children and adults can also respond to vagal stimulation with bradycardia.

Autoregulation of the Heart

Intrinsic autoregulation of cardiovascular function occurs in response to changes in blood volume flowing to the heart. As the heart fills, cardiac muscle fibers stretch. The degree to which these fibers stretch affects the force of contraction (contractility) and stroke volume.

The neonatal myocardium is less compliant and contains less contractile mass than the older child and adult myocardium. Because cardiac output is a function of heart rate and stroke volume, the pediatric patient's principle method of increasing cardiac output during a low output state is to increase his or her heart rate. However, cardiac output will fall when the heart rate exceeds 180 to 200 beats/min because ventricular filling time is compromised and during periods of sustained bradycardia because of limited stroke volume. Bradycardia is considered an ominous sign of impending cardiopulmonary arrest in the pediatric patient.

The Electrocardiogram (ECG)

ECG Paper

The ECG is a graphic representation of the normal cardiac cycle of depolarization and repolarization. The small lines are 1 mm apart, both horizontally and vertically, with each 5th horizontal and vertical line being darker to form a larger box of 25 small squares. The vertical lines measure time/rate. The interval between 2 light lines is 0.04 seconds, and the interval between 2 dark lines is 0.20 seconds. The slash marks at the top of the paper occur every 3 seconds.

The Basics of an ECG

Before you can diagnosis a dysrhythmia you must know the basics of the electrocardiogram. The ECG shows the relationship of the conduction system on paper. Each cardiac cycle consists of a P wave, a QRS complex, and a T wave. The P wave represents atrial depolarization. The PR interval represents the length of time required for the atria to depolarize and for the impulse to travel through the AV junction. It is measured from the beginning of the P wave to the beginning of the QRS complex. The normal interval is 0.12 to 0.20 seconds. The QRS complex represents depolarization of the ventricles with a normal interval of 0.08 seconds. Remember the QRS complex duration is short in children and increases with age. The Q wave is the initial negative deflection that precedes the R wave. The R wave is the first positive deflection followed by another negative deflection known as the S wave. The ST segment is normally an isoelectric line that begins with the end of the QRS complex and ends with onset of the T wave. The T wave represents ventricular repolarization[3] (**Figure 9-1**).

Analyzing the Rhythm Strip

The first step in analyzing a rhythm strip is to determine if the rate is fast, slow, or within normal limits for the pediatric patient's age. Normal heart rates can be found in **Table 9-2**. Once this is determined, you must

Table 9-2 Normal Pediatric Vital Signs

Age	Weight (kg)	Heart rate (avg/min)	Resp rate (avg/min)	BP (sys) (mm Hg)
Newborn	1	145	> 40	42 ± 10
Newborn	2-3	125		60 ± 10
1 month	4	120	38 ± 10	80 ± 16
6 months	7	130		89 ± 29
1 yr	10	125	39 ± 11	96 ± 30
2 to 3 yr	12 to 14	115	28 ± 4	99 ± 25
4 to 5 yr	16 to 18	100	27 ± 6	99 ± 20
6 to 8 yr	20 to 26	100	24 ± 6	105 ± 13
10 to 12 yr	32 to 42	75	21 ± 4	112 ± 19
> 14 yr	> 50	70	20 ± 4	120 ± 20

Reprinted with permission from Barkin R. M., & Rosen, P. (1999). *Emergency pediatrics: A guide to ambulatory care* (5th ed., inside cover). St. Louis, MO: Mosby.

Table 9-1

Characteristics	Clinical Significance
Myocardium has poor compliance (myocardial fibers are shorter and less elastic), contractile mass is less, stroke volume is limited (1.5 ml/kg/beat/min as compared to 75 to 90 ml/beat/min in an adult).	Heart rate rather than stroke volume increases to maintain cardiac output, which falls precipitously with bradycardia or heart rates exceeding 200 beats/min.
Infants have a higher cardiac output (200 ml/kg/min versus 100 ml/kg/min in the adult).	Provides for increased oxygen needs, but leaves little cardiac output reserve. Any stresses such as hypothermia or sepsis can lead to acute deterioration.
Circulating blood volume: Infant: 90 ml/kg; child: 80 ml/kg; adult: 70 ml/kg	Small blood losses can cause circulatory compromise.
Children are capable of maintaining adequate cardiac output for long periods due to strong compensatory mechanisms. Rapid deterioration can occur when compensatory mechanisms are exhausted.	Hypotension is a late sign of circulatory decompensation. Children may remain normotensive until 25% of their blood volume is lost. Assess capillary refill as an indicator of peripheral perfusion (capillary refill should be < 2 seconds).

then decide if this rate is regular or irregular. This can be done by measuring the distance between one R wave and the next two R waves of the rhythm strip that you are analyzing. Then ask the question: Are they evenly spaced? (If the rhythm is irregular, count the number of QRS complexes in a 6-second period and multiply by 10 to get the rate). Once you have determined the rate and its regularity, you need to determine if there are P waves present and, if so, whether they are regular or irregular. Is there a P wave for every QRS? What is the PR interval? What is the QRS interval? With this information you can now decide if this is a life-threatening rhythm or not.[3]

Figure 9-1 Relationship of the ECG to the heart and waveform

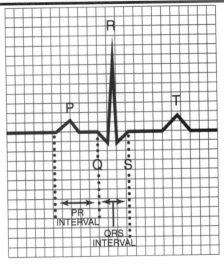

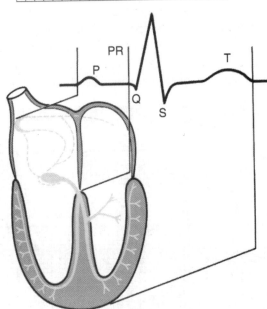

Reprinted with permission from American Heart Association. (2002). Rhythm disturbances. In *Pediatric advanced life support* (Provider manual) (pp. 185–228). Dallas, TX: Author.

Broad Classifications of Dysrhythmias

Dysrhythmias in the pediatric setting can be classified into three general categories: slow, fast, or not there at all (absent).

The most important concept with any of these dysrhythmias is to determine if the pediatric patient is stable or unstable. Those individuals with cardiovascular instability will display signs of shock (i.e., altered level of consciousness; respiratory distress; poor peripheral or end-organ perfusion; delayed capillary refill; pale, cool, clammy skin; and lastly, hypotension). Remember that hypotension is a very late sign, and these other signs and symptoms will become more profound before the hypotension is evident. If any of these rhythms are unstable, quickly determine the cause and provide treatment before total collapse and cardiopulmonary arrest occurs.

Note: The following sections related to specific dysrhythmias include the most current treatment recommendations from the American Heart Association's Pediatric Advanced Life Support course (2002) at the time of publication. Due to the continual evolution of treatment modalities and drug therapies these recommendations may be revised before the next revision of Emergency Nursing Pediatric Course. It is the responsibility of the health care provider to check with your health care institution regarding updated policies and procedures relating to medications and nursing practice.

Rhythm Recognition

"Too Slow"—Bradydysrhythmias

Case Presentation

A 10-month-old presents with her father who states that she has had a fever over the last day and he has noted over the last hour that she has become more listless and not wanting to eat. The father notes that she is breathing faster than normal and that her lips appear slightly blue tinged.

Hypoxemia is the most frequent cause of slow or bradydysrhythmias associated with the pediatric population. The symptomatic patient with a slow rhythm must have a patent airway established and be provided adequate oxygenation and ventilation. Many times this will be the only treatment that the pediatric patient needs. If the bradycardia persists despite adequate oxygenation and ventilation then cardiopulmonary resuscitation (CPR) and medications are indicated to improve the rate.

One important thing to remember is that in a pediatric patient a slow rhythm is any heart rate below the normal heart rate for that child's age, usually 60 beats/minute (bpm) or less. According to the American Heart Association 2001[2], "clinically significant bradycardia is defined as a heart rate less than 60 bpm associated with poor systemic perfusion." As was stated previously, hypoxemia is the leading cause of bradydysrhythmias in the pediatric population. So, if this dysrhythmia is recognized quickly and adequate oxygenation and ventilation is initiated immediately, you can take control of one of the most common prearrest rhythms in the pediatric population. Other characteristics of bradycardia are that the P waves may or may not be present, and the QRS complex will usually appear normal (**Figure 9-2**).

History

- Excessive suctioning secondary to increased secretions in the mouth
- Hypothermia
- Recently intubated
- Suspected overdose (especially calcium channel blockers, beta-blockers, or digoxin)
- Congenital heart disease
- Recent trauma (i.e., head or chest)

Signs and symptoms

- Heart rate < 60 bpm
- Delayed capillary refill
- Increased work of breathing
- Altered level of consciousness, listlessness

Interventions

- Administration of oxygen at 100% either by a nonrebreather mask or a bag-mask device.

- If these devices are not providing adequate ventilation, the airway must be secured by intubation.
- Establish IV access with either a peripheral intravenous (IV) or intraosseous (IO) access.
- Begin chest compressions if the heart rate remains < 60 bpm despite adequate oxygenation and ventilation.
- Look for potential causes for this dysrhythmia and treat.[2]
  - Hypoxemia: Adequate oxygenation and ventilation.
  - Hypothermia: Warmed fluids, oxygen, blankets, and overhead lights. The best way to warm the core is with warmed oxygen.
  - Head injury: Look for signs of increased intracranial pressure (change in the level of consciousness, bradycardia, and hypotension)
  - Ingestion of toxins: Treat the patient then the toxin if known.
- Consider pharmacologic agents (i.e., epinephrine, atropine).[2]
  - Epinephrine has alpha-adrenergic stimulating properties that cause vasoconstriction by increasing peripheral vascular resistance, which in turn increases blood flow to vital organs. It also has positive chronotropic properties that increase the heart rate along with inotropic properties that increase myocardial contractility, leading to an increase in the oxygen consumption by the heart. The usual dosage is 0.01 mg/kg of a 1:10,000 solution either IV or IO. Appendix A lists the usual drugs used in Pediatric Advanced Life Support (PALS) in the pediatric population with a cardiac dysrhythmia. Atropine is only considered in the pediatric patient when vagal stimulation or cholinergic drug toxicity is suspected. The IV/IO dose is 0.02 mg/kg with the minimum dose being 0.1 mg. Remember that oxygen followed by epinephrine is still the first-line

Figure 9-2 Sinus Bradycardia

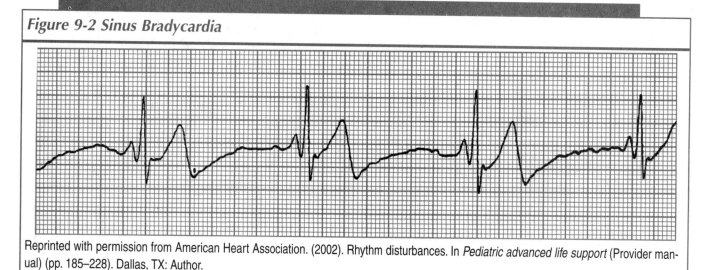

Reprinted with permission from American Heart Association. (2002). Rhythm disturbances. In *Pediatric advanced life support* (Provider manual) (pp. 185–228). Dallas, TX: Author.

treatment to consider in bradycardia with poor perfusion in pediatric patients.

- Early pacing (transcutaneous) may be considered with symptomatic bradycardia.

- Numerous sources[2] have noted that pacing can provide a bridge for improving the survival rates of those patients who have symptomatic bradycardia, especially when the bradycardia is due to a complete heart block or some type of congenital heart disease.

- Remember that transcutaneous pacing may be somewhat painful in the conscious patient, so you may want to reserve the use for those pediatric patients having a life-threatening event. You may even consider some sort of sedation prior to pacing.

- Pediatric-sized electrodes are recommended for a child who weighs less than 15 kg.[2] Adult-sized electrodes are recommended for the child who weighs more than 15 kg.[2]

- Pacing electrodes can be either placed anterior-anterior or posterior-anterior, with the latter being the most recommended positioning (see **Figure 9-3**).

- The initiation of transcutaneous pacing for a pediatric patient with symptomatic bradycardia includes setting the demand rate to 100 bpm, then adjusting the output to the maximum output that achieves capture. You may want to fine-tune this output by 10% to ensure that capture remains.

"Too Fast"— Tachydysrhythmias

A tachydysrhythmia is a heart rate that is faster than the normal heart rate for the child's age. Refer to Table 9-2 for normal values. These rhythms need immediate treatment to ensure that they do not decompensate into a state that results in shock and life-threatening (unstable) dysrhythmias. There are two categories of tachydysrhythmias: atrial and ventricular. These dysrhythmias will be addressed separately, but with any of these dysrhythmias the basic ABCs should not be forgotten in the initial assessment of these pediatric patients.

Atrial Case Presentation #1

*A father presents with his 2-year-old who has been fussy over the last 2 days with a decreased appetite. Because the child has also had vomiting and diarrhea for the past 12 hours, the father is not sure when the child last had a wet diaper. No fever has been noted but Dad states they do not have a thermometer at home. The child's skin is cool, dry, and pale. No retractions are noted but the child has some labored breathing with a rate of 30. Peripheral pulses are palpated, but are weak and thready. The child is brought back to the main department and has an apical pulse at 150 with a narrow QRS (**Figure 9-4**).*

History

- History of recent volume loss (i.e., vomiting, diarrhea or trauma)
- Poor feeding
- Suspected overdose
- Recent fever
- Excessive crying or agitation
- Decreased appetite

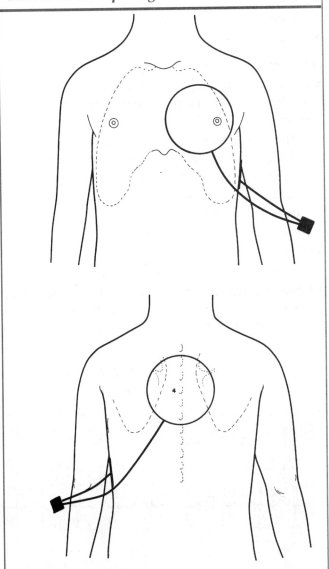

Figure 9-3 Location of pacing electrodes for transcutaneous pacing

Reprinted with permission from Erickson, C. C. (1997). Temporary cardiac pacing. In R. A. Dieckmann, D. H. Fiser, & S. M. Selbst (Eds.), *Pediatric emergency and critical care procedures* (pp. 312–322). St. Louis, MO: Mosby.

Signs and Symptoms of Sinus Tachycardia

- Delayed capillary refill
- Dry mucous membranes
- Decreased number of wet diapers
- Increased stooling or vomiting
- Pale/cool extremities; mottled skin
- Rapid heart rate
  - Does not have an abrupt onset
  - Rate is normally in the range of 180 to 200 bpm. (If above 200 bpm, think SVT.)
  - The QRS complex is narrow with P waves that are present.
- Change in the level of consciousness: alert to listlessness
- Rapid and thready peripheral pulses; strong central pulses
- Increased work of breathing
- Crying

Interventions for Sinus Tachycardia

- Initiate IV or IO access and then bolus with 20 mL/kg of a hypotonic crystalloid solution such as normal saline or lactated Ringer's.[2,4,5]
  - After the first bolus, reassess the pediatric patient for changes in skin color, capillary refill, and heart rate.
  - If these remain abnormal, initiate a second and maybe a third bolus and reassess the pediatric patient after each bolus.
- Look for the cause of the tachycardia.
- Obtain blood for complete blood count and any other studies that may be indicated.
- Obtain a urine specimen. If an infection is suspected, this must be a catheterized specimen and sent for a culture and sensitivity.

- Offer fluids by mouth, if appropriate.
- Monitor and maintain body normal temperature.

Atrial Case Presentation #2

A mother brings her 2-month-old child to the emergency department with a complaint that the child has been fussy and is only nursing for 2 to 3 minutes before stopping. Mother state that the child's color appears to be paler than normal. She had a normal delivery and has been healthy, but has not had her 2-month checkup or immunizations yet. She normally nurses for 10 minutes on each breast without any difficulties. She had normal stooling patterns. When you examine her, you see a pale, alert, but quiet 2-month-old female child. Her skin is cool and dry with mild retractions. Apical heart rate is too fast to count. When you place her on the cardiac monitor you see the rhythm shown in **Figure 9-5**.

Supraventricular tachycardia (SVT) is one of the most common tachydysrhythmias that produces cardiovascular compromise during infancy.[6] It is characterized as a fast rhythm, greater than 220 bpm in infants or greater than 180 bpm in a child. It may be as high as 300 bpm but regular and does not vary with agitation or crying.[6] In the child with SVT, you will not be able to distinguish the presence of P waves because they may be buried in the QRS complex. The QRS complex will be narrow and regular. Many times because this rhythm is so fast there will be systemic changes noted due to the decrease in the cardiac output (i.e., changes in skin color and temperature, change in level of consciousness, or a fast, thready pulse). This dysrhythmia has an abrupt onset and at times can be terminated with vagal maneuvers, such as coughing, bearing down as if they are having a bowel movement, venapuncture,[7] or even insertion of a rectal thermometer to simulate the bearing down. Some physicians still like to place a bag of

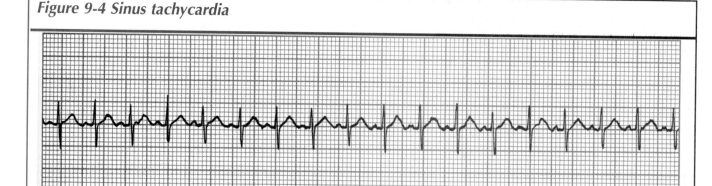

Figure 9-4 Sinus tachycardia

ice on the child's face to stimulate a diver's reflex and thereby slow down the heart rate.[8]

Additional History

- History of previous episode of SVT
- History of Wolff-Parkinson-White syndrome
- History of congenital heart disease
- Poor feeding

Signs and Symptoms of SVT

- Pale, cyanotic, or mottled skin
- Hypotension
- Faint or absent peripheral pulses
- Altered mental status
- Irritability

Additional Interventions for SVT

- Provide adequate oxygenation and ventilation with either a nasal cannula or nonrebreather mask.
- Obtain IV access, with the antecubital site being the preferred site due to its proximity to the heart.
- Synchronized electrical cardioversion must be used if IV access is not available and the pediatric patient is unstable (i.e., signs of poor perfusion and hypotension are present). The procedure for synchronized cardioversion is similar to defibrillation with the following modifications.[2,9]
  - The defibrillator and the cardiac monitor must be set so the delivery of the countershock can be synchronized to avoid delivery of the energy during the relatively refractory portion of the cardiac electrical activity.
  - Initial dose is 0.5 joules/kg; repeat doses are delivered at 1.0 joules/kg.
  - Discharge buttons must be held until the countershock is delivered.

- Consider administration of analgesics and sedation prior to cardioversion.
- Adenosine is the drug of choice for conversion of SVT in stable pediatric patients. In the unstable pediatric patient, adenosine must only be considered if IV access has been established.[2,6]
  - An initial dose of 0.1 mg/kg is recommended (with a maximum initial dose of 6 mg), with a subsequent dose of 0.2 mg/kg (maximum second dose is 12 mg).
  - Be sure that a continuous ECG is being run while the adenosine is being infused.
  - Adenosine must be given rapidly at the port closest to the infusion site and followed immediately by a 5 cc normal saline flush. It is not uncommon to administer both the drug and the flush at the same time.
  - If SVT persists, the initial dose may be doubled and repeated once (maximum doses 6 mg in children and 12 mg in the adolescent).
  - Adenosine interrupts the reentry circuits that involve the atrioventricular node, causing a brief period (up to 20 seconds) of asystole. Side effects are rare because the half-life of the drug is 10 seconds.[2,6]
  - Use with caution in children with heart transplants.[2,7]
  - Higher doses of the drug may be required in children receiving theophylline or caffeine.[3]

Ventricular Tachycardia

Ventricular tachycardia (VT) is very uncommon in the pediatric age group.[6,8] VT in children may have some type of underlying structural heart disease and cardiomyopathy, or it may be an isolated and completely benign finding. Other causes include hypoxia, acidosis, or toxin ingestion, such as cocaine or tricyclic antidepressants.[2] Large pediatric referral centers may

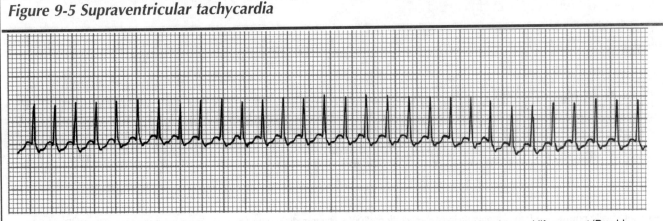

Figure 9-5 Supraventricular tachycardia

Reprinted with permission from American Heart Association. (2002). Rhythm disturbances. In *Pediatric advanced life support* (Provider manual) (pp. 185–228). Dallas, TX: Author.

encounter three to five patients with sustained VT each year.[10] In Europe, arrhythmogenic right ventricular dysplasia has been found to be a leading cause of sudden death and VT in young people.[10] Population-based studies in pediatrics are relatively small but have demonstrated a rise in simple ventricular ectopy in apparently normal infants, decreasing during preschool and elementary school ages, and increasing again with adolescence.[10,11] VT has a regular rate of 120, with a wide QRS complex (> 0.08) with a "tombstone" appearance. P waves cannot be identified (see **Figure 9-6**).

History
- Structural heart disease
- Myocarditis
- Prolonged QT syndrome
- Suspected overdose (i.e., tricyclics and cocaine)
- Electrolyte imbalance

Signs and Symptoms of VT
- Palpitations
- Increased work of breathing
- Decreased peripheral perfusion (delayed capillary refill, cool clammy skin, and decreased or absent peripheral pulses)
- Hypotension secondary to the ventricles not filling adequately and pumping blood normally
- Sustained VT can worsen until it becomes ventricular fibrillation
- Ventricular rate of at least 120 bpm and regular[6]
- Wide QRS complex (> 0.08 sec), "tombstone appearance"
- No identifiable P waves
- May or may not have palpable pulses
- Change in level of consciousness

Treatment of VT with a Pulse[2,6,10,12]
- If VT is present in an awake pediatric patient with a pulse and adequate perfusion, a consultation to a pediatric cardiologist may be warranted.
- Support the airway and provide adequate oxygenation with either a nasal cannula or nonrebreather mask.
- Obtain an ECG.
- Establish venous access.
- Consider the use of either amiodarone IV (5 mg/kg over 20 to 60 minutes), lidocaine IV bolus (1mg/kg), or procainamide IV (15 mg/kg over 30 to 60 minutes).
- Consider cardioversion at 0.5 to 1 joules/kg; be sure that you sedate the pediatric patient prior to cardioversion.

Treatment of VT without a Pulse[2,6,10,12]

Treat as if ventricular fibrillation. The treatment can be found in the following ventricular fibrillation section.

Ventricular Fibrillation (VF)

Ventricular fibrillation (**Figure 9-7**) and pulseless VT are not common dysrhythmias in the pediatric population but do occur.[6,11,13,15,16] Management is different from the adult patient in that defibrillation is administered at much lower joules than in the adult, and appropriately sized paddles must be available to perform effective defibrillation.[2,5,15,17]

Additional History
- Electrocution
- Recent viral illness
- History of cardiac surgery or heart transplant
- Ingestion of toxic substance
- Blunt impact to chest—especially in sports[16]

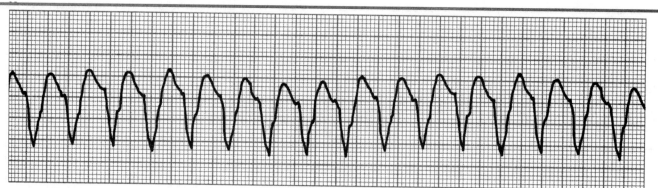

Figure 9-6 Ventricular tachycardia

Reprinted with permission from American Heart Association. (2002). Rhythm disturbances. In *Pediatric advanced life support* (Provider manual) (pp. 185–228). Dallas, TX: Author.

Signs and Symptoms of VF[2,6,15]

- Unresponsive child
- Absence of a palpable pulse
- VF or VT on the monitor without palpable pulses

Interventions for VF/Pulseless VT

If VT is present in a child with or without a pulse and inadequate perfusion (pallor, decrease central and peripheral pulses, and alterations in level of consciousness), the following interventions must be immediately initiated along with prompt defibrillation.[2, 6,15,17]

- Secure the airway and provide adequate oxygenation.
- Begin cardiac compressions.
- Defibrillate once with 2 joules/kg and immediately resume CPR for 5 cycles (about 2 minutes).
- If no change in the rhythm, defibrillate once at 4 joules/kg and resume CPR immediately.
- Administer a vasopressor agent such as epinephrine during chest compressions. Epinephrine is administered at 0.01 mg/kg (0.1 ml/kg of 1:10,000) IV or IO. Circulate for 5 cycles (about 2 minutes). May be repeated every 3 to 5 minutes.
- If unable to obtain IV or IO, may give epinephrine 0.1 mg/kg (0.1 ml/kg of 1:1000) via the endotracheal tube.
- If no change in the rhythm after circulating the epinephrine for 5 cycles (about 2 minutes) with CPR, attempt defibrillation at 4 joules/kg. Resume CPR immediately.
- If still no change in the rhythm, consider amiodarone (5 mg/kg) IV push or lidocaine (1 mg/kg) IV push if amiodarone is not available.
- Circulate with CPR for 5 cycles (about 2 minutes) and attempt defibrillation at 4 joules/kg and immediately resume CPR following defibrillation.
- Consider family presence during the resuscitation with an assigned staff member present at all times.
- Consider termination of resusitation efforts.

Pulseless Electrical Activity (PEA)

PEA is a display of electrical activity on the cardiac monitor (other than VT or VF) that does not produce a palpable pulse.[2,6] The electrical activity that can be seen on the monitor is too weak to produce an atrial pressure that can be detected by manually palpating peripheral or central pulses. It is critical that this dysrhythmia be identified early and treated before it degenerates to asystole.

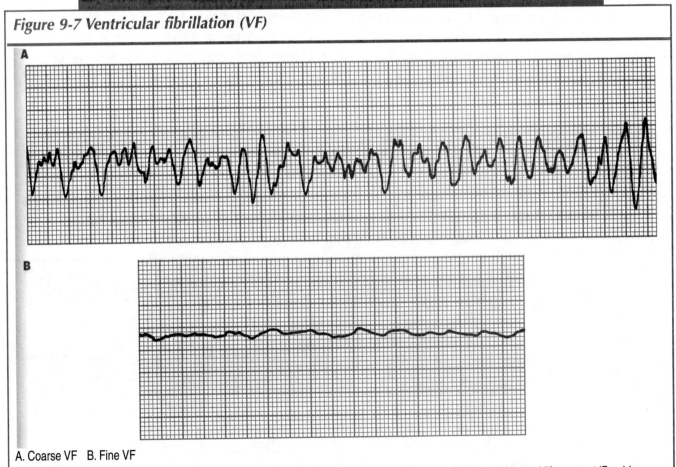

Figure 9-7 Ventricular fibrillation (VF)

A

B

A. Coarse VF   B. Fine VF

Reprinted with permission from American Heart Association. (2002). Rhythm disturbances. In *Pediatric advanced life support* (Provider manual) (pp. 185–228). Dallas, TX: Author.

Signs and Symptoms of PEA

- Electrical activity on the cardiac monitor (usually bradycardia) with no palpable pulses
- Change in the pediatric patient's level of consciousness
- Respiratory distress progressing to failure
- Signs of shock: pale, cool skin; delayed capillary refill

Interventions for PEA [2,6]

- Confirm pulselessness.
- Support airway and provide adequate ventilation with a bag-mask device or intubation.
- Monitor continuously with defibrillation or pacer electrodes.
- Begin cardiac compressions.
- Initiate IV or IO access.
- Consider the reversible causes and treatments.[2]
  - Hypoxia—provide adequate ventilation
  - Hypothermia—consider warmed fluids, warmed humidified oxygen, blankets, Bair Hugger®, or overhead lights
  - Hypovolemia—administer 20 mL/kg bolus of crystalloid solution, such as normal saline or lactated Ringer's solution
  - Electrolyte imbalances (especially hyper-/hypo-calcemia/kalemia/magnesemia)
  - Cardiac tamponade secondary to trauma—assist with pericardiocentesis (see Chapter 11, *Pediatric Trauma*)
  - Tension pneumothorax—perform needle thoracentesis (see Chapter 11, *Pediatric Trauma*)
  - Toxins/poisons—treat the patient, then the toxin if known
  - Thromboembolism
- Administer epinephrine 0.01mg/kg (0.1 ml/kg of 1:10,000) IV or IO. Repeat every 3 to 5 minutes.[2,6]
- If unable to obtain IV or IO, may give epinephrine 0.1 mg/kg (0.1 ml/kg of 1:1000) via the endotracheal tube.

Asystole

Pediatric cardiopulmonary arrest is uncommon.[6,14] However, when it does occur, it generally has dismal outcomes.[2] The most common cause of cardiac arrest in children is respiratory arrest. Unlike in the adult patient, cardiac arrest is usually not sudden in the child, but the end result of respiratory failure or shock.

Additional History

- Time child was found to be pulseless
- Description of event prior to pulseless event: Time last seen by the caregiver, last feeding, position in crib.
- Primary caregiver at the time of the event
- Time basic life support initiated: bystander, EMS
- Time advanced life support initiated

Signs and Symptoms of Asystole [2,6]

- Absent electrical activity on the cardiac monitor (**Figure 9-8**)
- Apnea
- Poor peripheral perfusion
- Absent heart tones
- No palpable pulses: absent central and peripheral pulses

Treatment of Asystole [2,6]

- Confirm asystole on cardiac monitor in two leads.
- Consider family presence with an assigned staff member.
- Look for causes and initiate treatment.
  - Hypoxia—provide adequate ventilation
  - Hypothermia—consider warmed fluids, warmed humidified oxygen, blankets, Bair Hugger®, or over head lights

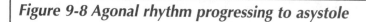

Figure 9-8 Agonal rhythm progressing to asystole

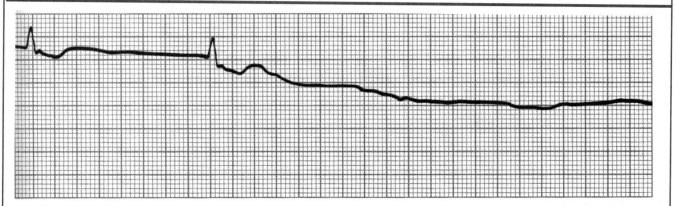

Reprinted with permission from American Heart Association. (2002). Rhythm disturbances. In *Pediatric advanced life support* (Provider manual) (pp. 185–228). Dallas, TX: Author.

Hypovolemia—administer 20 mL/kg bolus of crystalloid solution, such as normal saline or lactated Ringer's solution

- Electrolyte imbalances (especially hyper-/hypo-calcemia/kalemia/magnesemia)
- Cardiac tamponade secondary to trauma—assist with pericardiocentesis (see Chapter 11, *Pediatric Trauma*)
- Tension pneumothorax—perform needle thoracentesis (see Chapter 11, *Pediatric Trauma*)
- Toxins/poisons—treat the patient, then the toxin if known
- Thromboembolism

- Administer epinephrine 0.01mg/kg (0.1 ml/kg of 1:10,000) IV or IO. Repeat every 3 to 5 minutes.[2,6]
- If unable to obtain IV or IO, may give epinephrine 0.1mg/kg (0.1 ml/kg of 1:1000) via the endotracheal tube.
- Anticipate the need to decide to terminate resuscitative efforts by considering the following factors: duration of pulselessness.[12]

Summary

Evaluation of the pediatric patient with a cardiac dysrhythmia requires astute assessment of peripheral perfusion, vital signs, level of consciousness, and rhythm recognition. Shock and respiratory failure are common pathways to cardiovascular collapse and subsequent cardiac arrest in the pediatric patient. The outcome of cardiac arrest in the child is most frequently death or recovery with poor neurological outcome. Early recognition of the signs of cardiac dysrhythmias is critical to the initiation of prompt intervention and the prevention of adverse outcomes. The central piece of the puzzle in the care of the pediatric patient with cardiac dysrhythmias is the interlocking relationship between early recognition of the life-threatening dysrhythmias and the initiation of the rapid interventions.

References

1. Mott, S. (1994). Cardiac emergencies. In S. Kelly (Ed.), *Pediatric emergency nursing* (pp. 199–228). Norwalk, CT.: Appleton & Lange.
2. American Heart Association. (2005). Pediatric advanced life support. *Circulation, 112*(24)(Suppl.), IV167–IV187.
3. Aehkert, B. (1996). Rhythm disturbances. In *PALS: Pediatric advanced life support study guide* (pp. 151–172). St. Louis, MO: Mosby.
4. Castle, N. (2002). Paediatric resuscitation: Advanced life support. *Nursing Standard, 17*(11), 47–52.
5. Atkins, D. L., Chameides, L., Fallat, M. E., Hazinski, M. F., Phillips, B., Quan, L., et al. (2001). Resuscitation science of pediatrics. *Annals of Emergency Medicine, 37*(4 suppl.), S41–48.
6. Park, M. K. (2003). *The pediatric cardiology handbook* (3rd ed.). St. Louis, MO: Mosby.
7. Quan, L., Graves, J. R., Kinder, D. R., Horan, S., & Cummins, R. O. (1992). Transcutaneous cardiac pacing in the treatment of out-of-hospital pediatric cardiac arrests. *Annals of Emergency Medicine, 21*(8), 905–909.
8. Aydin, M., Baysal, K., Kucukoduk, S., Cetinkaya, F., & Yaman, S. (1995). Application of ice water to the face in initial treatment of supraventricular tachycardia. *The Turkish Journal of Pediatrics, 37*(1), 15–17.
9. Hatlestad, D. (2002). The benefits of electricity: Transcutaneous pacing in EMS. *Emergency Medical Services, 31*(9), 38–40, 42, 44–45.
10. Alexander, M. E., & Berul, C. (2002, April 10). Ventricular tachycardia. *eMedicine Journal.* Retrieved June 11, 2003 from http://www.emedicine.com/ped/topic2546.htm
11. Berul, C. I., Hill, S. L., Geggel, R. L., Hijazi, Z. M., Marx, G. R., Rhodes, J., et al. (1997). Electrocardiographic markers of late sudden death risk in postoperative tetralogy of Fallot children. *Journal of Cardiovascular Electrophysiology, 8*(12), 1349–1356.
12. Davis, A. M., Gow, R. M., McCrindle, B. W., & Hamilton, R. M. (1996). Clinical spectrum, therapeutic management and follow-up of ventricular tachycardia in infants and young children. *American Heart Journal, 131*(1), 186–191.
13. Alexander, M. E., & Berul, C. I. (2000). Ventricular arrhythmias: When to worry. *Pediatric Cardiology, 21*(6), 532–541.
14. Berger, S., Dhala, A., & Friedberg, D. Z. (1999). Sudden cardiac death in infants, children, and adolescents. *Pediatric Clinics of North America, 46*(2), 221–234.
15. Stephenson, E. & Berul, C. (2002, October 2). Ventricular fibrillation. *eMedicine Journal.* Retrieved June 11, 2003 from http://www.emedicine.com/ped/topic2398.htm
16. Maron, B. J., Poliac, L. C., Kaplan, J. A., & Mueller, F. O. (1995). Blunt impact to the chest leading to sudden death from cardiac arrest during sports activities. *New England Journal of Medicine, 333*(6), 337–342.
17. Mogayzel, C., Quan, L., Graves, J. R. Tiedeman, D., Fahrenbruch, C. & Herndon, P. (1995). Out-of-hospital ventricular fibrillation in children and adolescents: Causes and outcomes. *Annals of Emergency Medicine, 25*(4), 484–491.

Appendix 9-A
Drugs and Electrical Therapy Used in PALS for Rhythm Disturbances

Adenosine	*Indications:* Drug of choice for treatment of symptomatic SVT *Precautions:* Very short half-life (use rapid injection technique)	IV/IO: - Continuous ECG monitoring - 0.1 mg/kg rapid IV push, Follow with 5 mL NS flush - May double (0.2 mg/kg) for second dose - Maximum first dose: 6 mg - Maximum second dose: 12 mg
Amiodarone	*Indications:* Wide range of atrial and ventricular arrhythmias and shock-refractory VF/VT *Precautions:* May cause bradycardia and hypotension; may prolong QT interval and increase risk for polymorphic VT; do not routinely combine with other medications that prolong QT interval (e.g., procainamide)	*For perfusing VT and SVT:* 5 mg/kg IV/IO over 20 to 60 minutes (repeat as needed to maximum: 15 mg/kg per day) *For shock-refractory pulseless VT/VF:* 5 mg/kg rapid IV/IO bolus
Atropine Sulfate	*Indications:* Vagally induced symptomatic bradycardia; symptomatic bradycardia refractory to oxygenation, ventilation, and epinephrine *Precautions:* Low dose may cause paradoxical bradycardia; tracheal absorption may be unreliable	*IV/IO/tracheal:* 0.02 mg/kg per dose; may double for second dose - Minimum dose: 0.1 mg - Maximum single dose, child: 0.5 mg (maximum total dose: 1 mg) - Maximum single dose, adolescent: 1 mg (maximum total dose: 2 mg)
Calcium chloride (10% solution = 27.2 mg/mL of elemental calcium)	*Indications:* Symptomatic hypocalcemia, hyperkalemia, calcium channel blocker overdose *Precautions:* Rapid IV push may result in bradycardia or asystole; do not mix with buffer; infiltration may cause skin to slough	IV/IO: 20 mg/kg (0.2 mL/kg of 10% solution) slow push - Repeat for documented conditions
Calcium gluconate (10% solution = 9 mg/mL of elemental calcium)	*Indications:* Symptomatic hypocalcemia, hyperkalemia, calcium channel blocker overdose *Precautions:* Rapid IV push may result in bradycardia or asystole; do not mix with buffer; infiltration may cause skin to slough	IV/IO: 60 to 100 mg/kg (0.6 to 1 mL/kg of 10% solution) slow push - Repeat for documented conditions
Synchronized cardioversion attempt	*Indications:* Tachyarrhythmias (SVT, VT, atrial fibrillation, atrial flutter) with symptoms of cardiovascular compromise *Precautions:* Activate sync mode; provide sedation with analgesia when possible	Initial energy (shock) level: 0.5 to 1 J/kg - Second and subsequent energy levels: 1 to 2 J/kg

Drugs and Electrical Therapy Used in PALS for Rhythm Disturbances

Defibrillation attempt	*Indications:* VF/pulseless VT *Precautions:* Do not delay; use largest paddle size with good skin contact and no bridging	- Deliver 1 shock at 2 J/kg initially - Subsequent energy levels: 4 J/kg
Epinephrine for bradycardia*	*Indications:* Symptomatic bradycardia refractory to oxygenation and ventilation *Precautions:* May produce profound vasoconstriction, tachyarrhythmias, hypertension; do not mix with buffer	IV/IO: 0.01 mg/kg (0.1 mL/kg of 1:10,000) Tracheal: 0.1 mg/kg (0.1 mL/kg of 1:1,000)
Epinephrine for asystolic or pulseless arrest*	*Indications:* Pulseless arrest: asystole, PEA, shock-refractory VF/VT *Precautions:* May produce profound vasoconstriction, tachyarrhythmias, hypertension; do not mix with buffer; avoid use in cocaine-related VT	*First dose:* IV/IO: 0.01 mg/kg (0.1 mL/kg of 1:10,000) *Subsequent doses:* - Repeat every 3 to 5 minutes during CPR - Consider a higher dose (0.1 mg/kg, 0.1 mL/kg of 1:1,000) for special conditions
Epinephrine infusion	*Indications:* Refractory hypotension or persistent bradycardia *Precautions:* May produce profound vasoconstriction, tachyarrhythmias, hypertension; do not mix with buffer; avoid use in cocaine-related VT	0.1 to 1 mcg/kg per minute Titrate to desired effect
Lidocaine bolus*	*Indications:* Alternative treatment for wide-complex tachycardias or VF/pulseless VT *Precautions:* High doses may cause myocardial depression and seizures; do not use if rhythm is wide-complex bradycardia (ventricular escape beats)	IV/IO: 1mg/kg Tracheal: 2 to 3 mg/kg May repeat every 5 to 15 minutes Maximum dose: 100mg
Lidocaine infusion	*Indications:* Alternative for recurrent VT/VF or ventricular ectopy, especially if associated with ischemic heart disease *Precautions:* High doses may cause myocardial depression and seizures; do not use if rhythm is wide-complex bradycardia (ventricular escape beats)	IV/IO infusion: 20 to 50 mcg/kg per minute - Administer bolus of 1 mg/kg when initiating infusion if bolus has not been given within previous 15 minutes
Magnesium sulfate	*Indications:* Torsades de pointes VT or symptomatic hypomagnesemia *Precautions:* May cause hypotension with rapid bolus	Rapid IV/IO infusion: 25 to 50 mg/kg (maximum 2 g) over 10 to 20 minutes

Appendix 9-A (cont.)

Drugs and Electrical Therapy Used in PALS for Rhythm Disturbances

Procainamide	*Indications:* Alternative treatment for recurrent or refractory VT, SVT	Loading dose: 15 mg/kg IV over 30 to 60 minutes
	Precautions: Hypotension, bradycardia, and QT prolongation	
	Do not routinely administer with amiodarone	
Sodium bicarbonate	*Indications:* Hyperkalemia, sodium channel blocker toxicity, and severe metabolic acidosis (documented or suspected after prolonged arrest) with adequate ventilation	IV/IO: 1mEq/kg per dose Infuse slowly and only if ventilation is adequate
	Precautions: Infuse slowly; may produce CO_2; therefore, ventilation must be adequate; do not mix with catecholamines or calcium	

* For tracheal administration, dilute medication with normal saline to a volume of 3 to 5 ml and follow with several positive-pressure ventilations.

Reprinted with permission from American Heart Association. (2002). Rhythm disturbances. In *Pediatric advanced life support* (Provider manual) (pp. 185–228). Dallas, TX: Author.

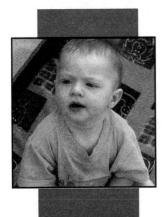

chapter 10

MEDICATION ADMINISTRATION

Objectives

On completion of this chapter, the learner should be able to:

1. Define medication.
2. Identify specific pediatric considerations related to the various routes of medication administration.
3. Describe the appropriate method for rapidly administering an intravenous fluid bolus.

Introduction

What is a medication? According to Webster's New World Collegiate Dictionary, a medication is "a substance for curing or healing, or for relieving pain." This includes both prescription and over-the-counter medications along with alternative medicines such as herbal remedies. Given this definition a full discussion of medication and pharmacology is beyond the scope of this chapter; therefore, only the key concepts related to medication administration in the pediatric patient population will be reviewed.

Medication Administration

The overriding principle related to medication administration is to provide the right patient with the right drug in the right dose by the right route at the right time.[1]

- Before any medications are administered, the pediatric patient's identification band should always be checked against the chart. The caregiver should also be asked to state the pediatric patient's name to verify the identity. If old enough, the pediatric patient may be asked to state his or her name. In some countries such as the United States, regulatory agencies may require two forms of identity verification.[1]

- All dosages are calculated based on weight. Ensure that the pediatric patient's weight is recorded accurately in kilograms.

- Check for medication interactions with over-the-counter or herbal remedies the pediatric patient may have been given.

- **Table 10-1** provides an overview of common routes of administration and tips to facilitate administration.

Positioning for an Injection

Consider using positioning-for-comfort techniques. Have the caregiver hold the child on his or her lap (chest to chest) and hug the child, or have the caregiver stand in front of the child who is sitting on the stretcher (chest to chest) and hug the child.

Intramuscular injections

- Prepare the injection out of the pediatric patient's sight.

- Position and secure the pediatric patient before the injection.

- Consider the pediatric patient's age, weight, and muscle mass, as well as medication volume and viscosity, when selecting an injection site. **Table 10-2** lists the recommended intramuscular injections sites and considerations for their use in pediatric patients.[2]

- Consider use of dermal anesthetic or local application of ice to the site prior to injection.

- Having the older child lie facedown on a table or stretcher with feet turned inwards (toe to toe) will make it harder for him or her to flex the gluteal muscles.

- The medication volume for injection per intramuscular site is limited to 0.5 ml to 1 ml in infants and 2.0 ml in older children.

- After the medication is drawn into the syringe, change the needle before administration. The insertion of the needle through a stopper dulls the tip, and residual medication on the needle may irritate the tissue or muscle.

- For the immunocompromised child, cleanse the site with povidone iodine and alcohol.
- After the injection, comfort the child and give him or her a reward such as a sticker or Popsicle®.

Subcutaneous Medication Administration[2]

- Sites used for the administration of subcutaneous medication include the upper lateral deltoid, anterior thigh, and anterior abdominal wall.

Table 10-1 Medication Administration

Route	Considerations
Ear	• In children younger that 3 years of age pull the pinna down and back. • In children older that 3 years of age lift the pinna up and back. • Have the child position his or her head to the side or on the caregiver's shoulder.
Nasal	• Have the caregiver hold the child across their lap with the child's head down. Place the child's arm that is the closest to the caregiver around the caregiver's back Firmly hug the child's other arm and hand with the caregiver's arm; snuggle the head between the caregiver's body and arm.
Eye	• Explain the procedure; tell the child the medication will feel cool. Prepare the child if the medication will sting. • Have the child lie on his or her back with their hands tucked under their buttocks. • Alternatively, have the smaller child sit on the caregiver's lap and have the caregiver hug the child securing their arms. • Have the child look up, then retract the lower lid and instill medication. • Provide distractions.
Oral	• Consider the child's age when determining the medication preparation (liquid, chewable, sprinkle, junior-sized pills). • Use an oral syringe or calibrated cup to ensure correct dosage. • To prevent aspiration, administer oral medication while the child's head is raised or the child is in a sitting position. • For infants, liquid medication can be administered through a nipple, followed by 5 ml of water. • When administering medication with an oral syringe, place the syringe between the gum and cheek. Administer slowly, no more than 0.5 ml at a time. • Do not administer chewable tablets to children without teeth; give children something to drink after the chewable tablet. • Do not crush enteric-coated tablets or caplets. • Do not open capsules if medication is sustained release; check with pharmacist before opening any capsule for administration. • Avoid mixing medication with formula because the infant may refuse formula thereafter. • When mixing medication with food or liquids, use as little diluent as possible. Masking the taste with food or fluid is often helpful; however, if the quantity is large, the child may not finish the entire amount and the full dose will not be given.
Rectal	• Consult a pharmacist prior to cutting a suppository since the medication is not necessarily distributed evenly through the suppository, (e.g., acetaminophen suppositories must be divided lengthwise but not widthwise). • Place the child in the knee-chest position on his or her side. • Lubricate the suppository with water-soluble lubricant prior to insertion. • It has been recommended to hold the buttock cheeks together until the urge to expel has passed. Consider eliciting the assistance of the caretaker. • Commercially available adult enemas and/or tap-water enemas should be avoided. Isotonic solutions should be used.
Inhaled	• Commercially available spacer devices are available with or without masks for MDI. For a parent that cannot afford a device a toilet paper roll can be used. • Nebulized medication may need to be given with a face mask adapter or with a "blow-by" technique. • Consider purchasing commercially available nebulizer sets. • Use distractions and stickers rewards to facilitate cooperation.
Dermal	• Pastes absorb moisture. Medications in pastes are released slower than medications that are in creams or ointment bases. • Bath treatments are helpful in widespread dermatitis but NEVER leave a child alone in a tub. Avoid rubbing the skin dry, pat instead. • Cover the ointment or medication as indicated.

- Volume of medication administered is limited to 0.5 ml to 1.0 ml. Maximum limitation is 1.0 ml in all age groups.
- The needle should be inserted at a 90° angle.
- Needle size: Infant or thin child–25- to 30-gauge 1/2-inch needle; larger child–25-gauge, 5/8-inch needle.

Intravenous Medication Administration

- Administration time may vary. Drugs and fluids may be given by intravenous bolus, constant infusion, or intermittent infusion.
- A syringe pump or infusion pump is used to deliver continuous to intermittent medication infusions to ensure accurate and timely delivery of medications. Administer medication following the guidelines for dilution and infusion of the specific drug. After drug administration, flush the intravenous tubing with normal saline to clear any residual medication from the line. Syringe pumps with low-volume tubing are available to minimize the amount of flush solution needed.
- Medications such as antibiotics can be administered using a burette. Following the infusion a 20-ml flush should be infused to flush the remainder of the medication from the chamber. Label the chamber device when flushing or administering medications.
- Caution should be used when administering infusions so that the total volume of medication and flushes does not exceed the recommended volume for the pediatric patient's weight.

- To administer an intravenous fluid bolus rapidly or when infusing via an intraosseous needle, a pressure bag may need to be applied to the intravenous solution bag in addition to using large-bore intravenous tubing because a small catheter may impede gravity flow. When more rapid administration is needed, the following stopcock technique may be used.
  - Attach a three-way stopcock between the T connector and intravenous tubing.
  - Attach a syringe to the stopcock; turn the stopcock off to the child (arrow toward the child).
  - Withdraw the syringe plunger, filling the syringe with intravenous solution.
  - When the desired amount is withdrawn, turn the stopcock off to the intravenous solution bag (arrow toward the bag) and push the solution from the syringe. Repeat this procedure until the desired fluid volume is administered.
  - If medications are administered through a stopcock, flush the stopcock with 3 to 5 ml of solution following the medication administration.

Endotracheal Administration[3]

- If vascular access is unavailable during resuscitation, the endotracheal route can be used to administer the following emergency drugs: lidocaine hydrochloride, epinephrine hydrochloride, atropine sulfate, and naloxone.

Table 10-2 Pediatric Intramuscular Injection Sites

Site	Recommended Age	Considerations

Vastus lateralis	• Infant
	• Preferred for children younger than 3 years of age
		• Larger muscle group in this age group
		• Can tolerate large injection volumes:
		  - Infants 0.5 ml to 1.0 ml
		  - Older children up to 2.0 ml
		• Area is free of important nerves and blood vessels
		• Use 22- to 25-gauge 5/8-inch to 1-inch needle

Ventrogluteal	• Child • Consider for children older than 3 years of age	• Can tolerate large injection volumes • Area free of important nerves and blood vessels • Easily accessible site • Health care professional often unfamiliar with this site • Injection volume up to 2.0 ml • Use 20- to 25-gauge 1-inch to 1.5-inch needle
Deltoid	• Infant	• Small muscle mass • Can tolerate only small injection volumes (0.5 ml to 1.0 ml) • Easily accessible site • Rapid absorption rate • Danger of radial nerve injury in young children • Use 22- to 25-gauge 1/2-inch to 1-inch needle

- The recommended dose of epinephrine hydrochloride during resuscitation via the endotracheal route is 10 times the intravenous or intraosseous dose.
- Delivery can be optimized in one of two ways.
  - Dilute the drug in 5 ml of normal saline and administer via the endotracheal tube followed by five manual ventilations; there are now commercially available endotracheal tubes with an integral medication injection port . Administer the drug through a small catheter threaded beyond the endotracheal tube tip followed by a normal saline flush.

Inhalation Administration[4]

Nebulized Pharmacologic Agents

- A face mask instead of a mouthpiece on the acorn (plastic cup) may be used for infants and children.
- Commercial pediatric nebulizer sets are available in a variety of pediatric-friendly characters.
- One end of the mouthpiece set can be occluded to use it as a blow-by method of delivery.
- Consider making it a game. For example, have the child take a deep breath in before pretending to blow out candles or use distraction techniques like watching the smoke go in and out.
- Monitor vital signs including respiratory status and oxygen saturation during and after administration. Document the results.
- Have primary caretaker hold the child during delivery.
- For effective medication delivery, a spacer should be used with metered-dose inhalers.
  - Allow several breaths between delivery puffs.
  - Proper technique is extremely important for effective delivery of the medication.

Dermal Administration

Topical Therapies

- Health care providers should use universal precautions to avoid exposure of the medication to his or her own skin.
- Make sure the area of application is clean prior to administration.
- Avoid overtreatment. Apply a thin layer of medication to the skin, spreading in the direction of hair growth.
- Prevent the pediatric patient from scratching by trimming nails or covering hands with socks or mittens.
- Use nondominant hand for anesthetic if possible to discourage the pediatric patients from putting their hand with medication in their mouth. Apply dermal patches out of reach.

- Lukewarm or tepid applications offer the most relief.
- Educate the primary caretaker on the appropriate method of applying topical medication, including what to look for and when to stop applying topical medications. Shampoos should be kept out of the eyes. Watch for central nervous system symptoms, such as a changing level of consciousness or seizures.

Occlusive Dressings

- For topical anesthetics apply a thick layer of medication and cover with a polyurethane dressing. Avoid thinning out the medication.
- Hydrocolloid dressings, such as DuoDerm®, protect superficial and small skin breakdowns or wound areas.
- Hydrogel dressings, such as Vigilon, are effective in treating superficial to moderately deep skin breakdown or wound areas.

Discharge Teaching for Caregivers Regarding Medication Administration

Caregivers and pediatric patients (when age appropriate) should be given information about the drug name, route of administration, action, dosage, and potential side effects.

Adequate discharge instructions promote compliance and the safe and accurate administration of medication at home. The following information should be included in the instructions.

- Time the medication should be given.
- Duration of drug therapy.
- Medication administration techniques, including methods of measuring suspensions. It is best to have a return demonstration by the primary caretaker when possible.
- When to seek additional medical care, such as when symptoms do not resolve or worsen.
- Educate primary caretaker about any expected or unexpected skin changes as a result of topical medications, such as blanching, thinning, increased redness, or hives
- Address any cleaning and maintenance issues related to nebulizers and spacers.
- Demonstrate methods for assessing metered-dose inhaler (MDI) volumes. For example, when an MDI canister is dropped in a cup of water, a full canister will drop to the bottom whereas an empty canister will float to the top. Recommend obtaining a refill when the canister bobs like a buoy.

References

1. Joint Commission on Accreditation of Healthcare Organizations. (2003). *2003 national patient safety goals.* Retrieved August 20, 2003 from http://www.jcaho.org/accredited + organizations/hospitals/standards/npsg_03.htm

2. Medication administration procedures. (1992). In N. Skale (Ed.), *Manual of pediatric nursing procedures* (pp.117–128). New York: Lippincott.

3. Chameidses, L, & Hazinski, M. F. (2002). Vascular access. In *Pediatric advanced life support* (Provider manual) (pp. 155–172). Dallas, TX: American Heart Association.

4. Layman, M. (1999). Nebulizer therapy. In J. Proehl (Ed.), *Emergency nursing procedures* (pp.124–128). Philadelphia: Saunders.

chapter 11

PEDIATRIC TRAUMA

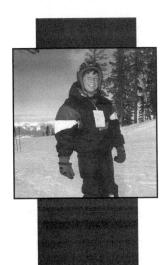

Objectives

On completion of this chapter, the learner should be able to:

1. Identify the anatomic and physiologic characteristics of the pediatric trauma patient that contribute to the signs and symptoms associated with trauma.

2. Identify the causes, types, mechanisms, and patterns of injury associated with pediatric trauma.

3. Describe how to systematically assess the pediatric trauma patient.

4. Determine the specific interventions needed to care for the pediatric trauma patient.

5. Evaluate the effectiveness of nursing interventions related to patient outcome.

6. Identify health promotion strategies related to pediatric trauma.

Introduction

Trauma has a greater impact on morbidity and mortality than all other diseases in the pediatric population. Death from unintentional injury accounts for 65% of all injury deaths in children younger than 19 years and is the number one killer of people ages 1 to 24 years. Approximately 20,000 deaths of those children who are killed each year are due to preventable injuries.[1] There are several factors that influence who are injured, with age, time of day, and sex being the most important factors for patterns of injury.[2] Mechanisms of injury are primarily caused by blunt trauma, with a small portion coming from penetrating trauma.

Fires and burns are the fifth leading cause of unintentional injury-related death among children ages 14 and younger.[3] The majority of burn-related injuries occur at home and are considered preventable. Children, especially those 5 years and younger, have the greatest risk from home fire-related deaths and injury. A less acute perception of danger, less control over their environment, and limited ability to react promptly and properly to a fire contribute to this excess risk.[3] Fortunately the number of deaths due to fire and burn injuries has declined by more than 50% between 1971 and 1998.[3] This decline coincides with the increased national attention to burn prevention, widespread use of smoke detectors, burn prevention education, regulation of consumer product safety, and establishment of burn centers.[4]

Anatomic, Physiologic, and Developmental Characteristics as a Basis for Signs and Symptoms

The mechanisms of injury are based on developmental milestones in a child's development, so practical knowledge of pediatric anatomy, physiology and the child's response to injury is of utmost importance in treating the traumatized child. Inherent in this process is the recognition of the distinct anatomic and physiologic characteristics of the pediatric patient.[5]

Cardiovascular Characteristics

- Children have a healthy cardiovascular system and physiologic ability to initially compensate for hypovolemia by vasoconstriction and tachycardia. By increasing their heart rate, children can increase their cardiac output with little if any change in the stroke volume.

- It is critical to remember that hypotension related to hypovolemia in the pediatric trauma patient is a late sign and may indicate a loss of at least 20% to 25% of the circulating blood volume.

- Children have a greater body surface area in proportion to their body weight and a higher extracellular to intracellular fluid volume ratio, and will require more fluid during resuscitation. Young children also require maintenance fluids, which are not usually accounted for in most burn resuscitation formulas.

Respiratory Characteristics

- The faster respiratory rate in children contributes to greater insensible pulmonary fluid loss.
- In closed-space fires, this increased respiratory rate may lead to increased uptake of toxic gases. Most pediatric victims (70%) of closed-space fires die as a result of inhalation of toxic gases such as carbon monoxide and cyanide rather than burns.
- Children have smaller airways. Inhalation of irritants and heated air may cause edema resulting in a decreased airway diameter. This leads to a greater resistance to airflow and more pronounced signs of respiratory distress. Interstitial fluid shifts occurring with major burns may also result in airway edema without inhalation injury.

Temperature Regulation

- Children have a less mature thermal regulatory mechanism.
- Children are susceptible to heat loss due to a high ratio of body surface area to body mass, large head in proportion to the rest of the body, and small amount of subcutaneous tissue.
- Hypothermia can impede the child's response to resuscitative measures.
- Factors that can lead to hypothermia in the pediatric trauma patient include
  - Prehospital environmental exposures
  - Leaving the child uncovered for even a short period of time
  - Cool ambient temperature of emergency vehicles and trauma rooms
  - Wet or moist dressings
  - Clothing saturated with blood, secretions, vomitus, perspiration, or other causes
- Young children can suffer significant burn injuries from exposure to lesser amounts of heat.
  - Exposure of tissue to temperatures at or below 44°C (111°F) can be tolerated for extended periods of time by children.
  - Exposure at 54°C (130°F) for 10 seconds produces more severe tissue injury.
  - Exposure at 60°C (140°F) causes tissue destruction in less than 5 seconds.[6]

Other Anatomic and Physiologic Characteristics

- The head is large and heavy, and the neck muscles are weak, predisposing the child to head and neck trauma. (Remember that the head is proportionally larger than the rest of the body until the child is 6 to 8 years old). Eighty percent of all pediatric trauma deaths are associated with head injury.
- The cranium is thin and more pliable in young children, with the scalp being very vascular.
- The protuberant abdomen, immature abdominal muscles, rib cage sitting higher in the abdominal cavity and small pelvis of the child offer little protection to the underlying solid and hollow abdominal organs. The kidneys are also larger and less protected. Therefore, abdominal organs are prone to injury.[5]
- Rib cage is flexible with a softer, thinner chest wall, allowing easier compression of the lungs.
- The disruption of the integumentary system as a protective barrier predisposes the child to infection or sepsis.
- Hypoglycemia is common in children; so it is important to monitor blood glucose routinely, especially in the burn patient.

Developmental Characteristics

- Children are easily distracted, impulsive, have little concept of cause and effect, and lack experience with similar situations.
- Children have difficulty determining the speed or the distance of an oncoming vehicle.
- It is often difficult for children to localize sound, and their visual field tends to focus on a single object similar to their own height.
- They often believe that because they see the car, the driver must see them.

Causes, Types, Mechanisms, and Patterns of Injury in Children

Blunt Injuries

Injury occurs by blunt trauma first to the outer skin and soft tissue, and then to the underlying structures. Initially, injury to one or more solid organs may be obscure in the pediatric patient.[1] Therefore, cautious evaluation with a high index of suspicion for intraabdominal injury is required for all children with blunt trauma.

Motor Vehicle Crashes

The largest number of trauma deaths in children is due to motor vehicle crashes. During a motor vehicle crash, three separate collisions occur. The first is the vehicle striking another object. Even though the vehicle has decelerated or stopped, the body continues to travel at the original speed. The second is the collision of the body with something in the car. The third collision involves the organs striking other organs, muscle, bone, or other supporting structures. A fourth collision can occur if there are loose objects in the vehicle that become projectile forces.

Head trauma is a common injury for unrestrained children involved in a motor vehicle crash. Until the age of 6 or 8, the head is significantly larger in proportion to the remainder of the child's body. When involved in a motor vehicle crash, the unrestrained child's large head acts like a missile, leading the torso throughout the vehicle cabin. In a front-end crash with a speed of 30 mph, an unrestrained child will hit the dashboard with the same force as the impact received after falling three stories to a solid surface. Although mechanisms of pediatric injury vary, the most common part of the child's body that comes in contact with an unyielding object is the head.

All states within the United States have mandated the use of car seats for young children. Regardless of geographic region, compliance and proper use of pediatric safety restraint devices continues to be a problem. Participation in safety restraint education programs is important for all health care workers who care for children.

Improper use of restraint systems can also lead to injury. These patterns of injury vary by the child's size, location in the vehicle, and the type and method of restraint used. The infant has a higher center of gravity. During a motor vehicle crash, infants have a greater risk of cervical fracture at the level of C-1 to C-3 when in a safety restraint seat that is positioned facing front in the vehicle. Placing the infant in a rear-facing restraint seat, secured in the backseat of the vehicle, can potentially prevent this type of injury by minimizing the fulcrum effect of the infant's head whipping forward.

The use of lap belts in children has been associated with a triad of injuries that include severe flexion-distraction injuries of the lumbar spine, abdominal wall bruising and hollow viscous injury. Children are prone to lap belt injuries because they often slouch with the belt loose and across the abdomen (rather than the hips). A booster seat corrects these problems by lifting the child up and forward, allowing better fit of both the lap and the shoulder belts. Recommendations for booster seat use extend to 27 kg (60 lb) or 8 years in Canada and to 36 kg (79 lb) or 11 years in the United States and the United Kingdom.[7-10] However, actual use is very low in most countries, and preventable lap belt injuries continue to occur, yet the use of lap belts has been proven to decrease the fatal injuries that could be sustained. The use of a shoulder belt and lap belt is even more effective in decreasing the incidence of injury.

Air Bag Injuries

Air bags are standard equipment in all new cars and are designed to supplement the protection provided by safety belts in frontal crashes. Federal safety standards require that all new passenger cars and light trucks be equipped with both driver and passenger side air bags beginning in1999. Although air bags have a good overall safety record and have saved an estimated 1,200 lives as of the end of 1995, they pose several risks for children. Children that are unbelted, are improperly belted, or are too close to the dashboard when an air bag inflates are at risk for injury. Due to an increasing number of child deaths related to air bag deployment, individualized deactivation measures are being explored. Children occupying the front seat have been killed or severely injured by front passenger air bags, even in minor crashes.[10,11] Children in the zone of air bag deployment can suffer facial trauma, upper extremity fracture, intraabdominal injury, abrasions and chemical irritation of the skin, cervical spine injury, and partial to complete decapitation. Several factors contribute to this problem including (1) children are poorly held by seat belts such as those available in the front seat, (2) children move around while the vehicle is moving; and (3) child safety seats are often erroneously used in the front seat.[11] Best practice indicates that children under 13 years of age must be seated in the rear, away from the air bags.

Side air bags in the rear seat are currently available in only a small number of luxury vehicles. There is little crash experience of their effect on child occupants. Transport Canada found that rear-seat air bags could cause injury—sometimes serious—to out-of-position 3- and 6-year-old child dummies.[7] Because most children are out of position for portions of any journey, it is wise to avoid rear-seat air bags in cars where children are the intended passengers. Current U.S. policy is that cars with rear air bags be sold with the bags deactivated, to avoid injury to children.[12,13]

To ensure that children ride safely, the National Traffic Highway Safety Administration (NHTSA) recommends the following.

- The best car safety seat is one that fits your child's size and weight and can be installed correctly in your car.
- Never place a rear-facing infant safety seat in the front seat of the vehicle with a front passenger airbag.
- Infants must be positioned rear facing until they have reached at least 1 year of age AND weigh at least 20 pounds (or more, depending on model). The American Academy of Pediatrics recommends that babies be kept in rear-facing seats until they reach the

maximum weight allowed, as long as the top of the head is below the top of the seat back.[9,10]

- The backseat is the safest place for children of any age to ride.

Pedestrian Injuries

In the United States, a pedestrian struck by a car is more likely to sustain left-sided injuries because cars are driven on the right side of the road. The structures most commonly injured, listed in the order of frequency, are the spleen, genitourinary system, gastrointestinal tract, liver, pancreas, pelvis, and major vessels.[13] Preschool children may be injured when they play around parked cars. Older children may be injured while running across the street.[14] Pedestrians who are struck by automobiles often have one or more injuries.[13-16] The biomechanics of the child pedestrian who is struck by a vehicle include the following.

- Classically, the injuries occur as the child impacts the vehicle and is thrown away from the vehicle. The child's physical size and the type of vehicle involved are the two factors that most affect the pattern of injuries sustained.
- Waddell's triad is a common pattern of injury sustained by children who are stuck by a motor vehicle. The triad generally involves injuries to the head, chest/abdomen, and lower extremities.[15]
- Toddlers and preschoolers may be knocked down and dragged under the vehicle. The vehicle's front bumper may cause chest, abdomen, pelvic, or femur injuries.
- Older preschool and school-age children may sustain femur fractures from the bumper and chest injuries from the hood.
- If the child is thrown onto the hood of the vehicle and strikes the windshield, head and facial injuries may occur. When the car decelerates or stops, the child slides or rolls to the street, usually striking his or her head on the pavement.

Children struck by motor vehicles are at high risk for multisystem injury. The pattern of injury sustained is dependent on the relationship among variables such as the speed of the vehicle, point of initial impact, additional points of impact, the child's height and weight, and landing surfaces. A thorough trauma assessment is essential to identify all injuries.

Falls

Falls account for greater than one third of childhood injuries requiring medical evaluation. The factors that contribute to the injuries sustained from a fall include (1) the velocity of the fall, (2) the child's body orientation at the time of impact, (3) the type of impact surface, and (4) the time that the force is applied to the body on impact.[17] In early childhood, children are prone to falls due to their higher center of gravity, increased mobility, and a limited perception of danger.

- Infants more commonly sustain falls from low objects such as high chairs, baby walkers, shopping carts, countertops, changing tables, beds, and tables.
- Toddlers and preschoolers sustain falls from low objects as well as falls from heights such as windows, balconies, and stairs.
- The school-aged child is often involved in a fall related to sports or recreational activity, such as tree climbing, bicycling, playground equipment, skating, and organized sports activities.

Recreational Injuries

Injuries related to sports are responsible for a significant number of emergency department (ED) visits. Those sports responsible for the highest number of emergency visits are basketball, biking, football, baseball, skating (ice or in-line), softball and soccer. The injuries that occur from these sports include extremity injuries, head trauma, abdominal injury (particularly in football and soccer), and spinal cord or vertebral column injury.

Biking has become a very popular sport among children and adults. The most common injury related to bicycle incidents is head injury. Bicycle-related injuries have risen in recent years. In 1997, an estimated 567,000 Americans sustained a bicycle-related injury that required ED care. Approximately two thirds of these cyclists were children or adolescents.[18] An estimated 140,000 children are treated each year in EDs for head injuries sustained while bicycling. This includes skull fractures, concussions, and subdural hematomas. The use of bicycle helmets has reduced the mortality related to bicycle incidents; however, compliance with wearing a helmet is reported at only 5%.[19] Compliance with wearing a helmet is enhanced by state legislation and municipal enforcement. By early 1999, 15 states and more than 65 local governments had enacted some form of bicycle helmet legislation. Most of these laws pertain to children and adolescents.[19] Accordingly, the national health goal for 2010 is for 50% of teenage bicyclists in 9th to 12th grade to wear helmets.[19]

Blunt abdominal trauma has been reported with bicycle incidents, including pancreatic injury, small bowel injury, and solid organ injury. About three quarters of all pediatric bicycle-related injuries to abdominal and pelvic organs involve the handlebars. University of Pennsylvania researchers and others extrapolated hospital discharge data from 19 states recorded in 1997 to determine national estimates of bicycle-related injuries in subjects younger than 20 years. They also used case series data from a pediatric trauma center to estimate the percentage of abdominal and pelvic injuries associated with handlebars and the cost of these injuries. They estimated that nationally, in 1997, 1,147 subjects under the age of 20 years had serious bicycle-related abdominal or pelvic organ injuries requiring hospitalization. Of these, 886 were likely associated with handlebars.[20]

The resurgence of skateboarding has been linked to an increase in extremity and head injuries. With the increase in popularity of the sport, the number of injured individuals younger than 20 years has increased from an estimated 24,000 in 1994 to approximately 51,000 in 1999.[21] In 1997, 1,500 children required hospitalization for an injury sustained while skateboarding. Of these injuries, 74% involved injuries to an extremity (ankle, wrist), and 21% were injuries to the head (face) or neck. Children in the 5- to 14-year-old age group are most frequently injured, with approximately 90% of all children and adolescents treated for skateboard-related injuries in 1999 being male.[21] Younger children more commonly sustain head trauma due to their higher center of gravity and limited ability to break the fall. Older children usually sustain extremity trauma as they try to break their fall. Death from skateboarding injuries is most commonly due to the child colliding with a motor vehicle.[21]

Nonpowered lightweight scooters have become very popular. Preliminary data from the U.S. Consumer Product Safety Commission indicates that an estimated 9,400 people (94% younger than 15 years) were injured while using nonpowered scooters between January and August 2000, with injuries increasing considerably during the summer months. Children younger than 8 years accounted for 31% of those injured.[21] Approximately one third of all injuries were fractures or dislocations. Head and face injuries accounted for 29% of all injuries, whereas wrist, elbow, lower arm, and knee injuries together accounted for 34%.[21]

Snowboarding is popular in many areas of the world. One study reported the age range of snowboarders was 10 years to 48 years with a mean age of 19.8 years.[22] The injuries associated with snowboarding include upper extremity injuries, particularly fractures and shoulder dislocations; concussion; spinal strain; abdominal injury; and lower extremity injuries. Injuries to the upper extremity are the most common.[22] In contrast, skiers have a higher incidence of lower extremity injury. Skiing injuries often are related to the collision of two skiers or with a stationary object. These collisions can result in severe injuries to the head, chest, or abdomen.

Trampolines have become popular and are a source of traumatic injuries in children. Most trampoline-related injuries occur on home trampolines when children land incorrectly while jumping or while performing stunts. Other injuries occur when children fall from the trampoline to the surface below or collide with another person on the equipment. Individuals are also injured when they contact the frame and/or springs while near the edge of the jumping surface.[23]

Asphyxiation and Submersion Injuries

Asphyxiation

Asphyxiation and suffocation are among the leading causes of death in children due to inhalation injuries during a fire, mechanical suffocation, foreign body obstruction or inhalation, or hangings. In addition to the hypoxia sustained during a hanging injury, the child may also sustain a spinal cord injury, cerebral injury, laryngeal edema, and pulmonary edema. Vertebral injury is uncommon in hanging incidents.

Submersion

Drowning is a common cause of death in the pediatric patient.[24,25] It occurs when a child is submerged and then attempts to breathe and either aspirates water or has laryngospasm leading to hypoxemia and neuronal death. Forty to fifty percent of deaths related to drowning occur in children ages 1 to 4 years.[24] Drowning is not isolated to pools and ponds, but it may include bathtubs, buckets, or water that is greater than 1 to 2 inches in depth. Males drown four times more often than females.[25]

Near drowning is defined as survival or temporary survival following asphyxia due to a submersion episode.[24,25] It is noted that the major reason for death in near drowning is due to hypoxemia and the decrease in oxygen delivery to vital tissues. Immersion in water with ice is associated with a better outcome than prolonged immersion in warm or cold (without ice) water. The length of time the child is submerged and the water quality will affect the length of resuscitation and the outcome.

Although the pathophysiology differs, similar symptoms occur with near drowning by salt-or freshwater because most only aspirate 4 ml. Aspiration of a minimum of 11 ml was found to be the point that alterations in blood volume occurred, and large amounts of fluid are rarely aspirated. One of the most important signs seen in these victims is hypovolemia, which is due to the decrease in capillary permeability from hypoxia and loss of fluid in the intravascular space. Other signs and symptoms may be delayed in onset and are associated with cerebral hypoxia and pulmonary injury. These may vary in severity from minimal or absence of symptoms to cardiopulmonary arrest.

Penetrating Injury

The incidence of penetrating trauma in the pediatric population is rising.[26] Mechanisms of injury causing penetrating trauma includes stabbings, firearms, and blast injuries. In 1998 there were approximately 2,570 deaths from firearms in the 10- to 19-year-old age group.[26] Homicide was the second-leading cause of death in this age group. The death rate is four times higher among males than females.

The injuries sustained from a penetrating force will depend on the location of the impact and the type of penetrating object. With firearms, the amount of tissue damage is related to the projectile, mass, shape, fragmentation, type of tissue struck, and the striking velocity. The injury sustained from a stabbing is dependent on the length of the instrument, the velocity at which the force was applied, and the angle of entry.

Burns

In 1999, approximately 99,500 children 14 years and younger were treated in hospital emergency departments for burn-related injuries in the United States. Of these injuries, 63% were thermal burns, 24% were scald burns, 9% were chemical burns, and 2% were electrical burns. In 1999, nearly 3800 children 14 years and younger were treated in emergency departments for fireworks-related injuries.

Children at greatest risk for fire-related death and injury include children in homes without smoke alarms; male children; children from low-income families; children living in rural areas; African-American children; and children with a physical or cognitive disability.[3]

Burn injury can occur through five mechanisms:[27]

1. Inhalation. Inhalation of products such as carbon monoxide or cyanide, from incomplete combustion, toxic products, or thermal injury to the respiratory tract. Symptoms may not begin until 24 hours after exposure.

2. Thermal. Dermal exposure to heat or flame.

3. Electrical. Contact with electrical current (e.g., children biting through an electrical cord). Injuries may include massive tissue necrosis of the muscles, nerves, viscera, and subcutaneous tissue.

4. Chemical. Dermal exposure to a corrosive agent.

5. Radiation. Ionizing burns can be seen in children receiving radiation therapy.

When burns occur, the integument of the body is disrupted. Intravascular capillaries become permeable and, as a result, proteins, electrolytes, and large amounts of fluids shift from the intravascular space to the interstitial space. This results in edema of the burned area and loss of circulating volume.

At the burn site, the vessels supplying the area are occluded, decreasing blood flow to the burn. The injured cells release vasoactive substances, causing vasoconstriction and the development of peripheral vessel thrombosis. Tissue necrosis can develop as a consequence of the decreased skin perfusion.

Electrolytes shift following a burn and can produce significant changes in serum potassium, sodium, calcium, and base bicarbonate levels. For example, the loss of cell wall integrity allows the extrusion of potassium from the cell into the extracellular fluid. Serum potassium concentration will reflect hyperkalemia, although intracellular potassium is depleted.

Approximately 24 to 36 hours after the initial burn trauma, the capillaries are repaired and fluid remobilization begins. Fluid then returns to the intravascular space, the kidneys excrete sodium, and potassium returns to the cells. The pediatric patient may develop hypernatremia, hypokalemia, and anemia from hemodilution and red blood cell destruction. Fluid administration in this phase must be closely monitored to prevent circulatory overload.[27]

Pediatric patients must be assessed for progressive edema of the soft tissue and mucosa, leading to an airway obstruction. The greater proportion of soft tissue in the child's airway predisposes children to the development of mucosal edema. Approximately 48 to 72 hours after a burn injury, the damaged mucosal layer may slough, producing an acute airway obstruction.

Initial Assessment of the Pediatric Trauma Patient

Primary Assessment

The primary assessment consists of assessment of the airway with simultaneous stabilization of the cervical spine, breathing, circulation, neurologic status, and exposure with environmental control. Interventions to correct any life-threatening conditions are performed before continuing the assessment. Refer to Chapter 4, *Initial Assessment*, for a review of a comprehensive primary assessment. Assessment and intervention components unique to the primary assessment of the pediatric trauma patient are delineated in the following section.

Airway

- Inspect the pediatric patient's airway while maintaining cervical spine stabilization.

  - Cervical spine stabilization includes holding the head in a neutral position, placing bilateral support devices, and using tape to secure the head and the devices. Do not hyperextend, flex, or rotate the neck during these maneuvers. If immediately available, apply a rigid cervical collar before applying the head supports and tape. The pediatric patient's body movement must be controlled before the head is secured; therefore, begin taping at the feet and maintain manual stabilization of the cervical spine until the head is secured. The tape must extend to the rigid surface beneath the child.

  - Because infants and young children have a large occiput, positioning them supine on a backboard causes their cervical vertebrae to flex and move anteriorly. Flexion may contribute to airway compromise and/or decreased effectiveness of the jaw thrust or the chin lift maneuvers. To provide neutral alignment of the cervical spine, place padding under the child's shoulders to bring the shoulders into horizontal alignment with the external auditory meatus.[28]

  - If the child is already in a rigid cervical collar and strapped to a backboard, do NOT remove any devices. Check that the devices are placed appropriately.

  - Spinal stabilization includes stabilization as defined previously with the application of a backboard and straps or tape.

  - Complete spinal stabilization with a backboard and straps must be done at the completion of the secondary assessment, depending on the degree of resuscitation required and the availability of team members.

  - Any pediatric patient whose mechanisms of injury, symptoms, or physical findings suggest a possible spinal injury must be stabilized or immobilized.

  - If the patient is awake and breathing, he or she may have assumed a position that maximizes the ability to breathe. Before proceeding with cervical spine stabilization, be sure that interventions do NOT compromise the pediatric patient's breathing status.

- Position the patient in a supine position.

  - If the patient is not already supine, logroll the patient onto his or her back while maintaining cervical spine stabilization.

  - Remove helmet, if necessary, while maintaining cervical spine stabilization

- Open and clear the airway while manually stabilizing the spine. The jaw thrust or chin lift may be done to manually open the airway and avoid manipulation of the neck. If the airway cannot be opened with this technique, use the head tilt - chin lift technique because you must establish a patent airway.

  - The mucous membranes lining the narrow passages are delicate and thereby easily traumatized. In a burn victim look for singed nasal hair, facial hair, or eyebrows; soot around nose or mouth; burns to face and neck; stridor; drooling; presence of increased secretions; decreased or absent cough reflex; and changes in voice or a hoarse cough.

  - A nasopharyngeal airway may be inserted if the child is conscious and without evidence of facial trauma or basilar skull fracture to eliminate obstruction of the airway by the large tongue.

  - An oropharyngeal airway may be inserted if the child is unconscious.

  - Be sure to have suction available, but use it sparingly to reduce the risk of gagging that may result in vomiting and aspiration.

- Consider endotracheal intubation for definitive airway control for patients who require manual positioning to maintain a patent airway or who meet other intubation criteria.

  - Due to the differences in pediatric anatomy, maintaining the airway of the pediatric patient who is immobilized on a backboard is more difficult. Intubation must be performed without manipulation of the cervical spine.

  - Preoxygenate the pediatric patient prior to endotracheal intubation. If the pediatric patient demonstrates ineffective or absent breathing, ventilate the pediatric patient with a bag-mask and 100 % oxygen prior to endotracheal intubation.

  - Rapid sequence intubation (RSI) technique may be needed.

Breathing

- Remember children have thin chest walls and breath sounds may be hard to assess; therefore, be sure to listen over the lateral portions and axilla regions.

- Administer oxygen via a nonrebreather mask to all multiple trauma patients. A flow rate of 12 to 15 L/min is required to keep the reservoir bag of the nonrebreather mask inflated. All multiple trauma patients must receive supplemental oxygen until a complete assessment of the oxygenation and perfusion status is completed.

- If the Glasgow Coma Scale (GCS) score is 8 or less, be sure to intubate while maintaining the pediatric patient's head in a neutral or "sniffing" position.

  - To be sure that the endotracheal tube is in the correct position you must: (1) observe for symmetrical rise and fall of the chest and (2) auscultate bilateral breath sounds. In addition you may observe for vapor in the endotracheal tube or observe the exhaled CO_2 detector for correct color change (after six manual ventilations). The mnemonic, "Yellow is mellow" confirms correct tracheal placement. However, if the child is in cardiac arrest, the color may not change on the exhaled CO_2 detector.

- Prepare for and assist with needle thoracentesis if a tension pneumothorax is present or evident, based on respiratory distress, inadequate or absent breath sounds, and/or asymmetrical chest wall movement.

- Apply an occlusive dressing taped on three sides if an open pneumothorax is present.

- Children swallow air when crying, which may impair diaphragmatic movement due to gastric distention, making it hard to ventilate the child. Consider a nasogastric tube to decrease diaphragmatic compromise.

- A full-thickness burn of the chest has the potential to impair respiratory function; anticipate escharotomy of the chest.

Circulation

- Identify, prevent, and treat shock during this portion of the primary survey.

- Control any uncontrolled external bleeding by:
  - Applying direct pressure over the bleeding site
  - Elevating the extremity
  - Applying pressure over arterial pressure points

- Establish two peripheral intravenous (IV) access sites in critically injured children
  - Obtain peripheral vascular access using the largest bore that the vessel can accommodate.
  - During pediatric resuscitation or with severe shock, establishment of intraosseous (IO) access must be initiated if peripheral vascular access cannot rapidly be achieved.[29]
  - A practical approach is to pursue IO and peripheral access simultaneously. You can use this technique in all individuals, from the preterm infant to the elderly. The preferred site for insertion is the anterior tibia, approximately two finger-breadths below the tibial tuberosity. Alternative sites include the distal femur, the medial malleolus, and the superior iliac crest.[29] You can infuse anything into the IO needle that you would infuse into a peripheral IV. Be sure that the fluid is flowing freely and that the IO needle is in the correct position by observing the posterior tibia/fibula area for extravasation of fluid.
  - If evidence of inadequate tissue perfusion is present, administer an initial 20 ml/kg fluid bolus. Repeat the bolus (up to three to four times) if

reassessment findings indicate inadequate tissue perfusion. If symptoms of shock persist after three bolus infusions of crystalloid solution, administer 10 ml/kg of warmed, packed red blood cells (type-specific or O-negative) as indicated.

- Crystalloid solutions such as lactated Ringer's or 0.9% normal saline are administered as rapidly as possible (usually over 5 to 10 minutes) using a syringe and stopcock or opening the flow rate mechanisms on the IV blood tubing and elevating the intravenous solution.
  - A pressure bag may be placed on the IV fluid bag to facilitate rapid administration.
  - If available, use a rapid infuser device as indicated. The child must be greater than 20 kg (requiring a fluid bolus of ~ 500 ml) and a 20 g or larger intravenous catheter must be in place.
  - Use "Y" tubing and normal saline when blood administration is anticipated.

- For burn victims a number of fluid administration formulas, such as Parkland, Brooke, or Caracal, are available to guide fluid resuscitation in the first 24 hours. The main concern with these formulas is that they do not differentiate between maintenance requirements and burn-related fluid losses.
  - The prescribed rate must be based on patient response. Adequacy of fluid administration is assessed by urine output, vital signs, level of consciousness, and peripheral circulation. Urine output should be greater than 0.5 to 2 ml/kg/hr. In addition, serum electrolytes, osmolarity, and albumin levels should be normal.[4]
  - Timing of the fluid resuscitation within the first 24 hours after the burn is critical to prevent shock and maintain organ function. The Parkland formula suggests that half of the first 24-hour fluid requirement be given in the first 8 hours. However a recent study reported that infusing the first half of the 24-hour fluid requirement over 4 hours instead of 8 hours demonstrated increased normalization of vital signs, increased urine output, normalization of urine specific gravity, and decreased need for ventilator support.[4]

- When venous access is secured, obtain blood samples for laboratory studies per your institution's policy.

- Prepare for and assist with emergency thoracotomy in the ED or resuscitation area. Emergency thoracotomies are rarely done for children and are associated with a dismal outcome. Patient history, patient presentation, and trauma protocol determine indications for emergency thoracotomy.

Disability

- Closed head injuries are very common in pediatric trauma due to a larger head in proportion to the rest of the body until they are 8 years of age.
- If the disability assessment indicates a decreased level of consciousness, conduct further investigation during the secondary assessment.
- Check response to the external environment using the AVPU (alert, verbal, pain, and unconscious) assessment tool.
- Check pupils for size, symmetry, and response to light. Observe motor function.
- Initiate pharmacologic therapy as ordered (i.e., dextrose, Narcan®).

Expose

- Any clothing that remains on the pediatric patient should be cut away to allow a complete assessment of all body areas. All clothing should be saved for forensic evidence, to identify the mechanism of injury or suspected injuries, or for the family. If this pediatric patient is a victim of a shooting, be sure not to cut through the area of entry or exit of the bullet.
- Warming methods must be initiated to maintain a normothermic state (radiant warmer, warmed blankets, overhead warmer, or warmed oxygen). Remember that infants and younger children are predisposed to hypothermia and take on the environmental temperature.
- In burn victims stop the burning process. Usually this is accomplished by the family or local emergency medical services. Remove all clothing and jewelry.
  - If the pediatric patient suffered a chemical burn, irrigate the wound immediately with copious fluids to limit tissue destruction.[30]
- Determine the depth and extent of the burn injury.
  - Depth of burn injury. The depth of the burn injury may not be completely determined in the emergency department. Burns that initially appear to be partial-thickness burns may be identified as full-thickness burns days after the initial injury.
    - Superficial burns involve only the dermis and are characterized by erythema, pain, a dry appearance, and blanching.
    - Partial-thickness burns are characterized by a moist appearance; blisters are usually present but may be disrupted; erythema; pain. Superficial partial-thickness burns involve the upper dermis and deep partial-thickness burns involve deeper portions of the dermis.
    - Full-thickness burns are characterized by a dry, leathery appearance; color ranging from white to brown to black; and decreased sensation to pain in the affected area.

Table 11-1 Modified Lund and Browder Chart

Burned Area	Age (years)					
	1	1 to 4	5 to 9	10 to 14	15 to 18	Adult
	Total Body Surface					
Head	19%	17%	`13%	11%	9%	7%
Neck	2	2	2	2	2	2
Anterior trunk	13	13	13	13	13	13
Posterior trunk	13	13	13	13	13	13
Right buttock	2.5	2.5	2.5	2.5	2.5	2.5
Left buttock	2.5	2.5	2.5	2.5	2.5	2.5
Genitalia	1	1	1	1	1	1
Right upper arm	4	4	4	4	4	4
Left upper arm	4	4	4	4	4	4
Right lower arm	3	3	3	3	3	3
Left lower arm	3	3	3	3	3	3
Right hand	2.5	2.5	2.5	2.5	2.5	2.5
Left hand	2.5	2.5	2.5	2.5	2.5	2.5
Right thigh	5.5	6.5	8	8.5	9	9.5
Left thigh	5.5	6.5	8	8.5	9	9.5
Right leg	5	5	5.5	6	6.5	7
Left leg	5	5	5.5	6	6.5	7
Right foot	3.5	3.5	3.5	3.5	3.5	3.5
Left foot	3.5	3.5	3.5	3.5	3.5	3.5

Adapted from the Emergency Nurses Association. (2000). Burns. In K. S. Hoyt, & B. B. Jacobs (Eds.), *Trauma nursing core course (Provider Manual)* (5th ed., pp. 207–232). Des Plaines, IL: Author.

- The extent of burn injury is expressed by the percentage of area burned in relation to total body surface area (TBSA). Several methods are available to calculate the percentage of BSA burned. Only partial- and full-thickness burns are included in the calculations.
    - Rule of Nines (see **Figure 11-1**)
    - Modified Lund and Browder Chart (see **Table 11-1**)
    - Rule of Palm. In children younger than 14 years of age, a rapid method to determine the extent of a burn injury is to use the size of the palmar surface of the child's hand (from the wrist crease to the finger crease). This area is approximately 1% of the total body surface area. Adding the number of times the child's palm would fit into the affected area will provide an estimation of the extent of the burn surface area.[4]

Secondary Assessment

Refer to Chapter 4, *Initial Assessment*, for a review of a comprehensive secondary assessment. Assessment and intervention components unique to the secondary assessment of the pediatric trauma patient are delineated in the following section.

Full Set of Vital Signs

- Palpate central and peripheral pulses and auscultate an apical pulse as a baseline rate. Compare bilateral peripheral pulses for strength and equality. There may be neurovascular compromise in an injured extremity; therefore, it is important to palpate pulses on an uninjured extremity when evaluating central perfusion.
- Auscultate an initial blood pressure. Remember that blood pressure in a pediatric patient may be normal despite significant blood loss. A noninvasive, automated blood pressure monitor must be used with caution on critically injured children. Some models are not accurate with extremely high or low blood pressures.[25]
- Obtain a temperature to monitor for hypothermia. The rectal route should be used in critically injured children unless otherwise contraindicated.

Family Presence

- Facilitate and support the family's involvement in the pediatric patient's care. Assign a staff member to remain with the family to provide explanations about procedures and to support the family while in the ED.

Give Comfort Measures

- Initiate pain control measures as soon as possible, including:
    - Use age-appropriate nonpharmacologic methods to facilitate coping and pain management (i.e., splint, elevation, ice).
    - Administer analgesics and other appropriate medications to control procedural pain and pain from injuries.
    - In addition, cover burns as quickly as possible to decrease air currents flowing across the burn area which can cause pain.

Head-to-Toe Assessment

Refer to Chapter 4, *Initial Assessment*, for a description of head-to-toe assessment.

History

- Obtain information from prehospital personnel as indicated by the injury event, using the MIVT mnemonic. This information often serves as a predictor of type and severity of injuries sustained.
    - **M**echanism and pattern of injury
        - If the mechanism of injury involved a motor vehicle crash, obtain information regarding the use of restraints, position in the vehicle, site of impact on the vehicle, vehicle speed, ejection, rollover, air bag deployment, and any fatalities in the vehicle. If the mechanism of injury is penetrating in nature, the type of object should be identified. If the mechanism of injury was a fall, the height from which the child fell is important. Falls over

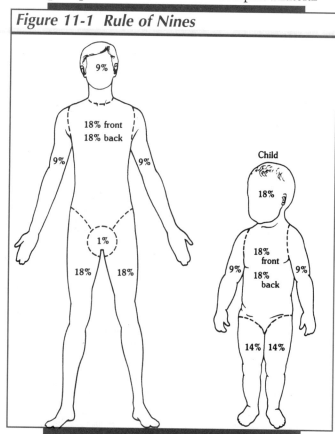

Figure 11-1 Rule of Nines

three times the child's height are significant. The history for a pediatric patient who is injured riding a bicycle should include what the bicycle collided with, was the child run over, was the child thrown from the bicycle, use of a helmet, and any damage to the vehicle. For the pediatric patient struck by a motor vehicle, obtain information regarding the speed the vehicle was traveling, was the child run over or caught under the vehicle, what type of surface did it occur on, and where was the child struck on the body. Additional history for burn victims: when, where, and how the burn injury occurred; place child was found (bedroom, closet); type of burn; duration of exposure; pattern of injury suggestive of child maltreatment

- **I**njuries suspected. Ask prehospital personnel to describe the patient's general condition, level of consciousness, and apparent injuries.
- **V**ital signs in the prehospital environment.

- **T**reatment initiated and patient responses.
  - ■ In burn victims, include measures that were taken to stop the burning process and type of dressing applied. Because of the risk of hypothermia, moist dressings must not cover greater than 10% TBSA. Dry sterile dressings or a sterile sheet must be used with burns that cover more than 10% TBSA.

- Obtain any additional history from caregiver, if available. The ENA recommends the use of the mnemonic, CIAMPEDS, to obtain additional information which is described in Chapter 4, *Initial Assessment*.
- Listen carefully to the history. It may reveal discrepancies or unlikely events to suggest nonaccidental trauma.

Additional Interventions

- Consider insertion of a gastric tube if abdominal injury is suspected, gastric distention is present, or the child has been intubated to decrease gastric distention.

Table 11-2 Pediatric Modification of the Glasgow Coma Scale (GCS) by Age of Patient

GCS Score	Pediatric modification	
EYE OPENING		
≥ 1 year	**0–1 year**	
4 Spontaneously	4 Spontaneously	
3 To verbal command	3 To shout	
2 To pain	2 To pain	
1 No response	1 No response	
BEST MOTOR RESPONSE		
≥ 1 year	**0–1 year**	
6 Obeys		
5 Localizes pain	5 Localizes pain	
4 Flexion withdrawal	4 Flexion withdrawal	
3 Flexion abnormal (decorticate)	3 Flexion abnormal (decorticate)	
2 Extension (decerebrate)	2 Extension (decerebrate)	
1 No response	1 No response	
BEST VERBAL RESPONSE		
> 5 years	**0–2 years**	**2–5 years**
5 Oriented and converses	5 Cries appropriately, smiles, coos	5 Appropriate words and phrases
4 Disoriented and converses	4 Cries	4 Inappropriate words
3 Inappropriate and converses	3 Inappropriate crying/ screaming	3 Cries/screams
2 Incomprehensible sounds	2 Grunts	2 Grunts
1 No response	1 No response	1 No response

* Score is the sum of the individual scores from eye opening, best verbal response, and best motor response, using age-specific criteria. GCS score of 13–15 indicates mild head injury, GCS score of 9–12 indicates moderate head injury, and GCS score of ≤ 8 indicates severe head injury. Reprinted with permission from Pons, P. T. (1999). Head trauma. In R. M. Barkin & P. Rosen (Eds.), *Emergency pediatrics: A guide to ambulatory care* (5th ed., pp. 412–425). St. Louis, MO: Mosby.

- Consider insertion of a urinary catheter to monitor fluid status and the effectiveness of fluid resuscitation.
- Initiate ongoing cardiac monitoring, pulse oximetry, exhaled CO_2 monitoring (with intubated patients) as soon as possible and as appropriate for the pediatric patient's condition. Pulse oximetry must be used with caution if carbon monoxide poisoning is suspected. The pulse oximeter cannot differentiate between carboxyhemoglobin and oxyhemoglobin.
- Facilitate laboratory studies if not done when initiating peripheral IVs. Blood typing is the highest priority in the critically injured patient. Consider carboxyhemoglobin and serum cyanide levels in burn victims.

Diagnostic Procedures

- Indications for laboratory and radiographic studies are determined by the pediatric patient's clinical presentation, pattern of injury, history, and specific institution protocols.

Planning/Implementation

Refer to Chapter 4, *Initial Assessment*, for a list of general interventions. Additional interventions specific to the pediatric trauma patient include the following.

- Consider the use of pneumatic antishock garment for suspected unstable pelvic fractures with shock. Inflation of the abdominal compartment may decrease respiratory excursion and result in ineffective ventilation due to increased abdominal pressure and elevation of the diaphragm.[5]

- Anticipate antidote therapy for toxic inhalants. This may include administration of 100% oxygen, hyperbaric therapy, and sodium thiosulfate for cyanide inhalation.
- Administer antibiotics as indicated, especially if open fractures are noted.
- Administer tetanus vaccine, as indicated.
- Provide psychosocial support to help the pediatric patient cope with the change in body image and fear of treatment procedures.
- Evaluate for indicators of child maltreatment.
- Calculate a pediatric GCS score which is the universal tool for rapid assessment of level of consciousness in the injured child (**Table 11-2**). A Pediatric Trauma Score should be calculated on admission to and discharge from the ED (**Table 11-3**).[31]
- Prepare for escharotomies if a full-thickness circumferential burn of the extremity is accompanied by inadequate neurovascular function.
- Contact the regional burn center for transfer as per policy or procedure (see **Table 11-4**)

Table 11-3 Pediatric Trauma Score

Category Component	+ 2	+ 1	− 1
Size	≥ 20 kg	10–20 kg	< 10 kg
Airway	Normal	Maintainable	Unmaintainable
Systolic BP†	≥ 90 mm Hg	50–90 mm Hg	< 50 mm Hg
CNS	Awake	Obtunded/LOC	Coma/decerebrate
Skeletal	None	Closed fracture	Open/multiple fractures
Cutaneous /wounds	None	Minor	Major/penetrating

If score < 8, refer to Pediatric Trauma Center.

†If proper size BP cuff is not available: + 2 = palpable pulse at wrist; + 1 = palpable pulse at groin; − 1 = no palpable pulse.

BP, blood pressure; CNS, central nervous system; LOC, loss of consciousness.

Reprinted with permission from Tepas, J. J., III, , Mollitt, D. L., Talbert, J. L., & Bryant, M. (1987). The pediatric trauma score as a predictor of injury severity in the injured child. *Journal of Pediatric Surgery, 22*(1), 14–18.

Table 11-4 American Burn Association Transfer Criteria[54]

- A burn unit may treat adults or children or both.
- Burn injuries that should be referred to a burn unit include the following:

1. Partial thickness burns greater than 10% total body surface area (TBSA).
2. Burns that involve the face, hands, feet, genitalia, perineum, or major joints.
3. Third-degree burns in any age group.
4. Electrical burns, including lightning injury.
5. Chemical burns.
6. Inhalation injury.
7. Burn injury in patients with preexisting medical disorders that could complicate management, prolong recovery, or affect mortality.
8. Any patients with burns and concomitant trauma (such as fractures) in which the burn injury poses the greatest risk of morbidity or mortality. In such cases, if the trauma poses the greater immediate risk, the patient may be initially stabilized in a trauma center before being transferred to a burn unit. Physician judgment will be necessary in such situations and should be in concert with the regional medical control plan and triage protocols.
9. Burned children in hospitals without qualified personnel or equipment for the care of children.
10. Burn injury in patient who will require special social, emotional, or long-term rehabilitative intervention.

Evaluation and Ongoing Assessment

Children involved in trauma require meticulous and frequent reassessment of airway patency, breathing effectiveness, perfusion, and mental status. Initial improvements may not be sustained and additional interventions may be needed. The pediatric patient's response to interventions and trending of the pediatric patient's condition must be closely monitored for achievement of desired outcomes. The following parameters must be monitored in the pediatric trauma patient.

- Airway patency
- Endotracheal tube placement as appropriate
- Breathing effectiveness and signs of respiratory distress
- Perfusion
- Vital signs including temperature
- Cardiac rhythm, oxygen saturation, and exhaled CO_2 as appropriate
- Pediatric coma scale or GCS as appropriate for age
- Volume of IV fluids and blood infused
- Output: Urine, gastric tube, and chest tube
- Ongoing blood loss

Selected Injuries

Assessment data and interventions specific to the pediatric patient with the particular injury being discussed are delineated in the following sections. Refer to Chapter 7, *Shock*, for specific shock management information.

Head Trauma

Head trauma (e.g., fracture of the vault, traumatic brain injury) is the most common type of pediatric trauma, occurring as a result of mechanisms associated with motor vehicle crashes, falls, assaults, and sports and recreation. Approximately 4,000 children die each year as a result of head injuries. Nearly 50% of these children die within 4 hours after injury.[32-37]

There are anatomical and physiological differences in children that increase the susceptibility to brain injury. These differences include

- The head is proportionally larger and heavier in regard to both body surface area and weight. This, along with the lack of strength in their neck muscles, places the pediatric patient at higher risk for head injury.
- In young children, the cranium is undergoing changes in thickness and elasticity. The child's brain may receive a greater insult due to the thinner and more pliable cranium.
- In young children, small changes in cerebral blood volume and/or cerebral tissue volume can result in significant insult to the brain and rapid decompensation.
- The brain is less myelinated in the infant and young child.
- Children are at greater risk for secondary brain injury due to intracranial hypertension and cerebral hyperemia (excess blood in brain). The initial increase in intracranial pressure is a result of the cerebral hyperemia, not brain edema.
- Young children can accumulate a significant percentage of their blood volume in their cranial vault and can lose relatively large amounts of blood from scalp lacerations and subgaleal hematomas and may present in hemorrhagic shock.

Specific brain injuries in pediatric patients differ by age. Infants less than 12 months of age with head trauma often sustain tears in the subcortical white matter of the temporal and frontal lobes. The white matter is not well myelinated and more susceptible to shearing injury and tears. In children under 2 years of age, there is a higher incidence of diffuse brain swelling and a lower incidence of subdural and epidural hematoma formation following head trauma. Other manifestations of head injury in pediatric patients includes impact seizures and diastatic fractures. Of all the pediatric patients seen for head injuries, approximately 5% to 15% also have associated neck injuries.[33]

With this in mind, management of pediatric patients brought to the ED with head trauma must have specific triage guidelines to provide a rapid and safe method of screening for the presence of risk of intracranial injury and management priorities set up according to the severity of the injury.

Nursing Care of the Pediatric Patient with Head Trauma

Obtaining a good history and physical exam are invaluable tools that will determine the severity of the intracranial injury and identify those at risk for secondary injury. These tools can also be useful in identifying injuries to other regions that may contribute to illness and death.

History

- Blood dyscrasia: Think hemorrhage.
- Loss of consciousness; but remember that reports may be inconsistent and hence unreliable.
- If comatose find out if sudden onset (think vascular catastrophe) or acute (ingestion of toxin).
- Temporary amnesia.
- Agitation, irritability, or listlessness.
- Inability to recognize caregivers.

- Nausea or vomiting since the injury. Many children will vomit two to three times after even a minor head injury. However, persistent vomiting and retching may be associated with other symptoms that may indicate a more severe head injury.
- Abnormal behavior for age.
- Prolonged seizure following injury. A brief seizure at the time of injury may not be clinically significant. Remember, infants do not exhibit the normal tonic/clonic movements that are noted in the older population. They may exhibit lip-smacking or bicycling movements.

Assessment

- Assess for signs of skull fracture, such as hemotympanum, periorbital ecchymosis (raccoon eyes), postauricular ecchymosis (Battle's sign), otorrhea, or rhinorrhea for presence of cerebrospinal fluid (CSF).
- Assess gait including width of base, stability, Romberg test, heel/toe/tandem for more alert, cooperative patient.
- Neurologic assessment in the secondary assessment should focus on sensorimotor deficits. Calculate a pediatric coma score or GCS as appropriate for age. Check pupillary responses and for presence of retinal hemorrhage.
- Test grip strength and equality in older children. In younger children and infants, test strength of extremity movement, withdrawal to touch, and tone assessment (resistance to passive movements).
- If the pediatric patient is comatose, additional assessment of reflexes associated with selected cranial nerves may indicate the integrity of brain stem function (see Appendix A).
- Assess for evidence of neurological deficit and signs of increased intracranial pressure (ICP). Remember that the Monro-Kellie doctrine states that an increase in the volume of one intracranial compartment (blood, brain, CSF) must be accompanied by a decrease in one or more of the other compartments if intracranial pressure is to remain unchanged. The CSF and cerebral blood volume are the two compartments best able to be manipulated to buffer changes in increased intracranial volume. Cerebral perfusion pressure (CPP) is the difference between the pressure of blood going to the brain (the mean arterial pressure or MAP) and the back pressure to this flow (the ICP). Thus: CPP = MAP – ICP.
- A normal ICP is 10 to 15 mm Hg or less. ICP will increase with agitation, coughing, and so on, but should rapidly return to baseline. Patients with sustained increases in ICP should be treated in a stepwise fashion to try to decrease their ICP, with the least

invasive means possible being employed first. Maintaining an adequate CPP is probably more important than keeping the ICP value normal. Our goal should be to maintain cerebral perfusion pressure at 50 to 70mm Hg.[32-37]

Signs and symptoms of increased intracranial pressure

- Decreased or altered level of consciousness
- Bradycardia
- Widened pulse pressure
- Pupil dilation with sluggish or absent reaction to light
- Bulging anterior fontanel in infants with an open fontanel
- Vomiting
- Slurred speech
- Sensorimotor deficits
- Posturing
- Seizures
- Inability to track objects
- Ataxia while sitting, crawling, standing, or walking

Additional Interventions

If Neurologic Deficit Present

- Elevation of the head of the bed 15 to 30 degrees and keeping the head midline may enhance cerebral venous drainage (**Figure 11-2**). Maintain spinal stabilization until all radiographs are obtained and cleared.
- Trend neurologic status and vital signs for signs of increases in ICP.
- Ensure adequate oxygenation and maintain blood pressure to enhance optimal outcome.
- Prepare for intubation and ventilation with 100% oxygen if pediatric GCS is eight or less. Pediatric patients who are unconscious or have signs of increased ICP must be intubated. Both hypoxia and

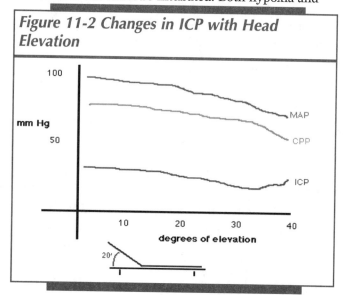

Figure 11-2 Changes in ICP with Head Elevation

hypercarbia have potent vasodilatory effects on the cerebral vasculature, resulting in an increased cerebral blood flow and, therefore, an increased ICP. Hyperventilation causes cerebral vasoconstriction and decreases the ICP. Ventilate the pediatric patient to keep the PaCO$_2$ at approximately 30–35 mm Hg.[32] Rapid sequence intubation (RSI) must be considered if the pediatric patient is awake, responsive to stimuli, or may gag during the intubation procedure. The medications used for RSI must be selected based on potential effects on ICP—avoid medications known to increase ICP. Prophylactic hyperventilation is no longer routinely employed; however, moderate hyperventilation (PCO$_2$ ~ 30 to 35 mm Hg) may be used for suspected increase ICP in the field or prior to computerized tomography (CT) scanning.

- Pediatric patients that are agitated or are possibly in pain should be sedated. Sedation can be accomplished by using Fentanyl at 1 to 3 mcg/kg every hour as needed as well as using Versed® at 0.1 to 0.2 mg/kg IV. Additional sedation and/or analgesia should be considered before suctioning, patient transfer, or procedures. In addition lidocaine 1 to 2 mg/kg IV before suctioning may blunt the increased ICP associated with this intervention. Refer to Chapter 17, *Procedural Preparation and Sedation*, for additional information.

- Administer osmotic and/or loop diuretics (e.g., mannitol or furosemide) as ordered to deplete water from the intracellular and interstitial compartments, ultimately resulting in a decrease in cerebral fluid volume and a decrease in ICP. Mannitol 0.25 Gm/kg is administered via a rapid IV push over ~ 5 minutes. Maintain euvolemia.

- Maintain normal body temperature. Hyperthermia and seizures cause elevations in ICP and should be anticipated, prevented if possible, and treated aggressively. Although anticonvulsants are not routine prophylaxis for all pediatric patients with a traumatic brain injury, pediatric patients with significant brain injury or mechanism of injury may be treated with Dilantin® prophylactically for 5 to 10 days.

- Avoid hyper- or hypoglycemia.

- Steroids are not indicated in the management of traumatic brain injury; however, they may have a role in the management of edema surrounding a brain tumor. In addition, steroids have shown to be of benefit in spinal cord injury.

If Neurologic Deficit Absent

- Observe for any changes in level of consciousness.
- Provide "head injury" discharge instructions to the caregiver.

Skull Fractures

Linear and Depressed Skull Fractures

A linear skull fracture can be described as a nondepressed fracture in any of the bones of the skull. Most children are asymptomatic except for swelling and tenderness over the site. This type of fracture usually heals spontaneously within two to three months and requires few interventions. Linear fractures associated with serious sequelae include[30-35]

- Fractures across the branches of the middle meningeal artery
- Occipital bone fractures that extend into the foramen magnum
- Basilar skull fractures

A depressed skull fracture is often associated with a significant direct force from a solid heavy object causing bony fragments to be displaced inward and toward the brain. Depressed skull fracture fragments may require surgical elevation if the depression depth is significant or if fragments pose a threat to underlying cerebral tissue and vasculature.

Signs and Symptoms

Signs and symptoms depend on the underlying injuries sustained from the blow.

- Fracture may or may not be palpable; a depression may be palpable with a depressed skull fracture
- Pain and tenderness over the fracture site when palpated
- Cephalohematoma over the fracture site
- Scalp laceration

Basilar Skull Fracture

A basilar skull fracture is a fracture of any bone that comprises the base of the skull: frontal, ethmoid, sphenoid, temporal, or occipital bones. A fracture of these bones creates a potential for infection and CSF leak, due to the potential for tears in the dura.

Signs and Symptoms

- Headache
- Decreased level of consciousness
- Otorrhea – if present suspect a CSF leak. Test the fluid by using a chemical reagent strip. If glucose is present, the drainage is CSF. Another indication of CSF in bloody drainage is the halo sign, in which CSF drainage on linen or gauze forms a dark inner ring and a light outer ring.
- Rhinorrhea
- Hemotympanum
- Unilateral hearing loss

- Battle's sign—hemorrhage in the posterior auricular area; may occur up to 24 hours after injury
- Raccoon eyes—orbital hemorrhage; may occur hours after injury
- Hypotension, tachycardia, or respiratory irregularity

Additional Interventions

If CSF drainage occurs, do not pack the ears or nose. Apply a nonocclusive sterile dry dressing below the draining nose and/or ear.

Cerebral Tissue Injury

Concussion

A concussion is a closed head injury usually associated with a blow to the head or rapid deceleration resulting in transient neurologic changes. Although symptoms are usually minor, permanent neurologic sequelae, often related to cognitive ability, may occur.

Signs and Symptoms
- Nausea or vomiting
- Headache, dizziness
- Brief loss of consciousness

Diffuse Axonal Injury (DAI)

Damage to the nerve axon can result from acceleration or deceleration forces that shear or stress the axon. This results in diffuse, microscopic, hemorrhagic lesions. Prolonged coma may result due to involvement of the brain stem and reticular activating system. The diagnosis of DAI may be delayed for several days. A magnetic resonance image (MRI) scan is used to confirm the diagnosis. The outcome varies ranging from minimal sequelae to permanent lifelong disability or death.

Signs and Symptoms
- Immediate unconsciousness that may last as long as several weeks to months
- Elevated blood pressure
- Excessive sweating due to autonomic dysfunction
- Abnormal posturing

Contusion

A contusion is a bruising of the brain tissue characterized by areas of hemorrhage and edema, commonly caused by a direct blow to the head. Areas of hemorrhage at the site of impact are referred to as a coup injury; contusions at sites opposite or distant from the site of impact are referred to as contrecoup injuries (**Figure 11-3**).

Signs and Symptoms

In addition to those listed for concussion, the pediatric patient may exhibit

- Transient or permanent neurological deficits
- Transient retrograde and/or antegrade amnesia

Intracranial Hemorrhage

Intracranial hemorrhages are uncommon in infants and young children, but may occur as a result of a fall, a direct blow to the head, or violent shaking. **Table 11-5** and **Figure 11-4** compares the various types of intracranial hemorrhages.

Dental Trauma

Fracture or Avulsion of a Tooth

Children may present with fractured or missing teeth due to a fall, sports injury, bicycle crash, or motor vehicle crash. The tooth may be in place but broken or it may be avulsed from the socket. In certain situations, a permanent tooth may be replanted. Primary teeth are generally not replanted due to the risk of damage to the permanent tooth bud. To insure optimal results, treatment of the avulsed tooth should begin within 30 minutes of the avulsion.

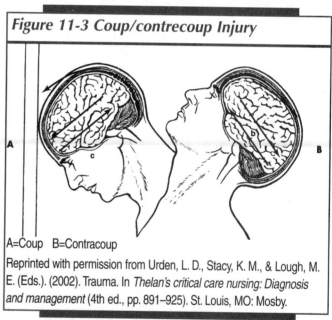

Figure 11-3 Coup/contrecoup Injury

A=Coup   B=Contracoup

Reprinted with permission from Urden, L. D., Stacy, K. M., & Lough, M. E. (Eds.). (2002). Trauma. In *Thelan's critical care nursing: Diagnosis and management* (4th ed., pp. 891–925). St. Louis, MO: Mosby.

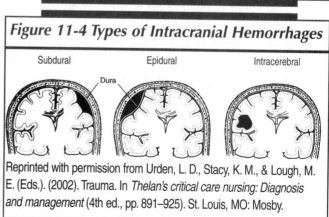

Figure 11-4 Types of Intracranial Hemorrhages

Subdural   Epidural   Intracerebral

Dura

Reprinted with permission from Urden, L. D., Stacy, K. M., & Lough, M. E. (Eds.). (2002). Trauma. In *Thelan's critical care nursing: Diagnosis and management* (4th ed., pp. 891–925). St. Louis, MO: Mosby.

Signs and Symptoms

- Jagged or broken tooth, loose or missing tooth
- Sensitivity to cold or fluids
- Bleeding
- Soft tissue lacerations, especially of the lower lip and tongue

Diagnostic Tests

- Panorex® film
- Mandible and maxilla films

Additional Interventions

- Assess airway patency as the tooth or tooth fragment may be aspirated and cause airway compromise.
- A fractured permanent tooth with pulp exposed or deeper dentin involvement is a dental emergency. Refer for immediate dental care.
- Procedure for handling an avulsed tooth
  - Find the permanent tooth.
  - Gently rinse the tooth with water or saline; do not scrub the crown or root.
  - Insert the tooth into the socket or place the tooth in milk until replantation.
  - Immediately refer to or contact a dentist or oral surgeon. If the consulting physician is coming to the ED, obtain the necessary supplies to replant the tooth.

Vertebral or Spinal Cord Trauma

Approximately 1,000 children sustain injury to the spinal cord each year, and many more sustain injury to the vertebral column.[38,39] Therefore, cervical spine injury must be presumed to be present until proven otherwise. The cervical spine of a child is less protected than the adult cervical spine for a variety of reasons. These differences include

- Children have relatively weak muscles of the neck.
- Neck ligaments are more lax.
- Facets of the upper cervical spine are flatter.
- Vertebral bodies are wedged anteriorly; they also have a tendency to slide forward with flexion.

The level at which spinal injuries occur varies with age. In children who are less than 8 years of age, injuries are more common to the upper cervical region (C-1 to C-3), whereas older children and adults more commonly have injuries of the lower cervical region. A phenomenon known as spinal cord injury without radiographic abnormality (SCIWORA) is unique among children due to the relative elasticity of a child's spine and supporting ligaments. Traumatic forces of hyperextension, flexion, and traction may cause SCIWORA. The clinical exam is the hallmark of this syndrome with documentation of neurologic deficit that may have changed or resolved by the time the child has arrived in the ED along with the absence of neck pain.[38-40] Although the overall prognosis for children with this injury directly relates to the severity of the spinal cord injury, long-term morbidity is common if it is left undiagnosed and reinjury to the area occurs.[38-40] Prognosis for functional recovery is considered to be poor.[38-40] It is important to remember that pediatric patients may sustain spinal cord injury without an associated vertebral fracture. The use of MRI has enhanced the diagnosis of spinal cord injury not detected on radiographs or other imaging studies.[38-40]

Interventions

The administration of methylprednisolone is indicated in the acutely injured pediatric patient with a spinal cord injury. The dosing schedule is the same as for an adult: 30 mg/kg IV over 15 minutes, followed by 5.4 mg/kg for the next 24 to 48 hours.[40]

Table 11-5 Types of Intracranial Hemorrhages

	Epidural Hematoma	Subdural Hematoma	Subarachnoid Hemorrhage
Definition	• Disruption of middle meningeal artery • Blood collects between skull and dura mater • Blunt trauma	• Venous bleeding • Blood collects between dura mater and arachnoid mater • May be caused by violent shaking • Consider child maltreatment or shaken impact syndrome	• Arterial disruption • Blood collects between arachnoid mater and pia mater • Frequently a result of child maltreatment
Signs and Symptoms	• Initial loss of consciousness, followed by transient consciousness, leading to unconsciousness • Ipsilateral pupil dilation • Contralateral paresis or paralysis	• Rapid deterioration in level of consciousness	• Stiff neck • Headache • Seizures • Irritability

Injuries of the Lumbar Spine Associated with Safety Restraints

Frontal impact motor vehicle crashes accompanied by rapid deceleration forces can cause midlumbar (flexion-distraction or Chance) vertebral fractures in children who wear lap safety restraints inappropriately. Children tend to wear the safety restraint around the abdomen versus the pelvis. Injuries usually occur between the second and fourth lumbar vertebrae. External abrasions across the lower abdomen are important clues to the injury.

Signs and Symptoms of Spinal Cord Injury
- Spinal deformity
- Neck pain
- Injuries to neck, face, head, and/or back
- Flaccid extremities
- Altered sensation in extremities and/or trunk
- Incontinence or absence of sphincter tone
- Abnormal breathing patterns, especially diaphragmatic breathing
- Bradycardia or hypotension
- Priapism

Interventions
- Maintain full spinal stabilization.
- Obtain immediate neurological consultation.
- Administer methylprednisolone, as indicated.

Cardiothoracic Trauma

Significant cardiothoracic trauma rarely occurs alone and is often a component of major multisystem injury. Cardiothoracic trauma in children can be caused either by blunt or penetrating mechanisms. Blunt trauma is more common and can often result in occult injuries to underlying structures. The presence of rib fractures in young children may indicate significant underlying injury. The ribs remain cartilaginous and pliable along with mediastinal mobility in children until approximately 8 years of age. A significant force may cause injury to underlying structures without concomitant rib fractures or external signs of trauma. Pulmonary contusions and pneumothoraces are frequently seen even though no rib fractures are present.[41] Penetrating injuries are not as common in children, but they may occur as a result of knives, firearms, and high-velocity mechanisms.

Nursing Care of the Pediatric Patient with Cardiothoracic Trauma

History
- Cardiothoracic trauma must be suspected in the child who has sustained the following mechanisms of injury.
  - Rapid deceleration incidents, such as motor vehicle crashes
  - High-velocity impact incidents, such as auto versus pedestrian crashes
  - Incidents involving firearms or any penetrating wound to the chest, neck, or abdomen
  - Significant fall or blow to the chest
- Chest pain

Assessment
- Presence of respiratory distress or increased work of breathing
- Tachypnea
- Agitation
- Physical signs of trauma such as tire marks, bruising, or open wounds (i.e., open pneumothorax)
- Paradoxical chest wall movement with breathing, decreased breath sounds, or decreases in oxygen saturation
- Distended neck veins. This symptom is associated with either a tension pneumothorax or pericardial tamponade. This may be difficult to evaluate in infants and small children due to their short, fat necks.
- Deviation of the trachea. Assess for tracheal deviation by palpating the trachea just above the suprasternal notch. It may be difficult to appreciate in infants and small children. In young children, a tension pneumothorax may be present without tracheal deviation.
- Percuss for hyperresonance or dullness to percussion; hyperresonance indicates air in the pleural space (e.g., pneumothorax), dullness indicates blood in the pleural space (e.g., hemothorax).

Pneumothorax

A simple pneumothorax is one of the most common forms of pediatric chest trauma and may result from a blunt or penetrating injury. It occurs when air accumulates in the pleural space. The severity of the signs and symptoms is dependent on the percentage of lung collapsed. Children with a small pneumothorax may be asymptomatic.

An open pneumothorax occurs when there is a loss in chest wall integrity and air enters the pleural space both through the wound and the trachea. This is most often associated with penetrating trauma. An open pneumothorax is easily recognized by the "sucking" heard with inspiration and the "bubbling" sound with expiration.

A tension pneumothorax develops when air enters the pleural space on inspiration but cannot escape on expiration. The intrathoracic pressure rises, causing collapse of the lung on the side of the injury and a mediastinal shift of the heart, great vessels, and trachea. When enough air accumulates, the unaffected lung collapses. Venous return is impeded, cardiac output falls, and hypotension results. Because of its impairment to the pediatric patient's ventilation and circulation, this injury can be classified as life threatening.

Signs and Symptoms

- Varying degrees of respiratory distress/increased work of breathing
- Diminished or absent breath sounds on the injured side. Auscultate the axilla areas along with the anterior and posterior lung fields. Because the chest wall of an infant or young child is so thin, breath sounds can be easily referred from other areas of the lung. As a result, decreased breath sounds may not necessarily be heard over involved areas of the lung; instead, a difference in the quality or pitch of the breath sounds over an area of pneumothorax may be noted.[39]
- Tachypnea and/or tachycardia
- Pale or cyanotic skin
- Asymmetrical chest expansion
- Hyperresonance to percussion
- In the event of a tension pneumothorax, the child may develop
  - Severe respiratory distress
  - Diminished or absent breath sounds on the affected side
  - Faint peripheral pulses
  - Signs of shock and hypotension (Remember hypotension is a late sign.)
  - Distended neck veins and tracheal deviation (also a late sign)
  - Bradycardia and altered level of consciousness
  - Agitation
  - Shift in the point of maximum impulse (PMI). Usually located at the left nipple line, but if the PMI is shifted laterally, it may indicate a right tension pneumothorax. If the PMI is shifted medially, it may indicate a left tension pneumothorax.

Additional Interventions

- If a tension pneumothorax is suspected, immediately prepare for or perform a needle decompression, which involves placing an IV or vascular catheter over the third rib into the second intercostal space, midclavicular line. This will relieve the pressure on the heart and lung. This pediatric patient will require insertion of a chest tube as soon as possible following needle decompression.
- Prepare for chest tube insertion to evacuate the air or blood from the pleural space. A pediatric chest drainage system provides a more accurate measurement of smaller fluid volumes.
- If an open pneumothorax is present, apply a nonporous dressing taped on three sides. Monitor for the development of a tension pneumothorax.

Pulmonary Contusion

A pulmonary contusion is a bruise of the lung tissue resulting in alveolar capillary damage. Interstitial and alveolar edema and hemorrhage decrease lung compliance and impair transport of oxygen and carbon dioxide. A pulmonary contusion is identified on a chest radiograph by consolidation and pulmonary infiltrates.

Signs and Symptoms

- Respiratory distress or tachypnea
- Localized rales or wheezes or decreased breath sounds
- Hemoptysis
- Hypoxemia
- Suspect in any child with a chest injury, especially if bruising on the chest is noted.

Additional Interventions

- Prepare for intubation and assisted ventilation if the contusion is severe; obtain the necessary intubation equipment and supplies.
- If the child is not in shock, restrict intravenous fluids. Overhydration during fluid resuscitation can extend the area of contusion.[39]
- If there is no cervical spine injury, elevate the head of the bed to a level of comfort.
- Administer high-flow oxygen.

Hemothorax

A hemothorax occurs when blood accumulates in the pleural space, eventually leading to collapse of the affected lung. In the adult patient, only 25 % of hemothoraces are large enough to produce shock. Children have a smaller circulating blood volume and the accumulation of smaller amounts of blood may be significant enough to produce signs of hypovolemic shock and respiratory distress. In addition, children can lose up to 40 % of their circulating blood volume into the pleural space.

Signs and Symptoms

- Signs of shock with mediastinal shifting
- Cyanosis
- Dyspnea, tachypnea, and/or ventilatory compromise
- Decreased chest wall movement
- Diminished or absent breath sounds on the injured side
- Dullness to percussion on the injured side

Additional Interventions

- Prepare for chest tube insertion.
- Ensure fluid resuscitation is initiated prior to chest tube insertion.
- Administer blood as indicated.

Myocardial Contusion

A myocardial contusion is a bruise of the myocardium caused by blunt trauma. Damage may range from mild muscular ecchymosis to infarction. The diagnosis is often difficult because of concurrent injury to the respiratory system and/or the presence of shock.

Signs and Symptoms

- Chest pain
- ECG abnormalities ranging from dysrhythmias (e.g., premature ventricular contractions) to ST and T wave changes. Dysrhythmia may be transient.
- Chest wall ecchymosis
- Signs of decreased cardiac output

Additional Interventions

- Cardiac monitoring for dysrhythmia.
- Perform 12-lead electrocardiogram.
- Administer antidysrhythmic medications as ordered.

Pericardial Tamponade

Pericardial tamponade is a collection of blood in the pericardial sac. This life-threatening cardiac injury most frequently occurs with penetrating injury but can occur with blunt trauma as well. As blood accumulates in the noncompliant sac, it exerts pressure on the heart and inhibits ventricular filling. Impairment of cardiac function is related to the rate and amount of fluid accumulation in the pericardial sac.

Signs and Symptoms

- Dyspnea
- Poor peripheral perfusion
- Cyanosis
- Penetrating chest wound, left-sided rib fractures, ecchymosis of the chest wall
- Signs of shock with hypotension with a narrow pulse pressure despite vigorous fluid resuscitation
- Distended neck veins and/or muffled heart tones
- Dysrhythmia (i.e., bradycardia, pulseless electrical activity, asystole)

Additional Interventions

- Prepare for pericardiocentesis if tamponade is suspected. This is a life-threatening event, so it must be treated immediately. Obtain a large spinal needle and attach a 30 cc syringe. The physician will insert this needle into the left subxiphoid area. Be sure to have the cardiac monitor running and observe for any ventricular dysrhythmias. Blood obtained from the pericardial sac should not coagulate.
- Prepare for possible ED pericardial window or thoracotomy.
- Prepare for operative intervention to identify the source of bleeding.

Abdominal Trauma

Abdominal trauma in children is related to a variety of causes, including sports, recreational activities, motor vehicle crashes, and bicycle crashes. Children who sustain any blunt trauma to the abdomen shortly after eating are at a greater risk for injury. There are many physiologic characteristics that increase the child's risk for developing injuries related to abdominal trauma. These include

- The abdominal muscles are thinner, weaker, and less developed than those of an adult.
- The chest wall is more pliable and does not provide as much protection to abdominal organs.
- The duodenum has an increased vascular blood supply, resulting in larger amounts of blood loss when traumatized.
- The liver, spleen, and kidneys are less protected by the ribs and overlying muscle and fat, which makes them more easily injured.

Nursing Care of the Pediatric Patient with Abdominal Trauma

History

- History of abdominal pain or tenderness
- History of nausea or vomiting
- Last intake of food or liquid
- Mechanism of injury (e.g., bicycle handlebars, motor vehicle crash with only lap safety restraint)

Assessment

- Location, quality, and radiation of abdominal pain
  - Pain and apprehension may cause children to tighten their abdominal muscles, making an adequate physical assessment difficult.
- Respiratory pattern and depth
  - Children are abdominal breathers. Therefore, abdominal pain such as that caused by peritoneal irritation may alter the breathing pattern.
  - Children with intraabdominal bleeding often exhibit an expiratory grunt.

- Rigidity, guarding, and abdominal distention (peritoneal signs)
- Evidence of external soft tissue injury (e.g., safety restraint marks)
- Bloody urinary drainage

Interventions

- If open abdominal wounds are present, cover with a sterile dressing moistened with sterile saline. Do not attempt to push abdominal contents back into the abdominal cavity.
- Consider use of the Focused Abdominal Sonography for Trauma (F.A.S.T.) exam. This procedure is becoming a resource in the diagnosis of free fluid in the abdomen.[42-46,50] However, CT is still being utilized for definitive diagnosis by most pediatric emergency attendings.[43]
- Prepare the pediatric patient for surgery. Pediatric patients with solid organ injury resulting in hemodynamic instability and unresponsive to fluid resuscitation may require operative intervention.

Splenic Injuries

Trauma of the spleen is often caused by a blunt impact sustained from a sports activity or a fall from a bicycle. Splenic injuries are associated with trauma to the left upper quadrant of the abdomen or left lower chest. Surgical management of splenic trauma is more conservative, with nonoperative management being the more common approach because of the risk of overwhelming sepsis following splenectomy.[51,52]

Signs and Symptoms

- Pain in the left upper quadrant of the abdomen that may radiate to the left shoulder
- Hypoactive or absent bowel sounds
- Dullness to percussion
- Signs of shock

Liver Laceration

Laceration of the liver is a major cause of morbidity and mortality in children with abdominal trauma.[41-46] Management varies, with isolated liver injuries responding well to a nonoperative approach. The use of the FAST exam can also be of benefit with this type of injury, although CT is still being utilized for definitive diagnosis by most pediatric emergency attendings.[41-46]

Signs and Symptoms

- Abrasions or contusions to the right upper quadrant of the abdomen or right lower chest
- Abdominal distention

- Right-sided rib fractures
- Guarding, tenderness, or rigidity to palpation
- Signs of shock
- Dullness to percussion

Safety Restraint-related Injuries

The possibility of thoracolumbar spine and abdominal injuries has been associated with the use of safety restraints in motor vehicle crashes with a significant impact. Although the number of reported injuries related to safety restraint use is low, there have been cases reported of concomitant spinal and abdominal injuries (duodenal and pancreatic injuries) in young children who were restrained using a lap safety restraint with or without a shoulder harness.

Signs and Symptoms

- Positive "safety belt sign": an area of ecchymosis correlating with the position of the safety restraint across the abdomen
- Back pain correlating to a lumbar fracture
- Possible sensorimotor deficits
- Peritoneal signs (rigidity, guarding, tenderness, and pain) related to hollow organ injury
- Fever may be present if presentation is delayed
- Rapid rise in amylase is suggestive of pancreatic trauma or perforation of the duodenum

Musculoskeletal Trauma

Approximately 30% to 45% of children seen have multiple injuries and have at least one skeletal fracture.[51] But children often sustain musculoskeletal injuries without multisystem injuries. These injuries are frequently related to sports and recreational activities, and they occur more often as a child's environment expands to include bicycles, skateboards, snowboards, trampolines, and automobiles.

Children may sustain a fracture, sprain, subluxation, or dislocation of a joint. Subluxations occur in children as a result of a sudden, forceful, longitudinal pull on extremity. The most common subluxation is known as "nursemaid's elbow," or dislocation of the radial head. The history is consistent with a sudden longitudinal pulling force on the extremity, such as a small child being pulled up by an extended arm.

Nursing Care of the Pediatric Patient with Musculoskeletal Trauma

History

- Mechanism of injury
- Treatment or splinting done prior to arrival

- History of previous orthopedic problems
- History of nonaccidental trauma

Assessment
- Deformity, shortness, or rotation of the affected extremity
- Edema or soft tissue injury (i.e., lacerations or contusions)
- Tenderness on palpation
- Reluctance or refusal to move or use an extremity
- Neurovascular status—assess for presence of the "5 Ps":
  - Pallor: Are the nailbeds and skin pink? Does blanching occur with pressure? Is the capillary refill less than 2 seconds?
  - Pain: Many children hesitate to complain of pain because they might have been injured while disobeying their caregivers.
  - Pulselessness: Are the peripheral pulses distal to the injury present, strong, and equal?
  - Paresthesia: What is the sensory status of the affected area and the area distal to the injury?
  - Paralysis: Can the child spontaneously move the injured extremity?

Interventions

Implement measures to provide optimal tissue perfusion. Always compare the peripheral circulation of the affected extremity to the unaffected extremity. What may appear to be impaired circulation in one extremity may actually be present in both extremities and throughout the body, indicating systemic circulatory problems such as hypovolemia.

- Evaluate peripheral circulation. If impaired, check the alignment of the extremity, assess the patient's hemodynamic status, and notify the physician. Proper alignment may be needed to restore adequate circulation to the affected extremity.
- Immobilize the injured extremity, including the joints above and below the site of injury, to avoid further injury or pain. This can be accomplished using
  - Rigid intravenous boards
  - Metal or plastic splints
  - Plaster or fiberglass splints
- Assess and document the neurovascular status of the affected extremity before and after stabilization.
- Obtain comparison view x-rays as warranted.

Fractures

Fractures are common in children, and the prognosis for healing is usually excellent. One of the more com-

mon types of fractures in children is the greenstick fracture, which is an incomplete fracture through the bone with a portion of the cortex and periosteum remaining intact. This type of fracture is common in very young children because their bones can sustain a larger amount of buckling and bending. Fractures are not always readily seen in the younger population, making it more difficult to diagnosis the fracture. Problems with healing and future bone growth can occur if the fracture extends through or involves the epiphyseal (growth) plate (**Figure 11-5**).

Signs and Symptoms
- Obvious angulation of the extremity
- If the fracture extends completely across the bone, shortening of the extremity may occur.
- Femur fractures may also have external rotation in addition to shortening.
- Signs of shock

Additional Interventions
- Prepare for possible closed reduction with conscious sedation.
- Fluid replacement if femur or hip are involved.
- Discharge teaching
  - If crutches are given, instruct the child on walking techniques, and assess the return demonstration for correct use.
  - If splints are applied, instruct the caregiver on the signs and symptoms of neurovascular compromise. If appropriate, teach the caregiver how to loosen and reapply the bandages or splints.

Figure 11-5 Types of Epiphyseal Injuries

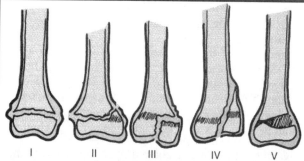

type I, separation or slip of growth plate without fracture of the bone; type II, separation of growth plate and breaking off a section of metaphysis; type III, fracture of the epiphysis extending through the joint surface; type IV, fractures of the growth plate, epiphysis, adn metaphysis; type V, crushing injury of epiphysis

Reprinted with permission from Hockenberry, M. J., Wilson, D., Winkelstein, M. L., & Kline, N. E. (2003). The child with musculoskeletal or articular dysfunction. In *Wong's nursing care of infants and children* (7th ed., pp. 1757-1831). St. Louis, MO: Mosby.

- Instruct the caregivers and pediatric patient to avoid putting sharp objects inside the cast or splint to relieve itching.

If pain continues or increases beyond 48 hours past the injury, the pediatric patient must be reexamined.

Amputations

Fingertip amputations are often caused by a closing door and are one of the most common amputations in children. Many amputated extremities can be successfully replanted if the elapsed time from injury to surgery is minimal. Most successful reattachments are guillotine-type amputations–a clean and complete severing of the tissue. Amputations caused by a crushing force are more difficult to replant. Curiosity, lack of coordination, and an inherent lack of understanding of danger predispose children to this type of injury.

Signs and Symptoms
- Partial to complete loss of a limb, hand, foot, finger, or toe
- Profuse hemorrhage from the limb if vessels are not completely transected
- Exposed tissue or bone (bones may be fractured)

Additional Interventions
- If profuse active bleeding is present, elevate the extremity and apply a pressure dressing.
- When bleeding is controlled, apply a sterile nonadhering dressing to the stump and wrap with sterile gauze. Once the area is covered, it will decrease the anxiety of the pediatric patient and parent.
- Care of the amputated part[48]
  - Gently rinse (avoid scrubbing) the part with sterile saline to remove gross dirt.
  - Wrap the part in gauze slightly moistened with sterile saline, and place the part in a sealable plastic bag.
  - After sealing the bag, place the bag on ice for transport to surgery or the closest replantation center. Remember to label the container.
  - If radiographs are done, include the part(s) and the stump.

Inhalation Injuries

Upper airway burns are often associated with facial burns and inhalation of hot gases. Edema produces rapid narrowing and obstruction of the airway. It is important to remember that children are very vulnerable to rapid occlusion of the airway because of their smaller airways and increased proportion of soft tissue.

Signs and Symptoms
- Carbonaceous sputum
- Singed nasal hair or eyebrows
- Mucosal redness
- Tachypnea or alteration in respiratory effort
- Tachycardia associated with inhaled toxin
- Hoarseness, cough, or hoarse cry
- Decreased ability to handle secretions or swallow
- Facial burns and swelling
- Wheezing, crackles, rhonchi, or stridor
- Oral or facial burns

Additional Interventions
- Determine the need for intubation based on the pediatric patient's level of consciousness, ability to protect airway, and oxygenation.
- Prepare for and assist with fiberoptic bronchoscopy to assess the degree of inhalation injury.

Health Promotion

Prevention measures have an impact on trauma-related morbidity and mortality. Current recommendations include
- Establish laws that prohibit children from riding in the cargo areas of pickup trucks.[49]
- Promote no extra seat or no extra rider on farm equipment ("Farm Safety for Kids").
- Develop community-based education and legislation to promote the use of bicycle helmets by all children as well as adults; educate caregivers and children on the importance of wearing bicycle helmets; and encourage state and local governments to pass legislation requiring helmet use by all bicyclists and mandating bicycle rental agencies to include helmets as part of the rental contract.
- Develop programs that support decreased availability of alcohol and drugs to young people.
- Increase enforcement of existing alcohol and drug use laws.
- Upgrade safety restraint and child passenger safety laws.
- Educate caregivers on firearm safety.
- Educate caregivers and children on the importance of wearing helmets when skiing or snowboarding. Encourage resorts and rental agencies to include helmets as part of the rental contract.
- Encourage state governments to ban the manufacturing and sale of mobile baby walkers and support efforts to redesign them. Educate caregivers on the

hazards of mobile baby walkers. Develop liaisons with other organizations (e.g., National Safe Kids Campaign®, American Academy of Pediatrics) to discourage the manufacture and sale of mobile baby walkers.

- Encourage the use of helmets, lightweight balls, and proper instruction for soccer players.
- Educate caregivers on the importance of installing smoke and carbon monoxide detectors in the home and setting water heaters at a safe temperature.
- Educate caregivers and children about fire safety and what to do in case of a fire (i.e., stop, drop, and roll).
- Identify appropriate prevention strategies for children with special needs (i.e., evaluating the status of the cervical spine of the child with Down syndrome prior to sports activities).

Injury prevention must include education, enforcement, and environmental interventions. Other suggested areas for injury prevention are listed in **Table 11-6**.

Summary

Care of the pediatric trauma patient requires a coordinated effort from the trauma team and the family. Collaboration by the multidisciplinary team facilitates optimal patient care and integrates the resources that are needed to care for the pediatric trauma patient. This is especially true when caring for pediatric burn patients who will need specialized acute and long-term care. Knowledge of normal growth and development, anatomy, mechanisms of injury, responses to injury (physiologic and psychosocial) are the foundations of providing trauma nursing care of the pediatric patient. Following a systematic approach to assessment and intervention contributes to positive patient outcomes through early identification of injuries and recognition of life-threatening conditions. Incorporating the family throughout the care process is important in meeting the psychosocial and emotional needs of the patient and his or her family.

References

1. Salomone, J. A., & Salomone, J. P. (2003). *Abdominal trauma, blunt*. Retrieved June 19, 2003 from http://www.emedicine.com/emerg/topic1.htm
2. Reinberg, O., Reinberg, A., Tehard, B., & Mechkouri, M. (2002). Accidents in children do not happen at random: Predictable time-of-day incidence of childhood trauma. *Chronobiology International, 19*(3), 615–631.
3. National Safe Kids Campaign. (2000). *Injury facts: Fire injury (residential)*. Retrieved January 12, 2004 from http://www.safekids.org/tier3_cd.cfm?folder_id = 540 &content_item_id = 1130
4. Perry, C. (2003). Thermal injuries. In P. A. Moloney-Harmon, & S. J. Czerwinski (Eds.), *Nursing care of the pediatric trauma patient* (pp. 277–294). Philadelphia: Saunders.
5. Emergency Nurses Association. (2000). Pediatric trauma. In B. B. Jacobs & K. S. Hoyt (Eds.), *Trauma nursing core course (Provider manual)* (5th ed., pp. 249–264). Des Plaines, IL: Author.
6. Nagel, T. R., & Schunk, J. E. (1997). Using the hand to estimate the surface area of a burn in children. *Pediatric Emergency Care, 13,* 254–284.
7. Howard, A. W. (2002). Automobile restraints for children: A review for clinicians. *Canadian Medical Association Journal, 167*(7), 769–773.
8. Winston, F. K., Durbin, D. R., Kallan, M. J., & Moll, E. K. (2000). The danger of premature graduation to seat belts for young children. *Pediatrics, 105*(6), 1179–1183.
9. Braver, E. R., Whitfield, R., & Ferguson, S. A. (1998). Seating positions and children's risk of dying in motor vehicle crashes. *Injury Prevention, 4*(3), 181–187.
10. National Highway Traffic Safety Administration. (n.d.). *Child passenger safety*. Retrieved June 19, 2003 from http://www.nhtsa.dot.gov/CPS/
11. Durbin, D. R., Arbogast, K. B., & Moll, E. K. (2001). Seat belt syndrome in children: A case report and review of the literature. *Pediatric Emergency Care, 17*(6), 474–477.
12. National Highway Traffic Safety Administration. (1999). *NHTSA issues consumer advisory on side air bags and child safety* [Press release]. Retrieved June 19, 2003 from www.nhtsa.dot.gov/nhtsa/announce/press/1999/ca10 1499.html.
13. Ziegler, M. M., & Templeton, J. M. (2000). Major trauma. In G. R. Fleisher & S. Ludwig (Eds.), *Textbook of pediatric emergency medicine* (5th ed., pp. 1089–1101). Philadelphia: Lippincott Williams & Wilkins.
14. Haley, K. & Mecham, N. L. (2003). Mechanisms of injury. In L. M. Bernardo, D. O. Thomas, & B. Herman (Eds.), *Core curriculum for pediatric emergency nursing* (pp. 401–407). Sudbury, MA: Jones & Bartlett.
15. Waddell, J. P., & Drucker, W. R. (1971). Occult injuries in pedestrian accidents. *Journal of Trauma, 11*(10), 844–852.
16. Orsborn, R., Haley, K., Hammond, S., & Falcone, R. E. (1999). Pediatric pedestrian versus motor vehicle patterns of injury: Debunking the myth. *Air Medical Journal, 18*(3), 107–110.
17. Wang, M. Y., Kim, K. A., Griffith, P. M., Summers, S., McComb, J. G., Levy, M. L., et al. (2001). Injuries from falls in the pediatric population: An analysis of 729 cases. *Journal of Pediatric Surgery, 36*(10), 1528–1534.
18. National Center for Statistics and Analysis. (1997). *Traffic safety facts 1997: Pedalcyclists*. Washington, DC: National Highway Traffic Safety Administration.
19. American Academy of Pediatrics Committee on Injury and Poison Prevention. (1995). Bicycle helmets. *Pediatrics, 95*(4), 609–610.
20. Winston, F. K., Weiss, H. B., Nance, M. L., Vivarelli-O'Neill, C., Strotmeyer, S., Lawrence, B. A., et al. (2002).

Table 11-6 Injury Prevention Interventions

Injury Mechanism	Education/Behavior Change	Enforcement/Legislation	Environment/Technology
Motor Vehicle	Implement media campaign about correct use and positioning of child safety seats; provide consumer training for correct child safety seat use.	Establish/enforce primary restraint laws; improve child safety seat laws, child safety seat check points, speed limit and DUI enforcement programs, and create "800" safety seat hotline for nonuse of restraints.	Distribute free child safety seats to low-income families; improve signals at problem intersections; reduce speed limits in neighborhoods with children and around schools.
Pedestrian	Motivate medical professionals to counsel parents about traffic dangers, and provide pedestrian safety programs at elementary schools.	Enact and enforce pedestrian right-of-way laws.	Improve lighting and crosswalks at problem intersections, and distribute reflector tape products.
Bicycle	Conduct bicycle safety rodeos at schools and community fairs; increase bicycle safety information in health curriculums.	Promote bicycle helmet legislation; enforce current bicycle helmet laws.	Distribute free bicycle helmets to low-income families; provide free bicycle repair workshops; increase bicycle lanes and trails.
Fires/Burns	Educate home owners and rental property owners about scald burn risks and smoke detectors; encourage firefighters to provide school assemblies on fire safety.	Enforce building codes for smoke detector use; encourage building code officials to require hot water heater settings under 120° F (49° C).	Promote the use of antiscald device products.
Home (falls, poisons)	Educate parents about gates and stairs, sharp-edged furniture, furniture near windows, proper crib construction, miniblind cords, and locking up poisons, medicines, and alcohol.	Prohibit the sale of baby walkers; inspect child care facilities and schools for all hazards.	Distribute no-choke tubes to determine safe objects for small children, encourage use of window guards, and distribute cabinet lock products.
Firearms/Violence	Develop media campaign promoting trigger locks and lock boxes; provide conflict resolution, anger management, and other violence prevention programs in schools.	Encourage restrictive licensing for handguns and enforcement of existing firearm laws.	Work with local police on community policing initiative; promote development of product modifications for handguns.
Child Abuse	Provide parent education programs to young and at-risk parents; develop self-help groups.	Work with local officials to maximize effectiveness of child protective services.	Support home visitor programs for new parents; provide affordable day care.
Playgrounds	Provide seminars on playground safety for school officials, park and recreation administrators, and child care providers.	Promote or mandate the use of U.S. Consumer Product Safety Commission standards for playground equipment and surfaces.	Support community development projects that improve playground equipment and surfaces.
Sports	Provide parents, students, and coaches with educational materials on proper sports equipment and physical conditioning.	Promote and mandate the use of proper safety equipment by school and community sports programs.	Promote the use of breakaway bases, mouth guards, and eye protection equipment.
Drowning	Provide information to pool owners about drown risks and appropriate pool barriers.	Enforce pool barrier codes for community and public pools.	Promote use of pool barriers, including 4-sided isolation fencing.

Reprinted with permission from Allen, K. (1997). *Preventing childhood emergencies: A guide to developing effective injury prevention initiatives.* Washington, DC: Emergency Medical Services for Children National Resource Center.

Estimates of the incidence and costs associated with handlebar-related injuries in children. *Archives of Pediatrics and Adolescent Medicine, 156*(9), 922–928.

21. Committee on Injury and Poison Prevention. American Academy of Pediatrics. (2002). Skateboard and scooter injuries. *Pediatrics, 109*(3), 542–543.

22. Chow, T. K., Corbett, S. W., & Farstad, D. J. (1996). Spectrum of injuries from snowboarding. *Journal of Trauma, 41*(2), 321–325.

23. American Academy of Pediatrics Committee on Injury and Poison Prevention and Committee on Sports Medicine and Fitness. (1999). Trampolines at home, school, and recreational centers. *Pediatrics, 103*(5 Pt 1), 1053–1056.

24. Phelan, A. (1994). Respiratory emergencies. In S. Kelly (Ed.), *Pediatric emergency nursing* (pp. 247–279). Norwalk, CT: Appleton & Lange.

25. Fiore, M., & Heidemann, S. (2003). *Near drowning.* Retrieved January 24, 2003 from http://www.emedicine.com/ped/topic2570.htm

26. Kaplan, L. (2003). *Abdominal trauma, penetrating.* Retrieved January 24, 2003 from http://www.emedicine.com/emerg/topic2.htm

27. Emergency Nurses Association. (2000). Burns. In K. S. Hoyt, & B. B. Jacobs (Eds.), *Trauma nursing core course (Provider manual)* (5th ed., pp. 207–232). Des Plaines, IL: Author.

28. Nypaver, M., & Treloar, D. (1994). Neutral cervical spine positioning in children. *Annals of Emergency Medicine, 23*(2), 208–211.

29. American Heart Association. (2002). Vascular access. In *Pediatric advanced life support (Provider manual)* (pp. 155–172). Dallas, TX: Author.

30. Cox, R., & Brooks, J. (2003). *Burns, chemical.* Retrieved January 12, 2004 from http://www.emedicine.com/EMERG/topic73.htm

31. Potoka, D. A., Schall, L. C., & Ford, H. R. (2001). Development of a novel age-specific pediatric trauma score. *Journal of Pediatric Surgery, 36*(1), 106–112.

32. Natale, J. E., Joseph, J. G., Helfaer, M. A., & Shaffner, D. H. (2000). Early hyperthermia after traumatic brain injury in children: Risk factors, influence on length of stay, and effect on short-term neurologic status. *Critical Care Medicine, 28*(7), 2608–2615.

33. Stock, A., & Singer, L. (2003). *Head trauma.* Retrieved June 23, 2003 from http://www.emedicine.com/ped/topic929.htm

34. Simon, B., Letourneau, P., Vitorino, E., & McCall, J. (2001). Pediatric minor head trauma: Indications for computed tomograhic scanning revisited. *Journal of Trauma, 51*(2), 231–238.

35. Tasker, R. L., Deshpande, J. K., & Carson, B. S. (1996). Head injury. In D. G. Nichols, D. G. Lappe, A. Haller, Jr., & M. Yaster (Eds.), *Golden hour—the handbook for advanced pediatric life support* (2nd ed.). St. Louis, MO: Mosby-Year Book.

36. Dickman, C. A., Hadley, M. N., Browner, C., & Sonntag, V. K. (1989). Neurosurgical management of acute atlas-axis combination fractures. A review of 25 cases. *Journal of Neurosurgery, 70*(1), 45–49.

37. Olson, D. A. (2002). *Head injury.* Retrieved May 19, 2002 from http://www.emedicine.com/neuro/topic153.htm

38. Frank, J. B., Lim, C. K., Flynn, J. M., & Dormans, J. P. (2002). The efficacy of magnetic resonance imaging in pediatric cervical spine clearance. *Spine, 27*(11), 1176–1179.

39. Hendey, G. W., Wolfson, A. B., Mower, W. R., Hoffman. J. R., & the National Emergency X-Radiography Utilization Study Group. (2002). Spinal cord injury without radiographic abnormality: Results of the national emergency X-radiography utilization study in blunt cervical trauma. *Journal of Trauma, 53*(1), 1–4.

40. Dare, A. O., Dias, M. S., & Li, V. (2002). Magnetic resonance imaging correlation in pediatric spinal cord injury without radiographic abnormality. *Journal of Neurosurgery, 97*(1 suppl.), 33–39.

41. Bliss, D., & Silen, M. (2002). Pediatric thoracic trauma. *Critical Care Medicine, 30*(11 suppl.), 409–415.

42. Carbon, R. T., Baar, S., Waldschmidt, J., Huemmer, H. P., & Simon, S. I. (2002). Innovative minimally invasive pediatric surgery is of therapeutic value for splenic injury. *Journal of Pediatric Surgery, 37*(8), 1146–1150.

43. Soud, T., Pieper, P., & Hazinski, M. F. (1992). Pediatric trauma. In M. F. Hazinski (Ed.), *Nursing care of the critically ill child* (2nd ed., pp. 829–873). St. Louis, MO: Mosby-Year Book.

44. Stylianos, S. (2000). Evidence-based guidelines for resource utilization in children with isolated spleen or liver injury. The APSA Trauma Committee. *Journal of Pediatric Surgery, 35*(2), 164–169.

45. Coley, B. D., Mutabagani, K. H., Martin, L. C., Zumberge, N., Cooney, D. R., Caniano, D. A., et al. (2000). Focused abdominal sonography for trauma (FAST) in children with blunt abdominal trauma. *Journal of Trauma, 48*(5), 902–906.

46. Yen, K., & Gorelick, M. H. (2002). Ultrasound applications for the pediatric emergency department: A review of the current literature. *Pediatric Emergency Care, 18*(3), 226–234.

47. Baka, A. G., Delgado, C. A., & Simon, H. K. (2002). Current use and perceived utility of ultrasound for evaluation of pediatric compared with adult trauma patients. *Pediatric Emergency Care, 18*(3), 163–167.

48. Nguyen, T. D., Raju, R., & Lee, S. (2002). *Considerations in pediatric trauma.* Retrieved June 23, 2003 from http://www.emedicine.com/med/topic3223.htm

49. Myers, J. G., Dent, D. L., Stewart, R. M., Gray, G. A., Smith, D. S., Rhodes, J. E., et al. (2000). Blunt splenic injuries: Dedicated trauma surgeons can achieve a high rate of nonoperative success in patients of all ages. *Journal of Trauma, 48*(5), 801–805.

50. Jacobs, I. A., Kelly, K., Valenziano, C., Pawar, J., & Jones, C. (2001). Nonoperative management of blunt splenic and hepatic trauma in the pediatric population: Significant differences between adult and pediatric surgeons? *American Surgeon, 67*(2), 149–154.

51. Sponseller, P. D. (1996). Orthopedic trauma. In D. G. Nichols, D. G. Lappe, A. Haller, Jr., & M. Yaster (Eds.), *Golden hour—The handbook for advanced pediatric life support* (2nd ed.). St. Louis, MO: Mosby-Year Book.

52. Fultz, J., & Bayer, G. (2000). Extremity trauma. In P. S. Kidd, P. Sturt, & J. Fultz (Eds.), *Mosby's emergency nursing reference* (2nd ed., pp. 362–392). St. Louis, MO: Mosby-Year Book.

53. Woodward, G. A., & Bolte, R. G. (1990). Children riding in the back of pickup trucks: A neglected safety issue. *Pediatrics, 86*(5), 683–691.

54. Committee on Trauma American College of Surgeons. (1999). Guidelines for the operation of burn units. In *Resources for optimal care of the injured patient: 1999* (pp.55–62). Chicago, IL: American College of Surgeons.

Internet Resources

National Highway Traffic Safety Administration
 http://www.nhtsa.dot.gov

National Youth Sports Safety Foundation
 http://www.nyssf.org

American Trauma Society http://www.amtrauma.org

Centers for Disease Control and Prevention
 http://www.cdc.gov

Insurance Institute for Highway Safety http://www.iihs.org

Transport Canada Road Safety
 http://www.tc.gc.ca/roadsafety/rsindx_e.htm

Appendix 11-A

Cranial Nerve Assessment

A gross evaluation of cranial nerve function can be completed relatively quickly. However, the pediatric patient's condition and developmental level may preclude evaluation of all cranial nerves. Basic cranial nerve evaluation should include eye movement and function, gag reflex, and facial symmetry.

Evaluation of Eye Movement and Function (Cranial Nerves II, III, IV, and VI)[1,2]

In the conscious child, evaluation of eye movement and function includes an assessment of extraocular movements and gross visual acuity. However, complete evaluation of all extraocular movements may not be possible in children younger than 2 to 3 years of age. The assessment includes evaluation for the presence of

- Equal rise of eyelids
- Equality of pupil size and reactivity to light and accommodation
- Ability to see and track an object
- Ability to identify color
- Ability to follow an object through the six fields of gaze

In conscious infants younger than 3 months of age, the assessment includes evaluation for the presence of

- Equal rise of eyelids
- Equality of pupil size and reactivity to light and accommodation
- Blinking in response to a bright light
- Ability to follow or track a dangling object, or moving the head to follow an object[3]

In infants and children with an altered level of consciousness, the position of the eyes at rest and the presence of abnormal spontaneous eye movement should also be noted.[4] The assessment includes evaluation for the presence of

- Equal rise of eyelids (if eye opening response present)
- Equality of pupil size and reactivity to light and accommodation
- Abnormal eye position
  - Deviation of the eyes toward one field of gaze
  - Dysconjugate gaze
- Abnormal movement (nystagmus)

Evaluation of Reflex Responses (Cranial Nerves IX and X [Gag, Cough, and Swallowing]; Cranial Nerves V and VII [Corneal Reflex]; Cranial Nerves III, VI, and VIII [Oculocephalic and Oculovestibular])[2,5,6]

The assessment of reflex responses includes evaluation for the function of

- Cranial nerves IX and X
  - Ability to swallow
  - Ability to cough
  - Presence of gag reflex
  - Presence of clear speech or alterations in speech pattern
- Cranial nerves V and VII
  - Spontaneous blinking
  - Blinking in response to corneal stimulus
- Cranial nerves III, VI, and VIII
  - Oculocephalic and oculovestibular responses are only tested for the evaluation of severe brain stem dysfunction in the unresponsive infant or child. This assessment includes evaluation for the presence of
    - Doll's-eyes reflex: when the head is turned but the eyes move in the opposite direction. If the eyes move in the same direction the head is turned, the doll's-eyes reflex is considered absent, and this is an abnormal finding.
    - Nystagmus in response to ice water caloric test. No eye movement or asymmetric eye movement in response to the ice water caloric test is considered an abnormal response.

Evaluation of Facial Movement and Expression (Cranial Nerves V and VII)[2,5,6]

The assessment of facial movement and expression includes evaluation for the presence of

- Facial symmetry with movement or during crying and sucking in infants
- Ability to raise eyebrows, smile, clench teeth, and chew
- Tears with crying
- Sucking reflex and strength of reflex in infants

Evaluation of Motor and Muscular Function (Cranial Nerves XI and XII)[2,5,6]

The assessment of motor and muscular function related to the cranial nerves includes observing for the presence of the pediatric patient's ability to

- Shrug shoulders
- Turn head and move upper extremities
- Stick out tongue. In infants, the position of the tongue when crying is observed; the midline position is the norm.

Basic Evaluation of Hearing (Cranial Nerve VIII)[3,6]

The assessment of hearing function includes observing for presence of the pediatric patient's ability to

- Respond to verbal commands and answer questions
- Repeat words

In infants younger than 3 months of age, the following behaviors are observed

- Spontaneous movements and/or sucking stop in response to voice or sounds. The infant should then resume the activity.
- Quieting to the sound of voice or soothing sounds
- Turning of head or eyes toward the sound
- Vocalization in response to sounds or voice

References

1. James, H. E. (1986). Neurologic evaluation and support in the child with acute brain insult. *Pediatric Annals*, *15*(1),16–22.
2. Hazinski M. F. (1992). Neurologic disorders. In M. F. Hazinski (Ed.), *Nursing care of the critically ill child* (2nd ed., pp. 521–628). St. Louis MO: Mosby.
3. Gordon, N. (1993). The neurologic examination. In N. Gordon (Ed.), *Neurologic problems in childhood* (pp. 1–24). Boston, MA: Butterworth-Heinemann.
4. Dolan, M. (1992). Head trauma. In R. M. Barkin (Ed.), *Pediatric emergency medicine: Concepts and clinical practice* (pp. 184–198). St. Louis, MO: Mosby.
5. Emergency Nurses Association. (1995). Consciousness. In *Course in advanced trauma nursing: A conceptual approach* (pp. 287–331). Park Ridge, IL: Author.
6. Brucker, J. M. (1996). Neurologic disorders. In J. M. Brucker & K. D. Wallin (Eds.), *Manual of pediatric nursing* (pp. 251–297). Boston, MA: Little, Brown and Company.

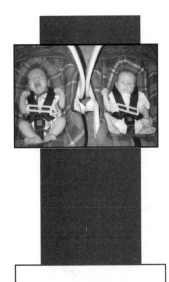

chapter 12

PEDIATRIC PAIN ASSESSMENT AND MANAGEMENT

Objectives

On completion of this chapter, the learner should be able to:

1. Identify misconceptions regarding the treatment of pain in the pediatric population.

2. Describe the pathophysiologic process of pain.

3. Determine physiologic and behavioral indicators of pain in the neonatal and pediatric populations.

4. Discuss methods and tools used to assess pain in infants and children.

5. Discuss nonpharmacologic nursing interventions used for relief of pain in infants and children.

6. Discuss pharmacologic pain management in infants and children.

Introduction

Pediatric patients experience pain as a result of illness, injury, and emergency intervention for treatment and diagnosis. Factors influencing a pediatric patient's experience with pain include underlying medical conditions; previous painful events; cultural, familial, and environmental influence; developmental level; body part involved; preparation for the procedure; type of medication administered; and use of nonpharmacologic intervention.

Pain management can be particularly challenging in the pediatric population in which patients may be unable or unwilling to express or specify the degree of pain they are experiencing. Emergency nurses must advocate for early pain assessment and appropriate interventions for the pediatric patients for which they provide care. Pain has both physical and emotional origins, which are interrelated. Attempts to treat physical and emotional pain separately may limit our ability to provide optimal pain management.

Pain and anxiety not only coexist but also often potentiate one another. Children may suffer from acute pain related to trauma or illness and be unable to benefit from the effects of analgesia due to high anxiety levels. Once relaxed, the analgesia takes effect, and the pain will ease. Children can also progress through uncomfortable experiences positively, without analgesia, using emotional support and cognitive-behavioral techniques. Optimal pain

management for the pediatric patient uses a combination of both pharmacologic and nonpharmacologic techniques.

Despite advances in understanding pain, common misconceptions, attitudes, and practice continue to contribute to inadequate pain management in children.[1] Personal views regarding pain management such as predetermination of pain levels and doubts about pain validity can influence our ability to provide adequate pain control. Research indicates that physicians continue to order inadequate amounts of sedation and analgesia and that health care providers continue to administer them insufficiently.[2] Misconceptions about neonatal pain related to neurologic immaturity and fears regarding respiratory depression in children also impact the frequency and amount of pain control administered.

Table 12-1 discusses facts and fallacies about pediatric pain.

Pain assessment and management in the pediatric population within the emergency environment are presented in this chapter. Chapter 17 discusses procedural preparation and sedation.

Types of Pain

The International Association for the Study of Pain defines pain as "an unpleasant sensory and emotional experience associated with actual or potential tissue damage, or described in terms of such damage."[2] Pain is generally grouped into two categories: (1) acute and (2) chronic.

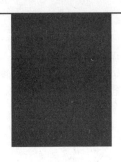

Acute pain is described as having a rapid onset and an identifiable cause. It varies in intensity from mild to severe, is self-limiting, and generally has a predictable course.[2] Examples of acute pain include postoperative pain and pain from injury or infection. Treatment of acute pain is often predictable and is most commonly managed using both pharmacologic and nonpharmacologic methods.

Chronic pain is defined as pain lasting a month beyond the usual course of illness or injury or pain that is present for more than three to six months in duration.[2,3] Management of chronic pain generally involves a complex plan of care including a multidisciplinary team and both pharmacologic and nonpharmacologic measures.

Pain associated with illness and injury is common in the emergency department (ED). It can also be the result of invasive procedures required to complete diagnostic testing, treat injury, and manage illness.

Pain Physiology

Acute pain occurs with tissue damage and the subsequent release of mediators including bradykinins, prostaglandin E, and histamine. These mediators stimulate peripheral afferent nerve endings or nociceptors. There are two types of nociceptors: (1) C-fibers that transmit slow, dull, chronic pain and (2) A-fibers that transmit fast, sharp, well-localized pain. In the dorsal horn of the spinal cord, these pain signals are modified and sent through the appropriate spinal pathway for transmission to the cerebral cortex. Once the stimulus reaches the brain, the cortex is then able to interpret it and elicit a response.

A common misconception regarding neonatal pain is that infants of that age are unable to feel pain and are therefore unable to remember painful experiences. Research has shown that nociceptive pathways are completely myelinated by 30 weeks of gestation indicating that infants of that age are able to transmit and feel pain. Even thinly or nonmyelinated fibers are capable of carrying pain stimuli. Although the conduction may be slower in neonates, the shorter distance between the fibers compensates for the conduction lag, and the pain is interpreted with the same intensity as with fibers that are fully myelinated.[4] In fact, it appears that cutaneous responses are exaggerated, they occur at lower thresholds, and muscle contractions are prolonged further in the neonate than in the adult.[5] Though previous views support neonates as being unable to remember pain, research studying the responses of neonates exposed to noxious stimuli in the neonatal intensive care unit showed that they can respond to previous stressors and

Table 12-1 Fallacies and Facts about Children and Pain

Fallacy	Fact
Infants do not feel pain.	Infants demonstrate behavioral, especially facial, physiologic, and hormonal indicators of pain. Neonates have the neural mechanisms to transmit noxious stimuli by 20 weeks of gestation.
Children tolerate pain better than adults.	Children's tolerance of pain actually increases with age. Younger children tend to rate procedure-related pain higher than older children.
Children cannot tell you where they hurt.	By 4 years of age, children can accurately point to the body area or mark the painful site on a drawing; children as young as 3 years old can use pain scales, such as FACES.
Children always tell the truth about pain.	Children may not admit to having pain to avoid an injection. Because of constant pain, they may not realize how much they are hurting. Children may believe that others know how they are feeling and not ask for analgesia.
Children become accustomed to pain or painful procedures.	Children often demonstrate increased behavioral signs of discomfort with repeated painful procedures.
Behavioral manifestations reflect pain intensity.	Children's developmental level, coping abilities, and temperament, such as activity level and intensity of reaction to pain, influence pain behavior. Children with more active, resisting behaviors may rate pain lower than children with passive, accepting behaviors.
Narcotics are more dangerous for children than they are for adults.	Narcotics (opioids) are no more dangerous for children than they are for adults. Addiction to opioids used to treat pain is extremely rare in children. Reports of respiratory depression in children are also uncommon. By 3 to 6 months of age healthy infants can metabolize opioids like other children.

Adapted from Hockenberry, M. J., Wilson, D., Winkelstein, M. L., & Kline, N. E. (2003). Family-centered care of the child during illness and hospitalization. In *Wong's nursing care of infants and children* (7th ed., pp. 1031-1100). St. Louis, MO: Mosby.

Table 12-2 Pediatric Responses to Painful Stimuli[7,8]

Age Group	Physical and Behavioral Response
Neonates & infants (< 6 months)	• Subcortical functioning • Unable to anticipate pain and localize response • Exhibits generalized body movements; facial grimacing; chin quivering; tightly closed fists and eyes; poor feeding; crying
Infants (6 to 12 months)	• Localization begins • Exhibits reflex withdrawal to stimulus; facial grimacing; irritability; physical resistance; loud crying
Toddlers (1 to 3 years)	• Able to localize and interpret pain • Exhibits localized withdrawal; resistance; aggressive behavior; pushing away; clinging to parent; reluctance to move injured or painful body part • Verbal toddlers may say they are in pain but are unable to elaborate therefore behaviors may manifest as crying, kicking, screaming
Preschool (3 to 5 years)	• Able to anticipate pain • Links unrelated events–may feel pain is punishment for bad deeds • Limited vocabulary; able to state "ouch," "owie," "boo-boo" • Can point to where it hurts. Expressive responses may include crying, screaming, verbal reprimands, such as "I hate you" • Exhibits active physical resistance, thrashing, guarding, or reluctance to move body part
School-age (6 to 10 years)	• Age of mastery and achievement. Likes to co-operate. Organized by rules; responds well to rituals. • Able to verbalize pain and describe intensity and location in detail • May engage in plea-bargaining or stall tactics; fears body mutilation, therefore may deny pain for fear of "getting a needle" • Nonverbal responses include fist and teeth clenching and body rigidity
Early to middle adolescents (11 to 18 years)	• Abstract and critical thinkers. Capable of "if-then" relationships • Able to identify type, onset, duration, and intensity of pain; may ignore, dismiss, or deny pain • May vacillate between adult and child behaviors including mood swings, crying, and regression • Nonverbal responses include muscle tension, clenching, guarding, decreased activity

Adapted from Hockenberry, M. J., Wilson, D., Winkelstein, M. L., & Kline, N. E. (2003). Family-centered care of the child during illness and hospitalization. In *Wong's nursing care of infants and children* (7th ed., pp. 1031-1100). St. Louis, MO: Mosby.

may be more fearful of pain than their peers during later childhood.[5,6] Though still in development, the newborn's nervous system is capable of transmitting, perceiving, remembering, and responding to painful stimuli.[5]

This evidence supports the need not only for adequate pain management in all age groups, but also for an increase in the understanding and use of pain assessment in the neonatal and pediatric populations.

Pain Assessment

Pain should be assessed using age-appropriate assessment tools and guidelines, including physical and behavioral responses and self-report indicators.

Physical Responses

Most pain states are characterized by a global pattern of physiologic arousal related to catecholamine release that can result in tachycardia, hypertension, increased respiratory rate, pupil dilation, diaphoresis, and pallor. However, if pain has persisted for several hours or days, these responses are often modified, and cardiovascular and respiratory measurement may be normal. Physiological indicators alone should be used cautiously when treating acute pain because this response is self-limited, and it may be perceived that pain has subsided when, in fact, it has not.

Physiologic expressions of pain may closely mimic agitation caused by other conditions, such as hypoxia and hypoventilation. The nurse caring for an agitated pediatric patient needs to be able to distinguish between these conditions and acute pain.

Behavioral Responses

Table 12-2 presents behavioral responses to pain by children at different developmental stages.

Verbal Report

Verbal statements of pediatric patients are the most reliable indicators of pain; however, not all pediatric patients are capable or willing to verbalize their discomfort.[7] Therefore, exploring past pain experiences with the parent will help identify the child's typical response to pain and identify methods that have previously provided comfort. At a minimum, a basic assessment must include the intensity and location of the pain. Other points to explore include pain quality, radiation, aggravating and relieving factors, and timing (onset, duration, constant or intermittent).

Pain Scales

Pain scales are simple and versatile tools to measure different dimensions of a pediatric patient's pain. They should be administered in a standard manner in order to provide quantitative and reliable ratings. Many pain assessment tools are available for use in the clinical setting. Choosing the appropriate pain scale is based on the age, developmental level, and ability of the child to

Table 12-3 Summary of Pain Assessment Tools for Infants

Tools and Authors/Ages of Use	Variables and Scoring Range	
Postoperative Pain Score (POPS) Barrier, G., Attia, J., Mayer, M. N., Amiel-Tison, C., & Shnider, S. M. (1989). Measurement of postoperative pain and narcotic administration in infants using a new clinical scoring system. *Intensive Care Medicine,15*(Suppl 1), S37-S39. *Ages of use:* 1 to 7 months	Sleep (0 to 2) Facial expression (0 to 2) Quality of cry (0 to 2) Spontaneous motor activity (0 to 2) Spontaneous excitability (0 to 2) Scoring range: 0 = worst pain, 20 = no pain	Flexion fingers/toes (0 to 2) Sucking (0 to 2) Tone (0 to 2) Consolability (0 to 2) Sociability (0 to 2)
Neonatal Infant Pain Scale (NIPS) Lawrence, J., Alcock, D., McGrath, P., Kay, J., MacMurray, S. B., & Dulberg, C. (1993). The development of a tool to assess neonatal pain. *Neonatal Network, 12*(6), 59-66. *Ages of use:* average gestational age 33.5 weeks	Facial Expression (0 to 1) Cry (0 to 2) Breathing patterns (0 to 1) Scoring range: 0 = no pain; 7 = worst pain	Arms (0 to 1) Legs (0 to 1) State of arousal (0 to 1)
Pain Assessment Tool (PAT) Hodgkinson, K., Bear, M., Thorn, J., & Van Blaricum, S. (1994). Measuring pain in neonates: Evaluating an instrument and developing a common language. *Australian Journal of Advanced Nursing, 12*(1), 17-22. *Ages of use:* 27 weeks gestational age to full term	Posture/tone (1 to 2) Sleep pattern (0 to 2) Expression (1 to 2) Color (0 to 2) Cry (0 to 2) Scoring range: 4 = no pain; 20 = worst pain	Respiration (1 to 2) Heart rate (1 to 2) Saturation (0 to 2) Blood pressure (0 to 2) Nurse's perception (0 to 2)
Pain Rating Scale (PRS) Joyce, B. A., Schade, J. G., Keck, J. F., Gerkensmeyer, J., Raftery, T., Moser, S., et al. (1994). Reliability and validity of preverbal pain assessment tools. *Issues in Comprehensive Pediatric Nursing, 17*(3), 121-135. *Ages of use:* 1 to 36 months	0-smiling, sleeping, no change when moved/touched 1-takes small amount orally, restless, moving, cries 2-not drinking/eating, short periods of cries, distracted with rocking or pacifier 3-change in behavior, irritable, arms/legs shake/jerk, facial grimace 4-flailing, high-pitched wailing, parents request pain medication, unable to distract 5-sleeping prolonged periods interrupted by jerking, continuous crying, rapid and shallow respirations Scoring range: 0 = no pain; 5 = worst pain	
CRIES Krechel, S. W., & Bildner, J. (1995). CRIES: A new neonatal postoperative pain measurement score. Initial testing of validity and reliability. *Paediatric Anaesthesia, 5*(1), 53-61. *Ages of use:* 32- to 60-weeks gestational age	Crying (0 to 2) Requires increased oxygen (0 to 2) Increased vital signs (0 to 2) Expression (0 to 2) Sleepless (0 to 2) Scoring range: 0 = no pain; 10 = worst pain	

Table 12-3 Summary of Pain Assessment Tools for Infants (cont.)

Premature Infant Pain Profile (PIPP)

Stevens, B., Johnston, C., Petryshen, P., & Taddio, A. (1999). Premature infant pain profile: Development and initial validation. *Clinical Journal of Pain, 12*(1), 13-22.

Ages of use: 28 to 40 weeks gestational age

Gestational age (0 to 3)	Eye squeeze (0 to 3)
Behavioral state (0 to 3)	Nasolabial furrow (0 to 3)
Heart rate (0 to 3)	
Oxygen saturation (0 to 3)	
Brow budge (0 to 3)	
Scoring range: 0 = no pain; 21 = worst pain	

Scale for Use in Newborns (SUN)

Blauer, T., & Gerstmann, D. (1998). A simultaneous comparison of three neonatal pain scales during common NICU procedures. *Clinical Journal of Pain, 14*(1), 39-47.

Ages of use: 0 to 28 days

CNS state (0 to 4)	Movement (0 to 4)
Breathing (0 to 4)	Tone (0 to 4)
Heart rate (0 to 4)	Face (0 to 4)
Mean BP (0 to 4)	
Scoring range: 0 = no pain; 28 = worst pain; average baseline score 10 to 14; a 2 represents normal or baseline value	

Neonatal Pain, Agitation, and Sedation Scale (NPASS)

Puchalski, M., & Hummel, P. (2002). The reality of neonatal pain. *Advances in Neonatal Care, 2*(5), 233-244.

Ages of use: Birth (23 weeks gestational age) and term newborns up to 100 days

Cry/irritability (0 to 2)

Behavior/state (0 to 2)

Facial expression (0 to 2)

Extremities/tone (0 to 2)

Vital signs-HR, RR, BP, SaO2 (0 to 2)

Scoring range: Pain score: 0 to 10 (0 = no pain; 10 = intense pain). Sedation score: 0 to 10 (0 = no sedation; 10 = deep sedation).

Reprinted with permission from Hockenberry, M. J., Wilson, D., Winkelstein, M. L., & Kline, N. E. St. Louis, MO: Mosby. (Eds.). (2003). The high-risk newborn and family. In *Wong's nursing care of infants and children* (7th ed., pp. 333-414).

understand the concepts related to the use of the scale. **Tables 12-3** and **12-4** summarize pain assessment tools for infants and children, respectively. Three examples of pain assessment tools are reproduced here (**Figure 12-1**, CRIES; **Figure 12-2**, FLACC; **Figure 12-3**, Oucher™ Scale; and **Figure 12-4**, FACES Pain Rating Scale).

The easiest and quickest method of evaluating pain using a scale is the verbal numerical scale (0 to 10). Children using this scale must understand rank and order as well as be able to count and understand numbers. This scale is often used at triage as part of a rapid assessment of pain levels.

Pain Management Interventions

Nonpharmacologic Interventions

Nonpharmacologic pain management has been recognized as an effective method for the reduction of pain, anxiety, and distress in children. Key principles regarding the use of this method of pain control revolve around early introduction of these methods and their use in addition to, and not as a replacement for, pharmacologic management. Interventions must be based on the child's age, the child's developmental level, and the desired outcome or task at hand. General strategies to consider are listed in **Table 12-5**.

Distraction

Distraction is a good way to keep a pediatric patient's mind from pain. The use of distraction requires little patient or caregiver preparation. The distraction techniques selected should be developmentally and age appropriate. The caregiver's participation with the distraction technique should be encouraged.   General distraction approaches include

• Playing soothing music, children's stories, or songs

• Playing a videotape for the pediatric patient to view

- Looking through a kaleidoscope

- Using soap bubbles, glitter wands, or puppets to engage the pediatric patient's attention

- Asking the caregiver to read or tell the pediatric patient a story

- Asking the pediatric patient to sing a song or count aloud slowly. The pediatric patient may be instructed to sing or count louder or faster if needed.

Other distraction or coping techniques require teaching the pediatric patient the strategy as well as providing an opportunity for the pediatric patient to rehearse the technique. These techniques are most useful in older children and adolescents. Examples of these techniques include the following.

- Deep breathing. The pediatric patient is coached in deep breathing, focusing on the inhalation and exhalation phases of each breath to initiate a relaxed breathing pattern.[9]

- Relaxation.
  - With an infant or child: Hold in a comfortable, well-supported position, such as vertically against the chest and shoulder; rock in a wide, rhythmic arc in a rocking chair or sway back and forth, rather than bouncing the child; repeat one or two words softly, such as "Mommy's here."

Figure 12-1 CRIES

Criteria	0	1	2
Crying	No	High pitched	Inconsolable
Requires O_2 for saturation > 95%	No	< 30%	> 30%
Increased vital signs	HR and BP less than or equal to preop	Increase in HR or BP < 20% of preop	Increase in HR or BP > 20% of preop
Expression	None	Grimace	Grimace/grunt
Sleepless	No	Wakes at frequent intervals	Constantly awake

Coding Tips for Using CRIES

Crying	The characteristic cry of pain is high pitched.
	If no cry or cry that is not high pitched, score 0.
	If cry high pitched but baby is easily consoled, score 1.
	If cry is high pitched and baby is inconsolable, score 2.
Requires O_2 for sats. > 95%	Looks for changes in oxygenation. Babies experiencing pain manifest decrease in oxygenation as measured by transcutaneous monitoring or pulse oximetry.
	If no O_2 is required, score 0. If < 30% O_2 is required, score 1.
	If > 30% O_2 is required, score 2. (Consider other cause of changes in oxygenation such as atelectasis, pneumothorax, oversedation).
Increased vital signs	Note: Measure BP last because this may wake child, causing difficulty with other assessments. Use baseline preoperative parameters from a nonstressed period.
	Multiply baseline HR X 0.2; then add this to baseline HR to determine the HR, which is 20% over baseline. Do likewise for BP. Use mean BP.
	If HR and BP are both unchanged or less than baseline, score 0.
	If HR and BP is increased but increase is < 20% of baseline, score 1.
	If either one is increased > 20% over baseline, score 2.
Expression	The facial expression most often associated with pain is a grimace. This may be characterized by brow lowering, eyes squeezed shut, deepening of the nasolabial furrow, open lips and mouth.
	If no grimace present, score 0. If grimace alone present, score 1.
	If grimace and noncry vocalization grunt present, score 2.
Sleepless	This parameter is scored based on the infant's state during the hour preceding this recorded score.
	If he or she is continuously asleep, score 0.
	If awakened at frequent intervals, score 1. If awake constantly, score 2.

Reprinted with permission from Krechel, S. W., & Bildner, J. (1995). CRIES: A new neonatal postoperative pain measurement score. Initial testing of validity and reliability. *Paediatric Anaesthesia, 5*(1), 53-61.

- With the older child: Ask the child to take a deep breath and "go limp as a rag doll" while exhaling slowly, then ask the child to yawn; help the child assume a comfortable position; begin progressive relaxation; allow child to keep his or her eyes open because children may respond better.

• Blowing away the pain. The child is instructed to blow out the pain, imagining he or she is blowing out candles slowly and steadily. Having the child blow bubbles or on a pinwheel also works with this technique.[10]

• Guided imagery. The older child is talked through a pleasant or enjoyable situation or activity. Developing the scenario requires the nurse to ask questions of the child and/or caregiver about an imagined situation.

Have the child describe details of the event; include as many senses as possible (i.e., "feel the cool breeze, see the beautiful colors, hear the pleasant sounds").

Figure 12-2 FLACC

Category	Scoring		
	0	1	2
Face	No particular expression or smile	Occasional grimace or frown, withdrawn, disinterested	Frequent to constant quivering chin, clenched jaw
Legs	Normal position or relaxed	Uneasy, restless, tense	Kicking, or legs drawn up
Activity	Lying quietly, normal position, moves easily	Squirming, shifting back and forth, tense	Arched, rigid or jerking
Cry	No cry (awake or asleep)	Moans or whimpers; occasional complaint	Crying steadily, screams or sobs, frequent complaints
Consolability	Content, relaxed	Reassured by occasional touching, hugging or being talked to, distractible	Difficult to console or comfort

Each of the five categories (F) Face; (L) Legs; (A) Activity; (C) Cry; (C) Consolability is scored from 0-2, which results in a total score between zero and ten.

Reprinted with permission from Merkel, S. I., Shayevitz, J. R., Voepel-Lewis, T., & Malviya, S. (1997). The FLACC: A behavioral scale for scoring postoperative pain in young children. *Pediatric Nursing, 23*(3), 293-297.

Figure 12-3 OUCHER™ Scale

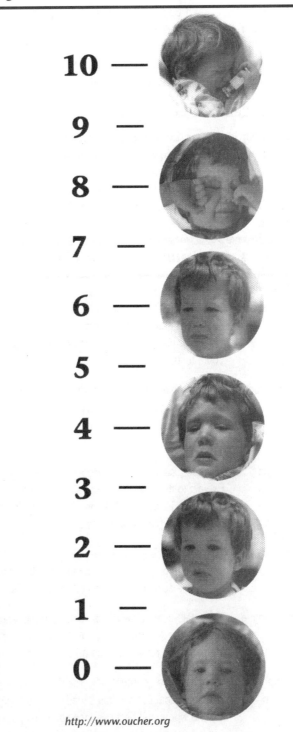

http://www.oucher.org

©The Caucasian version of the OUCHER was developed and copyrighted by Judith E. Beyer, PhD, RN, (University of Missouri-Kansas City), 1983. For information about the OUCHER, write to: Judith E. Beyer, P. O. Box 411714, Kansas City, MO 64141 or go to www.OUCHER.org

Encourage the child to concentrate only on the pleasurable event during the procedure or painful event; enhance the image by recalling specific details, such as reading the story or playing music.

- Positive self-talk. The child is coached to say positive statements, such as "I can do it," or "I'm doing great." Positive self-talk may also be combined with thought stopping to decrease anticipatory stress. The child stops thinking about the fearful or anxiety-provoking aspects of the procedure and substitutes a positive thought.[11]

Physical Comfort Measures

Physical positioning and comfort measures are components of nonpharmacologic pain management. Basic interventions are used to minimize pain and/or to prevent the exacerbation of pain. These measures may be initiated in response to illness or injury or as part of a procedure. There may be variations in these interventions based on cultural factors. Comfort measures include the following.

- Simple rhythmic rubbing, use of point pressure, massage

- Allowing the infant to suck on a pacifier, bottle, or breast as appropriate while providing physical comfort measures

- Applying splints or other immobilization techniques for suspected fractures or extremity injuries

- Applying ice or cold packs to an injury site

- Applying warm compresses

- Elevating an injured extremity

- Positioning the child in a comfortable position or support positioning with blankets or pillows

- Covering wounds with a dressing to decrease airflow across the wound

Table 12-4 Pain Rating Scales for Children

Rating Scale	Description
Oucher™ scale	This tool uses six pictures of a child's face representing from "no hurt" to "biggest hurt ever." It also includes a vertical scale with numbers from zero to 10 to use with older children. The child is asked to choose the face that best describes his or her pain. This scale can be used for children 3 to 13 years of age. The numeric scale can be used if the child can count to 10.
Poker chip tool	This tool uses four red poker chips placed in front of the child. The chips are placed horizontally, and the child is told that "these are pieces of hurt." Explain to the child that each chip represents a piece of hurt. Ask him or her how many pieces of hurt they have right now. Record the number of chips the child selected. This tool can be used for children over 3 years of age once they can count and understand numbers.
FACES pain rating scale	This tool consists of six cartoon faces ranging from a smiling face for "no pain" to a tearful face for "worst pain." Explain to the child that each face is for a person who feels happy because there is no pain or sad because there is some or a lot of hurt. Ask the child to pick the face that best describes his or her pain. This scale can be used for children as young as 3 years of age.
Numeric scale	This scale uses a straight line with end points that are labeled as "no pain" and "worst pain." Divisions with corresponding numbers from 0 to 10 are marked along the line. The child is asked to choose the number that best describes his or her pain. This scale can be used on children over 4 years of age once they can count and understand numbers.
Visual analogue scale	This scale uses a 10-cm horizontal line with end points marked "no pain" and "worst pain." The child is asked to place a mark on the line that best describes the amount of his or her pain. Measure the distance with a ruler from the "no pain" end and record the measurement as the pain score. This scale can be used on children over 4½ years of age.
Word-graphic rating scale	This scale uses descriptive words to describe varying intensities of pain. Examples of the words along the scale may include "no pain," "little pain," "medium pain," "large pain," and "worst possible pain." The child is asked to mark along the line the words that best describe his or her pain. Measure the distance with a ruler from the "no pain" end to the mark and record the measurement as the pain score. This scale can be used for children 5 years of age and over; however, they may need explanation of the words.
FLACC scale	This is a behavior scale that has been tested with children age 3 months to 7 years. Each of the five categories (Face, Legs, Activity, Cry, Consolability) is scored from 0 to 2, and the scores are added to get a total from 0 to 10. Behavioral pain scores need to be considered within the context of the child's psychological status, anxiety, and other environment factors.

Figure 12-4 FACES Pain Rating Scale

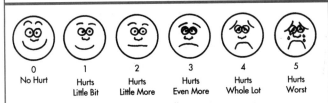

From Wong, D. L., Hockenberry-Eaton, M., Wilson, D., Winkelstein, M. L., & Schwartz, P: *Wong's Essentials of Pediatric Nursing*, 6/e, St. Louis, 2001, p. 1301. Copyrighted by Mosby, Inc. Reprinted with permission.

Table 12-5 General Strategies for Nonpharmacologic Pain Management

- Form a trusting relationship with child and family. Express concern regarding their reports of pain. Take an active role in seeking effective pain management strategies.
- Prepare the pediatric patient before potentially painful procedures, but avoid "planting" the idea. Use nonpain descriptors when possible.
- Avoid evaluative statements or descriptions.
- Stay with the pediatric patient during a procedure. Encourage parent/caregiver to stay with the pediatric patient if the patient and parent/caregiver desires.
- Educate the pediatric patient about pain, especially when explanation may lessen anxiety (e.g., pain is expected after surgery and does not indicate something is wrong).

Figure 12-5 Therapeutic Ladder for Pain Management

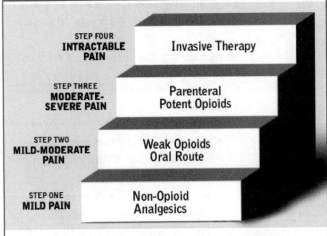

From World Health Organization. 1996. *Cancer Pain Relief and Palliative Care: Report of WHO Expert Committee* (3rd ed.). Geneva: WHO. Adapted with permission.

- Transporting the patient by wheelchair or stretcher to minimize movement associated with ambulation

Pharmacologic Interventions

The current standard for the management of pain in children consists of four concepts: "by the ladder," "by the clock," "by the mouth," and "by the child." This means that pain management in children should follow the World Health Organization (WHO) Analgesic Stepladder and be administered on a scheduled basis, be given by the least invasive route, and be tailored to the individual child's circumstance and needs.[12] The WHO Analgesic Stepladder (**Figure 12-5**) is a multistep approach to treating pain and is a guide for initiating analgesic drugs and dosages that correspond to the patient's reported level of pain. The ladder starts with nonopioid oral drugs for mild pain and progresses to strong opioids, adjuvants, and invasive therapies for severe and/or intractable pain. It is important to keep in mind that the potency of analgesia should be matched to the child's reported level of pain.[13] In other words, the key to pain management is providing the appropriate analgesia to meet the specific needs of the patient. For example, if children report severe pain, they should be started on a potent opioid such as morphine. It would be inappropriate to start a child with severe pain on ibuprofen or a weak opioid and progress up the ladder from that point.

Nonopioid Drugs

Nonopioids such as acetaminophen and nonsteroidal anti-inflammatory drugs such aspirin, ibuprofen, or ketorolac are used to control acute mild to moderate pain and chronic pain. These medications have a ceiling effect, and once maximal dosages are reached, the change to or addition of an opioid should be considered.

Opioids

Opioids bind with certain receptors in the central nervous system and peripheral tissues to provide analgesic effects. They may be given orally or parenterally. Administration of opioids by the oral route can be as effective as the parenteral route when the drug is given in an equianalgesic dose (i.e., one that achieves the same effect despite the change in route).[8] Moderate pain is most commonly managed with the use of oral opioids such as codeine, morphine, or fentanyl. Acute moderate to severe pain is usually best managed with intermittent intravenous administration of a narcotic analgesic. The most commonly used analgesics in the ED include morphine, fentanyl, and ketamine. Potential common complications of opioids include respiratory depression and cardiovascular collapse.

The route of administration is determined by the condition of the child, their developmental level, and their NPO status. Pain control should be administered as soon as an assessment is performed and the patient is stabilized. It should never be delayed while diagnostic testing or noncritical interventions are completed. Common routes of analgesia administration in the ED are listed in **Table 12-6**.

Adjuvant Drugs[13]

Adjuvant drugs are used in combination with nonopioid and opioid drugs to enhance pain management. Adjuvant drugs can by divided into two categories: (1) coanalgesic drugs and (2) drugs that treat side effects. Coanalgesic drugs include antidepressants, anticonvulsants, corticosteroids, and sedative/hypnotic drugs. Drugs used to treat side effects include antihistamines, psychostimulants, laxatives, neuroleptics, and antiemetics.

The majority of pediatric patients with pain will experience complete relief of pain using the previously discussed interventions. However, a small number of children may require more invasive pain management techniques. These children should be referred to specialists who are experienced in the management of pain in children.

Summary

Emergency nurses have an important role in the recognition, assessment, and management of pain in children. Early recognition of the physiological and behavioral responses children have to pain is the key to timely pain intervention. Appreciating the emotional and physical link in the response to pain is a vital component permitting us to incorporate both nonpharmacologic and pharmacologic pain interventions to provide effective and optimal pain management for the pediatric patient in the emergency environment.

References

1. Zeltzer, L. K., Bush, J. P., Chen, E., & Riveral, A. (1997). A psychobiologic approach to pediatric pain: Part I. History, physiology, and assessment strategies. *Current Problems in Pediatrics, 27*(6), 225–246.

2. Oakes, L. L. (2001). Caring practices: Providing comfort. In M. A. Q. Curley & P. A. Moloney-Harmon (Eds.), *Critical care nursing of infants and children* (2nd ed., pp. 547–576). Philadelphia: Saunders.

3. Kemp, C. (1995). *Terminal illness: A guide to nursing care* (p. 112). Philadelphia: Lippincott.

4. Stevens, B. J., Johnston, C. C., & Grunau, R. V. (1995). Issues of assessment of pain and discomfort in neonates. *Journal of Obstetric, Gynecologic, and Neonatal Nursing, 24*(9), 849–855.

Table 12-6 Common Routes of Analgesia Administration in the ED

Route	Description
Oral	• Preferred for mild to moderate pain if child is not NPO. • May require higher doses of oral medication as compared to the parenteral route in order to obtain equianalgesia.
Sublingual/buccal/ oral transmucosal	• More rapid onset than oral; however, few analgesics are available in this form. • One example is the Fentanyl Oralet®, which has been proven to reduce pain perception and initiate drowsiness in children undergoing procedures. Its side effects include vomiting and facial pruritus.[9]
Topical or transdermal	• May be used in a variety of preparations to provide both local anesthesia and systemic analgesia. • Examples of topical anesthetics include EMLA cream®, AMETOP, or LET gel • Examples of transdermal analgesics include Duragesic®, the fentanyl transdermal patch (not recommended for acute pain due to time required for absorption)
Intranasal	• Some medications, commonly midazolam and fentanyl, may be administered intranasally and can provide an effective method of pain and sedation relief for procedures.[9] Their administration may be frightening for young children, and absorption may be variable.
Intramuscular	• Not a preferred route of administration by children. This route is sometimes considered for a one-time dose that is required for quick relief of moderate to severe pain. • Its absorption can be both slow and variable.
Intravenous	• The most reliable and controllable method of pain relief. • Commonly administered by intermittent infusion for rapid relief of severe pain. Continuous infusions have less peaks and valleys and provide steady control of pain levels. • Patient-controlled analgesia (PCA) with continuous infusion may be initiated in the ED for patients with chronic conditions in an effort to control severe pain.

5. Agarwal, R., Enzman, H., & Gardner, S. (1998). Pain and pain relief. In G. Merenstein & S. L. Gardner (Eds.), *Handbook of neonatal intensive care* (pp. 173–196). St. Louis, MO: Mosby.

6. Anand, K. J., & International Evidence-based Group for Neonatal Pain. (2001). Consensus statement for the prevention and management of pain in the newborn. *Archives of Pediatrics and Adolescent Medicine, 155*(2), 173–180.

7. Hockenberry, M. J., Wilson, D., Winkelstein, M. L., & Kline, N. E. (Eds.). (2003). Family-centered care of the child during illness and hospitalization. In *Wong's nursing care of infants and children* (7th ed., pp. 1031-1100). St. Louis, MO: Mosby.

8. Ball, J. W., & Bindler, R. C. (2003). Pain assessment and management. In *Pediatric nursing: Caring for children* (3rd ed., pp. 287–307). Upper Saddle River, NJ: Prentice Hall.

9. Salantera, S., Sirkka, L., Salmi, T., & Helenius, H. (1999). Nurses' knowledge about pharmacological and nonpharmacological pain management in children. *Journal of Pain and Symptom Management, 18*(4), 289–299.

10. Kennedy, R., M., & Luhmann, J. D. (1999). The "ouchless emergency department." Getting closer: Advances in decreasing distress during painful procedures in the emergency department. *Pediatric Clinics of North America, 46*(6), 1215–1247, vii–viii.

11. Fanurik, D., Koh, J., Schmitz, M., & Brown, R. (1997). Pharmacobehavioral intervention: Integrating pharmacologic and behavioral techniques for pediatric medical procedures. *Children's Health Care, 26*(1), 289–299.

12. McGrath, P. A. (1996). Development of the World Health Organization guidelines on cancer pain relief and palliative care in children. *Journal of Pain and Symptom Management, 12*(2), 87–92.

13. Hockenberry-Eaton, M., Barrera, P., Brown, M., Bottomley, S. J., & O'Neill, J. B. (1999). *Cancer pain management in children.* Retrieved September 11, 2003 from http://www.childcancerpain.org/frameset.cfm?content = pharm01

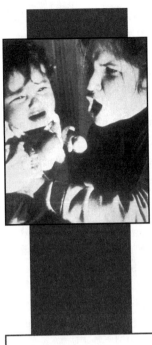

chapter 13

CHILD MALTREATMENT

Objectives

On completion of this chapter, the learner should be able to:

1. Define the five forms of child maltreatment.
2. Discuss risk factors for child maltreatment.
3. Describe key points to the history and physical examination of child maltreatment.
4. Describe nursing interventions for maltreated children and their families.
5. Identify key concepts in collecting evidence for the maltreated child.
6. Describe injuries and inflictions suspicious or diagnostic of child maltreatment.

Introduction

Child maltreatment is a serious threat to the health and well-being of children of all ages. The recognition of child maltreatment can be difficult and requires careful assessment by health care providers. In the United States, approximately three million referrals for child maltreatment were made to child protective service agencies in the year 2001, resulting in 1,300 deaths. Children younger than 1 year accounted for 41% of child fatalities, and 85% were younger than 6 years of age.[2] The reason for increased information on child maltreatment is more a reflection of changes in awareness, recognition, and reporting.[1]

Mandated reporters are required by law to report child maltreatment if there is reasonable suspicion that abuse or neglect has occurred. State statutes define who mandated reporters are as well as the conditions for reporting maltreatment; therefore, it is important to be knowledgeable of child abuse laws in the jurisdiction in which one practices. Failure to report a case of suspected child maltreatment could result in civil or criminal charges.[3] In most states, standard mandated reporters include, but are not limited to, physicians, nurses, paramedics, psychiatrists, social workers, teachers, child care providers, and law enforcement personnel.

More times than not, maltreated children present to the health care system without a declaration of abuse or neglect. This, along with a caregiver's false presentation of the child's history or intentionally withholding information, may contribute to the difficulty in identifying child maltreatment. A thorough physical examination and a detailed history are the diagnostic tools needed in identifying maltreatment. Nurses play a special role in caring for these patients because they may be the first to see the child and caregiver and are the consistent health care provider if the child is hospitalized.

Definitions

Definitions of *child maltreatment* differ by community, culture, and country. The broad term child maltreatment includes any recent act or failure to act on the part of a parent or caregiver that results in death, serious physical or emotional harm, sexual abuse or exploitation, or an act or failure to act that presents an imminent risk of serious harm.[2]

- Neglect: Characterized by failure to provide for the child's basic needs. Neglect can be physical, emotional, or educational.[2]
  - Physical neglect includes refusal of, or delay in, seeking health care, abandonment, expulsion from the home, and inadequate supervision.
  - Emotional neglect includes inattention to the child's needs for affection, refusal or failure to provide needed psychological care, and spousal abuse in the child's presence.
  - Educational neglect includes the allowance of chronic absenteeism, failure to enroll a child of mandatory school age in school, and failure to attend to a special educational need.
- Emotional: The deliberate attempt to destroy or impair a child's self-esteem or competence. Psychological maltreatment occurs when a person

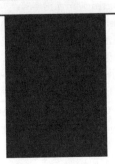

conveys to a child that he or she is worthless, flawed, unloved, or unwanted.[4] All forms of child maltreatment involve some emotional or psychological abuse.

- Physical abuse: The deliberate infliction of physical injury on a child, usually by the child's caregiver.

- Sexual abuse: The American Academy of Pediatrics defines sexual abuse as "the engaging of a child in sexual activities that the child cannot comprehend, for which the child is developmentally unprepared and cannot give informed consent, and/or that violate the social and legal taboos of society."[7]

Types of sexual abuse include, but are not limited to, digital manipulation; fondling; actual or attempted oral, vaginal, or anal intercourse; exhibitionism; and pornography.

- Munchausen syndrome by proxy: A rare form of child maltreatment in which the caregiver-perpetrators exaggerate, feign, or induce symptoms and/or illness in children and are motivated by the need to assume the sick role by proxy or to gain another form of attention.[5]

Conditions Mistaken for Child Maltreatment

There are a number of circumstances or conditions that can be confused for child maltreatment, including cultural, physical, and medical conditions. As stated earlier, a health care provider who discovers signs of child maltreatment is legally required to report these findings to child protective service agencies. Because the diagnosis of child maltreatment has serious consequences for the child, the family, and the suspected perpetrator, it is important not to arrive at the diagnosis of child maltreatment hastily, but to take a careful history, perform a thorough physical exam, and obtain necessary tests to rule out conditions other than abuse.

The health care team must maintain an awareness of cultural and religious health practices in the evaluation of potential maltreatment. This is a complex issue that requires balancing the parent's rights with keeping the child healthy and safe. Certain cultural practices or remedies can be misdiagnosed as child maltreatment by uninformed professionals.[11]

- Cupping—used in Asia, Europe, Russia, and the Middle East. A heated cup containing steam is applied to specific points on the body to "draw out the poison" or other evil elements. When the heated air within the container cools, a vacuum is created that produces circular ecchymotic areas on the skin. Cupping is often used for headaches and respiratory ailments.

- Coining—a Vietnamese practice that may produce weltlike lesions on the child's back when a coin is repeatedly rubbed lengthwise on the oiled skin to rid the body of disease. The intent is to promote the release of toxins that may be causing the illness. This practice is often used for respiratory ailments.

- Burning—a Southeast Asian practice whereby small areas of the skin are burned to treat pain, cough, diarrhea, failure to thrive, enuresis, and temper tantrums.

- Moxibustion—a Southeast Asian practice in which a stick of burning mugwort, incense, or yarn is placed over an affected area of the body. This may produce lesions that resemble cigarette burns, usually in a pattern of four, six, or eight marks, in a pyramid formation.

- Topical garlic application—a practice of the Yemenite Jews in which crushed garlic is applied to the wrists to treat infectious diseases. This can result in blisters or garlic burns.

- Traditional remedies that contain lead—greta and azarcon are used in the Mexican culture to treat digestive problems, paylooah is used in the Southeast Asian culture to treat rash or fever, and surma is used in India to improve eyesight.

The preceding practices are those of well-intentioned caring parents who are attempting to relieve pain and suffering for their children in the way their culture has taught them. It is important to explain to the caregivers why these types of remedies may be considered harmful (e.g., those that contain lead). This may require collaboration with a folk healer to explore different options or modifications to these practices that would cause less injury to the child such as not rubbing so hard during the practice of coining.

In some ethnic groups, normal skin pigmentations have also been frequently confused with bruising. Mongolian spots are benign bluish-gray areas of pigmentation. They are found in about 95% of African-American infants, 80% of Asian infants, 70% of Latino and Native American infants, and 10% of Caucasian infants. These areas of pigmentation are usually found over the sacral area and buttocks but may also be located on the legs, shoulders, upper arms, and face. Mongolian spots typically fade during childhood.[6,12]

Some medical conditions that may be mistaken for child maltreatment may include erythema multiforme, Henoch-Schönlein purpura, idiopathic thrombocytopenic purpura, leukemia, or hemophilia, which may cause bruising or lesions resembling a burn. Glutaricaciduria type 1 is a rare disorder of amino acid metabolism that can result in subdural and retinal hemorrhages after minimal trauma. Osteogenesis imperfecta results from abnormal collagen synthesis and is characterized as the "brittle bone" disease due to frequent fractures.[6]

Predisposing Factors

Multiple dynamics lead to situations that result in the maltreatment of children. There are factors that place the child at risk for maltreatment and the caregiver at increased risk for becoming abusive. Younger children, children with an irritable temperament, excessively demanding children, and children with developmental disabilities are more often victims of physical abuse than older children and children without these characteristics.[9] Although caregivers across the socioeconomic spectrum abuse their children, younger parents and those with a low income are at greater risk to abuse their children. **Table 13-1** lists the risk factors for child maltreatment.

The number of children surviving disabling medical conditions is increasing due to technological advances. The rates of child maltreatment have been found to be high in children who are blind, deaf, chronically ill, developmentally delayed, and behaviorally or emotionally disordered. In addition, child maltreatment may result in a disability, which in turn can precipitate further abuse. Several elements increase the risk of maltreatment for children with disabilities. Children with chronic illnesses or disabilities often place higher emotional, physical, economic, and social demands on their families. Parents with limited social and community support may be at especially higher risk for maltreating children with disabilities. Lack of respite or breaks in child care responsibilities can contribute to an increased risk of abuse and neglect.[13] Refer to Chapter 16, *Children with Special Health Care Needs*, for additional information.

General Assessment and Interventions

Indicators of Maltreatment

When a pediatric patient presents to the emergency department (ED) with an injury, the historical data and physical findings must be compared and evaluated in terms of congruency. The interactions among the pediatric patient, caregivers, and staff are also important to evaluate. Pediatric patients or caregivers may exhibit some of the following behaviors listed in **Table 13-2** that could indicate that the pediatric patient is suffering from child maltreatment.

Obtaining a Comprehensive History

It is essential to obtain a comprehensive history when maltreatment is suspected. It is also important to coordinate the collection of the complete history with all health care professionals who will be involved in the patient's care. This may include nurses, physicians, and social workers. Ideally, the interview should be led by a health care professional who has been specifically

Table 13-1 Risk Factors for Child Maltreatment

Child	Caregiver	Environmental
• Crying	• Childhood history of abuse	• Domestic violence or instability
• Prematurity	• Unmet emotional needs	• Poverty
• Prenatal drug exposure	• Belief in use of corporal punishment	• Unemployment
• Developmental or physical disability	• Rigid or unrealistic expectations of the child	• Poor housing
• Chronic illness	• Negative perceptions of the child	• Homelessness
• Recent illness	• Lack of parenting knowledge	• Frequent relocation
• Hyperactivity (ADHD)	• Single parent	
• Product of multiple births	• Social isolation	
• Product of an unwanted pregnancy	• Psychological distress	
• Toilet training or difficulty with developmental milestones	• Low self-esteem	
	• Acute and chronic stressors	
	• Health problems	
	• Divorce	
	• Alcoholism or substance abuse	
	• Recent arrest	

Table 13-2 Indicators of Child Maltreatment

Child	Caregiver
• Extremes of behavior (excessive compliance and passivity or overly aggressive)	• Inappropriate response to seriousness of child's condition
• Wary of physical contact with caregiver	• No explanation or changing explanation for injury
• Clingy and indiscriminate in his or her attachments	• Explanation does not match clinical findings
• Shows no expectation of being comforted, flat affect	• Concealment of past injuries
• Does not cry during painful procedures	• Delay in seeking medical attention
• Sexualized behavior toward adults or other children; has specific knowledge beyond developmental level	• Bypass hospitals closer to home
• Sudden and severe drop in school performance	• Caregiver exhibits psychologically destructive behaviors toward child
• Delinquency	• Hostility toward hospital staff
• Regressive behaviors	• Uncooperative
• Child appears malnourished, inappropriately dressed, or unkempt	• Tension between caregivers

trained in forensic interviewing. The following are general guidelines to assist in obtaining a comprehensive history when child maltreatment is suspected.

- Use a nonjudgmental and nonaccusatory approach, even when it is apparent that the caregiver has injured the pediatric patient. Convey a genuine concern for the pediatric patient.
- Conduct the interviews in a private setting.
- Interview the verbal pediatric patient alone, if possible. If separating the pediatric patient and caregiver is too distressing for the pediatric patient, allow the caregiver to remain in the room while cautioning them that they are to observe and support the pediatric patient without answering questions.
- Interview the caregivers separately.
- Use open-ended, nonleading questions. Begin with "What happened?" and follow with more specific questions.
- Do not promise not to tell anyone.
- Document what the pediatric patient says as direct quotes whenever possible.
- If a language barrier is present, utilize professional interpreters or staff fluent in the language.
- Complete a cultural assessment, as appropriate.
- Obtain pertinent history for the current problem using the CIAMPEDS format, which is discussed in Chapter 4, *Initial Assessment*.
- Elicit other pertinent information:
  - Developmental milestones the pediatric patient has achieved
  - Social history, including who cares for the pediatric patient routinely, who lives in the home, and who cared for the pediatric patient over the last several days
  - Family history of chronic disorders
  - Past medical history, including previous illnesses or injuries, hospitalizations, and ED visits

Along with a comprehensive history, it is imperative to complete a thorough physical examination to ensure that no injuries are missed. The physical exam should include a full head-to-toe examination with the pediatric patient unclothed. Height and weight should also be measured and plotted on a standard growth chart. Identify and document all injuries, old and new, comparing historical information to clinical evidence.

General Nursing Interventions for the Maltreated Child

Refer to Chapter 4, *Initial Assessment*, for a description of the general nursing interventions for the pediatric patient. After the primary assessment has been completed, the following interventions are initiated, as appropriate, for the pediatric patient's condition.

- Provide a safe environment.
- Provide appropriate treatment for injuries or identified medical needs.
- Provide emotional support to the pediatric patient and family. Assign one staff member to care for the family.
- Explain and prepare the pediatric patient and caregiver for all procedures and interventions.
- Provide information to caregivers regarding normal growth and development, and alternatives to corporal punishment as appropriate.
- Refer caregivers to appropriate social and community agencies for support and therapy.
- Report suspected child maltreatment in accordance with state or local guidelines.

Documentation and Evidence Collection

Medical records of evaluation for child maltreatment frequently become legal documents with important implications. Careful documentation of the reported history and physical findings can determine legal outcomes. Statements made by the pediatric patient to a health care provider may be admissible as evidence, depending on the jurisdiction.

The following should be documented when child maltreatment is suspected.

- The date and time of the interview. The information gathered during the interview, including the names of those present.
- The questions asked, the responses (verbatim), and emotional reactions observed during the interview.
- All relevant verbal statements made by the pediatric patient and caregivers should be documented verbatim, using direct quotations whenever possible.
- Date, time, and place of occurrence. Presence of witnesses.
- Sequence of events with recorded times.
- Description of the parent-child interactions.
- The physical examination should be documented with great detail. All injuries must be documented carefully and consistently on the pediatric patient's medical record.
  - Location, size, shape, and color of all cutaneous injuries including a drawing of a body outline
  - Distinguishing characteristics indicating a pattern injury
  - Symmetry or asymmetry of injury

- Evidence of past injuries, general state of health and hygiene

Table 13-3 is one example of a child abuse documentation template.

Proper evidence collection is an essential component of the care of the maltreated child. The evidence collected during the exam may be used in court and can drastically affect the outcome of such proceedings and the future safety of the pediatric patient.

- All visible external injuries, such as bruises and burns, should be photographed in color. If a 35-mm camera is being used, an instant, back-up photograph must also be taken. Forensic photographs must include a ruler, standard color chart in the field (if available), and patient data such as name, birth date, and medical record number. The acceptance of digital photography varies by jurisdiction. Forensic photography may also be deferred to local law enforcement specialists.

- All injuries must be carefully and consistently documented on the patient's medical record. Document shape, exact size, location, and appearance of all cutaneous injuries.

- In cases of sexual abuse, specific medical and forensic evidence may be collected. Protocols and equipment used for collecting and preparing medical evidence may vary from setting to setting; therefore, it is important to know what is used by each state and local jurisdiction.

- Psychosocial preparation for the examination is essential and increases the likelihood of cooperation.

Table 13-3 Child Abuse Documentation Monitor	
Consistency of injury with developmental stage	• Is the incident as described plausible for age and development of the child?
History inconsistency with injury	• Does the medical history of the child or the incident history change from person to person? • Is there a previous history of fractures, ingestions, or injuries? • Is the injury consistent with the presenting history?
Inappropriate parental concerns	• Do parents/caregivers: -Ask pertinent questions? -Seem concerned about outcomes? -Offer comfort measures to the child?
Lack of supervision	• Question family member/caregiver as to -What happened? -When it happened? -How it happened? -Where it happened? -Who was present?
Delay in seeking care	• Is the time frame between when the injury occurred and when medical care was sought reasonable? Note unusual delays.
Affect	• Document reaction of child to all family members/caregivers present. • Document response and behavior of family members/caregivers present.
Bruises of varying ages	• Document findings or absence of findings of head-to-toe exam with pediatric patient unclothed. • In documenting bruises note location, pattern, size, color, and number.
Unusual injury patterns	• Describe injury characteristics and diagnostic testing performed. Try to differentiate between nonintentional and inflicted patterns.
Suspicions	• Remember that a report to a child protective service team is just for a suspicion of abuse or neglect. You do not have to prove it. Photograph suspicious areas.
Environmental cues	• If a run report from EMS is present, does it contain any contributing information about the environment in which the injury occurred? Gather information from EMS personnel prior to their departure from the ED.

Reprinted from *Illinois Emergency Medical Services for Children's Child Abuse and Neglect Policy and Procedure Guidelines.* (2001). Retrieved July 29, 2003 from www.luhs.org/emsc.

- Pediatric patients who are unable to cooperate must never be physically restrained for an examination. Forced restraint for the examination could further traumatize the pediatric patient. In such cases, the pediatric patient may be examined under sedation in the ED or general anesthesia later in the operating room.
- The specimens and other evidence collected are determined based on whether the suspected sexual assault occurred within the last 72 hours and the nature of the sexual acts committed. The primary goal is to not only collect the offender's DNA, but also to corroborate the pediatric patient's story by linking the offender to the scene. The offender's DNA can be found in blood, semen, saliva and hair. Types of specimens or items that may be collected for evidence include the following.
  - Clothing to look for hair, fibers, semen, and other DNA that may be detected. If not laundered, DNA may be detectable for years. The integrity of the clothing may also be evaluated (e.g., torn areas, dirt, or fibers).
  - Hair samples to look for any loose hairs from the offender.
  - Oral, vaginal or penile, and rectal swabs to look for the presence of semen and to perform DNA typing of the offender.
  - Fingernail scrapings may be collected. If the victim scratched his or her offender or scraped his or her fingernails on the offender's clothing or items at the scene, valuable evidence might be found under the nails.
  - Miscellaneous stains or bite marks may be swabbed in an attempt to collect the offender's DNA. Examination under a Wood's lamp may be helpful in finding semen on the pediatric patient's body.
  - Blood may be collected from the victim to accompany the preceding evidence in order to provide a DNA standard for comparison.

All evidence must be sealed and stored securely to maintain the integrity of the evidence until released to law enforcement personnel. A written record of chain of evidence must be maintained.

Assessment and Interventions for Specific Types of Child Maltreatment

Neglect and Emotional Abuse

Neglect is the most common form of child maltreatment and accounts for about 58% of all reported child mal-treatment cases in the United States.[2] Emotional abuse is often suspected, but is very difficult to substantiate. Physical signs are often nonspecific, and health care providers must rely on behavioral indicators such as depression or acting-out behaviors to help identify a possible abusive situation. Any persistent and unexplained change in the child's behavior is an important clue to possible emotional abuse.

History

The history of a pediatric patient who has been neglected may include

- Delay in seeking health care for an injury or illness or poor health care, such as no immunizations
- History of previous injuries, ingestions, or exposures to toxic substances
- Self-stimulating behaviors, such as finger sucking, biting, or rocking
- Excessive absenteeism from school
- Substance abuse
- Delinquency
- History of being left alone, abandoned, or inadequately supervised

Signs and Symptoms

- Malnourishment or nonorganic failure to thrive (weight below the fifth percentile)
- Inactivity or extreme passiveness
- Poor hygiene and/or inappropriate attire
- Untreated dental caries and periodontal diseases that can lead to pain, infection, and loss of function. This can adversely affect learning, communication, nutrition, and other activities necessary for normal growth and development.[10]
- Lags in emotional and intellectual development, especially language

Diagnostic Procedures

- Consider toxicology screen if suspect ingestion or exposure to toxic substances.

Physical Abuse

Physical abuse may result in injuries from single or multiple episodes and can range from minor bruising to death. Inflicted injuries may involve the skin and soft tissues, bones, and/or all major organ systems.

History

The history of a pediatric patient who has been physically abused may include

- History inconsistent with developmental milestone achievements or abilities
- No explanation for the injury
- Vague, unclear, or changing account of how the injury occurred
- Discrepancy between the caregiver's and pediatric patient's accounts
- Inappropriate reaction to injury, such as failure to cry with pain
- Unreasonable delay in seeking medical attention
- Unrealistic expectations of the pediatric patient
- History of previous ED visits or hospitalizations for an injury

Signs and Symptoms

Bruises

Characteristics of noninflicted bruises

- On extensor surfaces and bony surfaces such as the elbows, knees, and shins
- Forehead and chin of a toddler

Characteristics of potentially inflicted bruises

- Unexplained bruises or welts
- Multiple or symmetric bruises or marks
- Bruises and welts to the face, mouth, neck, chest, abdomen, back, flank, thighs, or genitalia
- Bruises and welts with patterns descriptive of an object such as a looped cord, belt buckle, shoe or boot pattern, wire hanger, chain, wooden spoon, hand, or pinch marks (crescent-shaped bruises)
- Bruises in various stages of healing. See **Table 13-4** for dating of bruises by color.[15]

Burns

Chapter 11, *Pediatric Trauma*, includes the assessment and treatment of burn injuries. Correlation of the severity and pattern of the burn injury with the history provides a basis for the identification of inflicted burns.

Characteristics of noninflicted burns

- Asymmetric and/or splash pattern congruent with history
- Contact burn not uniform
- Treatment sought immediately

Characteristics of potentially inflicted burns

- Immersion burns: Circumferential and often symmetric "stocking" pattern burns to the feet, "glovelike" pattern burns to the hands, doughnut pattern burn to the buttocks

- Burns with sharply demarcated edges without splash patterns and/or symmetric burns
- Patterns descriptive of an object used such as cigar or cigarette burns; rope burns on wrists, ankles, torso, or neck from being bound; or uniform burns in the shape of an iron, radiator, or electric stove burner
- Burns to dorsum of the hand
- Splash patterns indicative of hot liquid being thrown on the pediatric patient
- Delay in seeking treatment

Bite Marks

Bite marks are lesions that may indicate abuse. Bite marks should be suspected when ecchymosis, abrasions, or lacerations are found in an ovoid pattern. The normal distance between the canine teeth in adult humans is 2.5 to 4.0 cm. The canine marks in a bite will be the most prominent or deepest parts of the bite. If the distance is > 3.0 cm, the bite was probably from an adult.[10] Forensic dentists can make impressions from the bite mark to help identify the perpetrator. DNA may also be obtained from the bite mark before cleaning the wound.

Head Injuries

The following are head injuries suggestive of physical abuse.

- Skull fractures: Multiple fractures, depressed occipital fracture, or any skull fracture in an infant. All skull fractures should have a history of appropriate severity.
- Subdural hematomas or subarachnoid hemorrhages are the most common types of inflicted head injury in children. If associated with retinal hemorrhage, shaken impact syndrome should be suspected.
- Scalp bruises and traumatic alopecia
- Dislocated lens, hyphema, corneal or conjunctival abrasion, laceration, or ulceration

Table 13-4 Dating of Bruises	
Color	**Age**
Red	0 to 1 days
Blue, purple	1 to 4 days
Green, yellow	5 to 7 days
Yellow, brown	8 to 10 days
Cleared	1 to 3 weeks

Reprinted with permission from Schwartz, A. J. & Ricci, L. R. (1996). How accurately can bruises be aged in abused children? Literature review and synthesis. *Pediatrics, 97*(2), 254–257.

- Bruising to the eyelid or periorbital tissue; orbital fracture
- Low-velocity or short vertical falls rarely result in serious head injuries (e.g., from a sofa or changing table)[8]

Shaken Impact Syndrome

Shaken impact syndrome is a serious form of child maltreatment most often involving children younger than 2 years but may be seen in children up to 5 years of age. Shaking by itself may cause serious or fatal injuries, but in many instances, there may be other forms of head trauma, such as impact injuries. Shaken impact syndrome is unlikely an isolated event, and evidence of prior child abuse is common.[18]

Signs of shaken impact syndrome may vary from mild and nonspecific to severe.

- History of poor feeding, vomiting, lethargy, and/or irritability
- Respiratory depression, apnea
- Altered level of consciousness or coma
- Seizures, abnormal posturing, hypotonia, full fontanel
- Fixed dilated pupils and/or retinal hemorrhages
- Subdural hematoma, subarachnoid hemorrhage, and/or depressed skull fracture from impact
- Bruising or fractures of the upper extremities or ribs (grip marks/injuries)

Skeletal Fractures

Any fracture can be caused by abuse. A fracture that results from abuse may be single or multiple, recent or old, or a combination and may be found in one or more sites. If one fracture is noted, total body films may be obtained when appropriate. The humerus is one of the most frequently injured bones in abuse as a result of being violently grasped by the arm, pulled, swung, or jerked.[1] Suspicious fractures include

- Multiple fractures in various bones, different stages of healing
- Metaphyseal-epiphyseal fractures at the end of long bones
- Rib fractures; scapular or sternal fractures usually resulting from a direct blow
- Transverse, oblique, and spiral shaft fractures
- Bilateral or symmetric fractures

Abdominal Injuries

Abdominal trauma may result from a kick or punch, and injury to gastrointestinal as well as solid organs may result. Abdominal injuries are very difficult to identify as abuse. There may be no signs of external injury, although the patient's condition may be poor, and shock may be present.[1] Abdominal injuries may have occurred several days prior to presentation because signs and symptoms are subtle, so it is important to extend your history to days prior.

Types of injuries seen in abuse cases include[1]
- Perforation of the gut
- Hemorrhage
- Laceration, contusion, hematoma: liver, spleen, duodenum, pancreas, mesentery, kidney

Symptoms associated with abdominal injury may include
- Abdominal distension; rigidity
- Vomiting and abdominal pain
- Bruising to the abdomen
- Fever, septic shock
- Hypovolemic shock
- Hematuria

Diagnostic Procedures

The differential diagnosis of child abuse includes nonabusive injuries and medical conditions that may mimic abuse. Ancillary tests may provide additional evidence of abuse or uncover further injury. These tests may also provide important medico-legal information.

Laboratory Studies

- Consider obtaining a complete blood count (CBC), platelet count, bleeding time, prothrombin time, and partial thromboplastin time when contusions or hematomas are found to rule out bleeding disorders.
- Consider obtaining a urine sample for glutaric-aciduria, a spinal tap, and blood cultures with central nervous system dysfunction.
- Consider obtaining liver enzymes, amylase, blood cultures, CBC, and urine for blood with abdominal injuries.

Radiographic Studies

Radiographic screening is indicated in children younger than 2 years with evidence of abuse and in infants with evidence of abuse and/or neglect. This screening may detect multiple and/or old fractures and should include multiple views of the skull, thorax, long bones, hands, feet, pelvis, and spine. However, fractures in children can be difficult to visualize, and serial radiographs are often advised. Radiographs should be obtained in radiology versus portable because the quality of the film is much better.

Some types of radiographic studies that may be obtained in suspected maltreatment include

- X-rays of any suspected injury. Fractures should be documented with at least two views.
- Computerized tomography (CT) for children with abusive head injuries and/or shaken impact syndrome to detect intracranial hematomas and cerebral edema. CT of the abdomen to uncover damage to the abdominal organs.
- Magnetic resonance imaging (MRI) or ultrasound.

Sexual Abuse

Sexual abuse presents in many ways, and because children who are sexually victimized generally are coerced into secrecy, a high level of suspicion may be required to recognize the problem.[7] The primary portal of entry into the health care system for many children who have been sexually abused is the ED.

Sexual Development in Children

Sexual abuse can be differentiated from sexual play by determining whether there is a developmental asymmetry among the participants and by assessing the coercive nature of the behavior.[7] Sexual play can be characterized by the following.[6]

- Children of the same developmental age and/or stage looking or touching genitalia
- No coercion or force
- No intrusion of body or orifices
- Nonabusive

An understanding of normal development of sexual behavior is helpful for distinguishing between normal and abnormal sexual activities. Genital self-stimulation is evident by 18 months in both sexes. Children learn to identify themselves as boys or girls by age 2 to 3 years and enjoy displaying their nude bodies. Between the ages of 3 and 6 years, children understand the differences between boys and girls, and masturbation is common. By the age of 6 or 7 years, children become more modest, although they remain curious about sex, dirty words, and pornography. As children enter adolescence, interest turns more toward the opposite sex. Up to one fourth of adolescents initiate sexual intercourse by 12 years of age.[6]

History

A behavioral history may reveal events or behaviors relevant to sexual abuse, even without a clear history of abuse in the child. An appropriate history should be obtained before performing the physical exam.[7]

The history may reveal the following characteristic behaviors.

- Sexualized activity with peers, adults, animals, or objects; seductive behaviors
- Age-inappropriate sexual knowledge or curiosity; excessive masturbation
- Regressive (e.g., wetting bed, sucking thumb) and/or aggressive behavior
- Sudden onset of phobias or fears
- Sleep disorders or nightmares
- Depression, withdrawn behaviors, and/or suicidal gestures
- Poor school performance, running away, and/or substance abuse
- Self-mutilation and/or eating disorders

In addition to the interview guidelines for child maltreatment stated earlier in this chapter, the following techniques may also be used with a pediatric patient who has been sexually abused.

- Use clear, simple language. Determine and use the pediatric patient's own terminology for describing body parts.
- Use age-appropriate media such as anatomic drawings and anatomically correct dolls to facilitate verbal communication.
- Avoid multiple interviews and limit the interview to one hour or less.

The following information should be gathered when obtaining the history of the sexual abuse incident(s):

- Date, time, and location of the attack(s).
- Description and/or name of the offender if known by the pediatric patient. Do not document "unknown assailant" if the pediatric patient does not know the offender's name but is familiar with the offender (e.g., janitor at school).
- The number of assailants, statements made by the offender(s) including threats, bribes, or intimidation.
- Physical force or other violent activity; involvement of other children or adults.
- Knowledge of photographs or movies taken of the child.
- Loss of consciousness and/or amnesia of the incident, which may indicate use of date-rape drugs.

Signs and Symptoms

Physical findings are often absent, even when the perpetrator admits to penetration of the pediatric patient's genitalia.[7]

- Vaginal, penile, or rectal pain, discharge, or bleeding
- Bruises, lacerations, or irritation of external genitalia, anus, mouth, or throat

- Chronic dysuria, enuresis, constipation, or encopresis
- Sexually transmitted disease, nonspecific vaginitis, or venereal warts
- Difficulty walking or sitting
- Pregnancy in young adolescents

Diagnostic Procedures

- Cultures obtained from the mouth, anus, and genitalia for *Neisseria gonorrhoeae*, *Chlamydia trachomatis*, and herpes simplex virus
- Wet preparation for *Trichomonas vaginalis* and the presence of sperm
- Blood for the Venereal Disease Research Laboratory (VDRL), which tests for syphilis.
- Blood for hepatitis B and HIV testing
- Pregnancy test

Additional Interventions

Current recommendations are to provide prophylactic treatment for *Chlamydia trachomatis* infection and *Neisseria gonorrhoeae* to sexual assault victims with a history of penetration (oral, vaginal, penile, or anal) and to provide prophylaxis for pregnancy prevention as appropriate. HIV prophylaxis is not universally recommended but should be considered.[7]

Drug-Facilitated Rape

Alcohol or drug use immediately before a sexual assault has been reported by more than 40% of adolescent victims and adolescent assailants.[15] The recent increase in the rate of adolescent acquaintance rape has been associated with the illegal availability of date-rape drugs such as Rohypnol® (flunitrazepam) and gamma-hydroxy-butyrate (GHB).[15,16] These drugs can go undetected if added to any drink. Date-rape drugs cause sedation and amnesia to the extent that victims cannot resist or may not be aware of a sexual assault. Other more common date-rape drugs include alcohol, marijuana, benzodiazepines, cocaine, heroin, and amphetamines. Any substance that is administered to lower sexual inhibition and enhance the possibility of unwanted sexual intercourse is potentially a date-rape drug.[16]

In a sexual assault involving a date-rape drug, the history may include[16,17]

- Awakening in strange surroundings with disheveled clothing and/or a feeling of being sexually violated.
- If some memory of the event remains, the victim may describe feeling paralyzed, powerless, and a disassociation of mind and body.
- Symptoms may be similar to alcohol intoxication, although the severity may not match the amount consumed.
- Sudden onset of symptoms after consuming a drink (15 to 20 minutes after ingestion). Symptoms can range from drowsiness, confusion, and impaired memory to coma.

Evidence Collection

- The sooner a urine specimen is collected after the event, the more likely that rapidly excreted drugs such as alcohol and GHB will be detected.
- Rohypnol and GHB are not detected on most urine toxicology screens. If a date-rape drug is suspected, a urine specimen should be sent to the local crime lab while maintaining the chain of evidence.

Munchausen Syndrome by Proxy

Munchausen syndrome by proxy (MSBP) occurs when a parent, usually the mother, simulates disease in her child for the gratification or attention she receives from having the child undergo medical diagnosis and treatment. This form of abuse includes both falsifying history to make it appear as if the child has an illness and actually producing illness in the child. The history provided is often elaborate and sophisticated and may also include falsified family history. The mother often demands extensive medical evaluation and appears to be very concerned for her child.

History

Warning signs of MSBP are listed in **Table 13-5**.

Signs and Symptoms

The most common chief complaints, or presentations, of MSBP include

- Apnea and seizures: May be falsified or created by partial suffocation.
- Vomiting or diarrhea: May be created by administering syrup of ipecac or laxatives.

Table 13-5 Warning Signs of Munchausen Syndrome by Proxy

- Unexplained, prolonged, recurrent, or extremely rare illness
- Discrepancies between clinical findings and history
- Discrepancy between the child's apparent good health and history of grave symptoms
- Illness is unresponsive to treatment
- Signs and symptoms occur only in parent's presence
- Parent is knowledgeable about illness, procedures, and treatments
- Parent is very interested in interacting with health care team
- Parent is very attentive toward child
- Signs and symptoms subside once separated from the parent

- Simulated or actual hemorrhage, bacteremia, rash, and fever.

Additional Interventions

Hospitalized children should be under constant surveillance.[14] This may include hidden video monitoring in coordination with law enforcement. All cases should be reported promptly and with careful documentation to child protective service agencies. The consequences of MSBP include persistence of abuse, emotional problems, chronic disability, and death. Other siblings may also be at risk for abuse. There is an association of this syndrome with unexplained infant deaths.

Evaluation and Ongoing Assessment

Children who have been maltreated require careful and frequent reassessment of airway patency, breathing effectiveness, perfusion, and mental status. Appropriate medical, surgical, and psychiatric treatment should be promptly initiated. Hospital admission is indicated for children whose medical or surgical condition requires inpatient management, in whom the diagnosis is unclear, and when no alternative safe place for custody is immediately available. If the safety of the child is in doubt, health care professionals should always err on the side of protecting the child. No matter how severe the abuse, children will usually grieve the separation from their parents. They need help to understand why they cannot return home and that it is in no way their fault or a punishment.

The parents should be told by the health care team why an inflicted injury is suspected, that the team is legally obligated to report the circumstance, that the referral is being made to protect the child, that the family will be provided with services, and that child protective services and law enforcement will be involved. Consider informing the family after security or law enforcement personnel is available to prevent possible removal of the child prior to further evaluation. Siblings and children cared for by the suspected abuser should have full examinations within 24 hours because they too are at risk for child abuse.

Health Promotion

Prevention

It is essential that health care providers are able to recognize children and families at risk for abuse. Prevention of child maltreatment has been an extremely difficult task.

Some interventions that may assist in prevention include

- Having educational and informational materials on parenting techniques, child abuse prevention, and domestic violence readily available in the ED waiting and treatment areas.
- Providing information on normal child growth and development and routine health care needs.
- Making referrals to appropriate services when the need for assistance is identified. Nurses need to know what kinds of community services are available, including self-help groups.
- Unlike preventive efforts for physical abuse and neglect, prevention of sexual abuse focuses on educating children to protect themselves. Sexual abuse prevention is more than teaching a child to say "no" or to recognize their right not to be touched in "private places." It is just as important to teach safety in terms of potential risk situations and to notify an adult no matter what the other person says or does.

Summary

Child maltreatment is a serious threat to the health and well-being of children of all ages and all socioeconomic backgrounds. Recognizing and reporting child maltreatment is essential in preventing subsequent injury. Most child abuse fatalities have already experienced some form of maltreatment before the severe or fatal injury is incurred. Nurses play a key role in prevention through early identification of children and caregivers at risk and initiation of appropriate referrals. Nursing care for the maltreated child includes providing a safe environment for the child, appropriate treatment for injuries, and emotional support to the child and family. Reporting all suspected child maltreatment cases to the appropriate child protective agency and law enforcement is critical in preventing further maltreatment.

A thorough physical exam and a comprehensive history are essential in diagnosing child maltreatment and should be documented in great detail. The physical examination should include a full head-to-toe assessment, paying special attention to any injuries noted. These injuries should be carefully and consistently documented, including the location, size, color, distinguishing patterns, symmetry, and evidence of past injuries. Ideally, the child and caregiver should be interviewed by a health care professional trained in forensic interviewing. The child should be interviewed alone and the caregivers separately. Careful documentation of both the history and physical examination can determine legal outcomes. All evidence that is gathered by health care professionals must be sealed and stored securely along with a written record of chain of evidence.

The health care team must be knowledgeable about the variety of conditions that may be mistaken for child maltreatment, including cultural, physical, and medical conditions. The diagnosis of child maltreatment requires obtaining a thorough history and physical examination as well as ancillary tests to rule out conditions that may mimic abuse.

Internet Resources

ARCH National Respite Network and Resource Center http://www.archrespite.org/index.htm

National Information Center for Children and Youth with Disabilities (NICHCY) http://www.nichcy.org

National Clearinghouse for Alcohol and Drug Information (NCADI) http://www.health.org

EPOCH-USA (End Physical Punishment of Children) http://www.stophitting.com/disathome

National Children's Alliance http://www.nca-online.org/features.html

National Coalition for the Protection of Children and Families (NCPCF) http://www.nationalcoalition.org.

"Never Shake a Baby" Campaign (in each state of the Unites States); National Clearinghouse on Child Abuse and Neglect Information http://www.calib.com/nccanch/pubs/prevenres/organizations/shake.cfm

Parents Anonymous http://www.parentsanonymous.org

References

1. Hobbs, C. J., Hanks, H. G. I., & Wynne, J. M. (1999). *Child abuse and neglect: A clinician's handbook* (2nd ed.). London: Harcourt Brace and Company.

2. United States Department of Health and Human Services. Administration for Children and Families. National Clearinghouse on Child Abuse and Neglect Information. (2001). *Child maltreatment 2001.* Retrieved August 5, 2003 from http://www.acf.hhs.gov/programs/cb/publications/cm01/cm01.pdf

3. Myers, J. E. B. (1992). *Legal issues in child abuse and neglect practice.* Newbury Park, CA: Sage.

4. Kairys, S. W., Johnson, C.F., & Committee on Child Abuse and Neglect. (2002). The psychological maltreatment of children: Technical report. *Pediatrics, 109*(4), e68.

5. Hettler, J. (2002). Munchausen syndrome by proxy. *Pediatric Emergency Care, 18*(5), 371–374.

6. Reece, R. M., & Ludwig, S. (2001). *Child abuse: Medical diagnosis and management* (2nd ed.). Philadelphia: Lippincott Williams and Wilkins.

7. American Academy of Pediatrics Committee on Child Abuse and Neglect. (1999). Guidelines for the evaluation of sexual abuse of children: Subject review. *Pediatrics, 103*(1), 186–191.

8. Tarantino, C. A., Dowd, M. D., & Murdock, T. C. (1999). Short vertical falls in infants. *Pediatric Emergency Care, 15*(1), 5–8.

9. Giardino, A. P., & Giardino, E. R. (2002). *Recognition of child abuse for the mandated reporter* (3rd ed.). St. Louis, MO: G. W. Medical Publishing, Inc.

10. American Academy of Pediatrics Committee on Child Abuse and Neglect in collaboration with the American Academy of Pediatric Dentistry Ad Hoc Work Group on Child Abuse and Neglect. (1999). Oral and dental aspects of child abuse and neglect. *Pediatrics, 104*(2), 348–350.

11. Ratliff, S. S., & Nguyen, H. (1989). *Southeast Asian healing practices, birthmarks, and amulets* [Poster]. Columbus, Ohio: Children's Hospital.

12. Bays, J. (1994). *Child abuse: Medical diagnosis and management.* Philadelphia: Lea & Febiger.

13. American Academy of Pediatrics Committee on Child Abuse and Neglect and Committee on Children with Disabilities. (2001). Assessment of maltreatment of children with disabilities. *Pediatrics, 108*(2), 508–512.

14. Hall, D. E., Eubanks, L., Meyyazhagan, S., Kenney, R. D., & Johnson, S. C. (2000). Evaluation of covert video surveillance in the diagnosis of Munchausen syndrome by proxy: Lessons from 41 cases. *Pediatrics, 105*(6), 1305–1312.

15. Kaplan, D. W., Feinstein, R. A., Fisher, M. M., Klein, J. D., Olmedo, L. F., Rome, E. S., et al. (2001). Care of the adolescent sexual assault victim. *Pediatrics, 107*(6), 1476–1479.

16. Weir, E. (2001). Drug-facilitated date rape. *Canadian Medical Association Journal, 165*(1), 80.

17. Schwartz, R. H., Milteer, R., & LeBeau, M. A. (2000). Drug-facilitated sexual assault ("date rape"). *Southern Medical Journal, 93*(6), 558–561.

18. American Academy of Pediatrics Committee on Child Abuse and Neglect. (2001). Shaken baby syndrome: Rotational cranial injuries-technical report. *Pediatrics, 108*(1), 206–210.

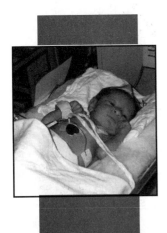

chapter 14

THE NEONATE

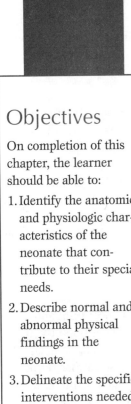

Objectives

On completion of this chapter, the learner should be able to:

1. Identify the anatomic and physiologic characteristics of the neonate that contribute to their special needs.

2. Describe normal and abnormal physical findings in the neonate.

3. Delineate the specific interventions needed to manage the neonate.

4. Identify health promotion strategies related to the neonate.

Introduction

Approximately 65% of all deaths in the first year of life occur during the neonatal period.[1] The term neonate is used to describe term infants (38 to 42 weeks gestation) from birth to 28 days of age.[2] However, the neonatal period for preterm, or premature, infants (delivered prior to 37 weeks gestation) is extended due to delays in or slower progression of development. The premature infant is considered a neonate until the expected due date plus 28 days is reached. The terms neonate and newborn will be used interchangeably.

Emergencies in the neonatal period may arise from either congenital or acquired conditions. The nurse's systematic examination of the neonate requires knowledge of normal growth and development of the neonate to identify subtle signs of illness or injury. The initial assessment, combined with a comprehensive history, is needed to determine the appropriate nursing diagnoses and needed interventions. Some information presented in this chapter may also apply throughout infancy.

The neonate may be brought to the emergency department for a variety of reasons and caregiver concerns. Common concerns include irritability or increased crying, poor feeding, fever, perceived constipation, vomiting, diarrhea, and jaundice. More severe concerns include decreased responsiveness, episodes of apnea, respiratory distress or tachypnea, seizures, and precipitous delivery.

Anatomic, Physiologic, and Developmental Characteristics as a Basis for Signs and Symptoms

Transitional Physiology of the Newborn

The transition from intrauterine life to extrauterine life begins as the newborn takes the first breath and the umbilical cord is cut. As the lungs fill with air and the alveoli fully expand, the partial pressure of oxygen (PaO_2) increases from fetal levels of approximately 25 mm Hg to a level of 50 to 70 mm Hg. Because oxygen is a potent pulmonary vasodilator, the arterioles in the lungs open. The pulmonary vascular resistance is decreased, and pulmonary blood flow is enhanced. This change from high to low pulmonary vascular resistance must occur in the first few minutes of life to establish normal neonatal circulation.[3] Newborns who are unable to elevate their PaO_2 to appropriate levels risk a continuance of fetal circulation (decreased blood flow to the lungs) called persistent pulmonary hypertension of the newborn.

Approximately 90% of neonates begin breathing spontaneously at birth and make the transition with minimal assistance, needing only warming, clearing of the airway, and mild stimulation. When intervention is required, neonates usually respond to positive pressure ventilation with a bag-mask device. Of the 10% requiring assistance, only about 1% require involved resuscitative measures.[4] Neonates rarely have primary cardiac arrest. Cardiac arrest in neonates generally follows a sequence of events that begins with respiratory distress and progresses to respiratory failure, respiratory arrest, and cardiac arrest.[5]

Preterm infants or those born small for their gestational age (SGA) are at greater risk for complications at the time of delivery and during the neonatal period. Perinatal mortality is the lowest in newborns who weigh between 3000 and 4000 grams (g) with an accompanying gestational age greater than 36 weeks.[6]

Thermoregulation

Neonates are highly susceptible to the development of cold stress, both from increased heat loss as well as from a diminished ability to produce heat. The newborn's proportionally large head, increased body surface area to weight ratio, and minimal subcutaneous fat allow for rapid heat loss with exposure. A cool ambient environment or a draft blowing across the newborn will increase the newborn's rate of heat loss. Additionally, these factors, in combination with the neonate's limited ability to produce heat, make this population particularly vulnerable to the development of hypothermia and cold stress.

Older children and adults produce heat through shivering, but neonates less than 6 months of age are unable to shiver and are dependent on nonshivering thermogenesis to produce heat.[7] When the infant is exposed to a cool environment, nonshivering thermogenesis begins, which causes an increase in the infant's metabolic rate and subsequent increases in oxygen and glucose consumption. The ill infant's ability to compensate for these additional physiologic demands is limited. As a result, cold stress can lead to hypoxia or accentuate existing hypoxia. Hypoglycemia, increased renal excretion of water and solutes, and metabolic acidosis may also develop. Pulmonary vasoconstriction may also occur, worsening any existing cardiovascular dysfunction and increasing the risk for heart failure.[6,7,8] Additionally, the presence of cold stress can impede the infant's ability to respond to resuscitative efforts.

To prevent the deleterious effects of cold stress, a neutral thermal environment that keeps the neonate's core temperature within normal range with minimal heat production must be provided. The use of an overbed radiant warmer is critical for the neonate who is already hypothermic or requires significant body exposure for resuscitation or other procedures.

Elevations in body temperature may also be seen in the neonate. Fever, defined as a rectal temperature > 38°C (> 100.4°F), may result from a number of conditions including infection, alteration in heat production, or exposure to extreme heat. Additionally, the neonate is less able to dissipate excess heat than the older infant;

therefore, overbundling in combination with a warm or hot ambient environment may elevate the neonate's body temperature.[6,9,10] As with hypothermia, fever increases physiologic demands due to the resulting increase in metabolic rate.

Pulmonary System

Anatomic and physiologic characteristics of the infant's pulmonary system are described in Chapter 6, *Respiratory Distress and Failure* (see Table 6-1). The neonate's higher respiratory rate fluctuates with crying (increases) and sleep (decreases). The slightly irregular respiratory rate of the neonate is normal and should not be confused with apnea, which is an episode of non-breathing for greater than 20 seconds or for less if accompanied by cyanosis or bradycardia. Term infants will often exhibit periodic breathing, a period of rapid respirations that are not labored followed by a pause of less than 20 seconds. Periodic breathing is not accompanied by cyanosis or bradycardia.[6]

The small and immature pulmonary system affects the neonate's ability to respond to increased physiologic demands. Increased oxygen consumption quickly leads to hypoxia in the ill neonate due to the limited ability to increase gas exchange. Due to limited respiratory reserves, increased respiratory demands may precipitate rapid progression from respiratory distress to respiratory failure.[7] Apneic episodes may occur as the neonate in respiratory distress fatigues.

Cardiovascular System

The neonate has a less compliant myocardium and a smaller contractile mass. The limited contractility in combination with a small stroke volume (1.5 ml/kg) affects the neonate's ability to increase cardiac output. Therefore, cardiac output is maintained by increasing the heart rate rather than stroke volume.[7,8] The neonate's resting functional heart rate is higher than in older children and will vary with crying and sleep. Transient bradycardia may occur with sleep or vagal stimulation during suctioning or defecation. However, a sustained bradycardia (< 100 beats/min) is most commonly a result of hypoxemia.[4]

Blood pressure measurement should be obtained in the ill neonate, although auscultation of the blood pressure may be difficult due to the lower systolic blood pressure. Utilizing an appropriately sized neonatal cuff, the blood pressure may be assessed by palpation, the use of a Doppler ultrasound, or oscillometry (e.g., mechanical recording). The preferred site for blood pressure measurement is the arm; however, other sites, such as the forearm, calf, or thigh, may be used with an appropriately sized cuff. The thigh is the most uncomfortable site and if used may agitate the neonate. Additionally, thigh blood pressures may be 4 to 8 mm Hg higher than the arm or calf.[6] Normal vital signs for neonates are listed in **Table 14-1**.

The neonate has vasomotor instability and sluggish peripheral circulation that may persist for hours, days, or weeks after birth. This may result in peripheral cyanosis or mottling of the hands and feet (acrocyanosis) related to transient changes in skin temperature. Central color, however, should be pink with strong central pulses. Persistent central cyanosis that does not respond to 100% oxygen and adequate ventilation may be due to a congenital defect that interferes with pulmonary or cardiac function.

Growth

Neonates usually lose up to 10% of their birth weight by the third to fifth day of life due to the excretion of excessive extracellular fluid by the kidneys. Breastfed neonates may lose slightly more weight than bottle-fed neonates because it may take several days for the mother's milk supply to begin. Most neonates have stopped losing weight by day five and will again reach their birth weight by day 10.[11] Normal neonatal weight gain is 0.5 to 1.0 ounce per day.

Other Characteristics

Other anatomic and physiologic characteristics of the neonate described in **Table 14-2**.[6]

Nursing Care of the Neonate

Assessment

The initial assessment of the neonate is the same as for any other pediatric patient. Refer to Chapter 4, *Initial Assessment*, for a review of a comprehensive primary and secondary assessment. However, the unique developmental characteristics of the neonatal period dictate some adjustments in the approach to the assessment and the incorporation of some additional components during the secondary assessment.

Approach to the Assessment of the Neonate

- Make the observational assessment prior to touching the neonate if possible. When disturbed, the neonate's normal reaction is to be startled and cry, thus changing the assessment of baseline respiratory and heart rates.

- Perform the most intrusive aspects of the assessment last, and use a toe-to-head approach to the secondary assessment.

- Protect the neonate against heat loss during the examination.

- Use sensorimotor and tactile comfort measures to soothe the neonate (i.e., swaddling, rocking, stroking skin, or speaking with a calm soothing voice).

- Allow the neonate to use a pacifier if desired. The normal neonate will have a strong sucking reflex.

- Observe the general condition of the neonate, including nutritional status, quality of cry, neonate and caregiver interaction, and behaviors and responses to comforting measures.

Additional History

Assessment of the neonate includes obtaining information about the pregnancy and delivery. This data, as outlined in **Table 14-3**, may yield information that is significant regarding pathology as well as the social setting.

Assessments Specific to the Neonate

Tables 14-4, 14-5, and **14-6** summarize various assessment findings that are specific to the neonate. Pain assessment of the neonate can be found in Chapter 12, *Pediatric Pain Assessment and Management*.

Diagnostic Procedures

A variety of radiographic and laboratory studies may be indicated based on the suspected etiology of the neonate's condition.

Radiographic Studies

- Chest film should be done for any neonate with a history of respiratory symptoms or any febrile neonate.

- Abdominal film should be done for the neonate with gastrointestinal symptoms or a positive abdominal examination.

- Combined chest and abdominal film, encompassing the torso from the neck to the pelvis, should be done

Table 14-1 Normal Vital Signs for Neonates	
Temperature	36.5°C to 37°C (97.7°F to 98.6°F) axillary
Respiratory rate	40 to 60 breaths/minute
Heart rate	110 to 160 beats/minute
Systolic blood pressure	65 to 86 mm Hg (60 is lower limit of normal for term newborn)

Reprinted with permission from Landry, N. (1999). Uncomplicated antepartum, intrapartum, and postpartum care. In J. Deacon & P. O'Neill (Eds.), *Core curriculum for neonatal intensive care nursing* (2nd ed., pp.2-17). Philadelphia: Saunders.

for the neonate with obvious abdominal distention. This particular film allows the practitioner to evaluate the effect of the abdominal distention on the lungs. In some institutions, this film may be referred to as a babygram.

- In order to obtain a good film, the neonate is held on the x-ray plate, maintaining good position without rotation. A pacifier may help to calm the neonate during the procedure.

Laboratory Studies

- Glucose. A whole blood or serum glucose test must be performed on all ill neonates. Due to decreased stores of glycogen in the liver, the stressed neonate may be unable to meet metabolic demands and may present with hypoglycemia. A bedside glucose test must be performed in addition to laboratory specimens. Serial bedside glucose testing is needed when the ill neonate requires correction of hypoglycemia.

- Total and direct bilirubin. Obtained on neonates who appear jaundiced. The jaundiced coloration of the skin progresses from head to toe as bilirubin levels increase. High levels should be suspected if the neonate's entire body is yellow-orange.[7]

Planning/Implementation

Refer to Chapter 4, *Initial Assessment*, for a description of the general nursing interventions performed during the initial assessment.

Table 14-2 *Additional Anatomic and Physiologic Characteristics of Neonates*

Neurologic system	The healthy term infant will have flexed arms and legs. Primitive reflexes are present, and movements are often uncoordinated. Neonates do feel pain, although they are unable to localize pain. Both the CRIES neonatal postoperative pain measurement score and the Premature Infant Pain Profile can be used to assess the infant in pain.
Renal system	Although all renal structures are present at birth, the kidneys are immature and not able to concentrate urine to conserve body water. Urine output is approximately 2 ml/kg/hr, and the bladder empties with a volume of 15 ml, resulting in frequent voiding (as many as 20 per day) of colorless, odorless urine. The kidneys also cannot dilute urine, conserve or excrete sodium, or acidify urine. This makes the neonate more prone to dehydration if given concentrated formula or overhydration if given too much free water.
Gastrointestinal system	Decreased stores of glycogen in the liver make the neonate especially prone to hypoglycemia, particularly when stressed. Due to immature liver function, physiological jaundice may occur when the liver's ability to excrete bilirubin from red cell hemolysis is exceeded. Regurgitation is common due to delayed gastric emptying and a relaxed lower esophageal sphincter.
Fluid and electrolytes	The newborn has a high ratio of extracellular fluid, resulting in higher total body sodium and chloride levels and lower levels of potassium, magnesium, and phosphate. The rate of fluid exchange is greater in the neonate than older children, resulting in minimal fluid volume reserve. The rate of metabolism is also increased, resulting in more acid formation and making the neonate more prone to the rapid development of acidosis when stressed.
Integumentary system	The epidermis and dermis are thin and loosely bound together, making the epidermis more prone to injury from friction such as removing tape too fast. Melanin levels are low at birth so that, regardless of race, skin color may be very light. This also makes infants more prone to the harmful effects of the sun.
Skeletal system	The newborn's skeleton is made up more of cartilage than ossified bone. The skull bones are soft and not fully joined at the sutures until around 18 months of age.
Endocrine system	The immature posterior pituitary gland produces limited amounts of antidiuretic hormone. With the inability to inhibit diuresis, the newborn is prone to dehydration.
Hemopoietic system	The venous hematocrit peaks at 2 to 4 hours of age and may be as high as 60 to 75%. Then, with normal red blood cell breakdown, the level will fall to 55% by day three and 52% by day 14. Capillary blood samples may show higher levels due to peripheral vasoconstriction. The circulating blood volume of the term infant is approximately 80 to 100 mL/kg and of the preterm infant is 90 to 105 mL/kg.[12]

Additional Interventions

- Assess need for admission. Prepare for admission or transfer to a neonatal intensive care unit, pediatric intensive care unit, or pediatric floor equipped to care for neonates.

- Prevent heat loss/correct hypothermia. Use commercial radiant warmer or heat lamps for neonates requiring invasive procedures, resuscitation, or exposure for close observation. Cover the neonate's head and wrap in a blanket when exposure is not required for procedures or observation. Monitor temperature.

- Obtain weight. Completely undress (including diapers) the neonate and obtain a weight if possible.

- Keep the base of the umbilical stump dry and exposed to air. The diaper should be folded down so that the umbilical stump is exposed. Although historically

Table 14-3 Pregnancy and Delivery History

Prenatal history	• Mother's health before and during pregnancy • Singleton versus multiple gestation (e.g., twin, triplet) births. If multiple gestation, health status of sibling(s). • Drug use during pregnancy • Prenatal care (started during which week of pregnancy) • Maternal age • Other children in family (e.g., Is this the first baby for both parents?)
Delivery history[13]	• Type of delivery (vaginal, cesarean section). If cesarean section, emergent or planned. • Problems associated with labor • Problems at birth • Birth weight • Gestational age at birth • Length of hospital stay (of both mother and infant). Ask, "Did your baby come home from the hospital with you?" If the answer is no, further inquiry is necessary as to why the infant stayed in the hospital. • Problems or interventions during hospital stay. Particularly ask about oxygen delivery and intubation.
Diet	• Breast milk • Formula—If formula, ask what type (name), which form (premixed, liquid concentrate, or powder), and how it is mixed (e.g., number of scoops of powder to ounces of water).
Feeding patterns	• Length of time neonate nurses at each feeding or amount taken per feeding • Typical time required to complete feeding • Interval between feedings • Awakens self for feedings. Neonates should awaken to feed every two to three hours. Infants will not sleep through the night until 2 to 6 months of age. A neonate who sleeps through the night is cause for concern. • Quality of suck • Eagerness to feed • Does neonate finish each feeding without prompting (or does neonate fall asleep partway through and need repeated stimulation to finish feeding)? • Color change with feeding • Changes in feeding behavior
Sleep patterns	• Has caregiver noted any changes in sleep patterns? • How do parents place neonate for sleeping? On the back is the recommended position.
Urine	• Usual number of wet diapers per day • Number of wet diapers in previous 24 hours • Last wet diaper • Changes noted
Stool[11]	• Usual number of bowel movements per day. Breastfed infants typically have more bowel movements per day than bottle-fed infants. • Color, consistency, and odor • Changes noted

alcohol has been used for daily cord care, current research does not support this practice.[15]

- Provide circumcision care. Apply a petroleum gauze dressing over the healed circumcision site and apply diaper loosely to prevent friction against the penis.

- Offer the option of family presence. Encourage caregivers to remain with the neonate and to hold and comfort the neonate. Promote sensory soothing interventions (i.e., rocking, stroking skin, or sucking on pacifier).

- Support the breastfeeding mother. The neonate may need to be NPO during the assessment and initial treatment period. Provide the mother access to a breast pump with disposable fittings and privacy as needed.

- Treat hypoglycemia. Administer 15 to 30 ml of 5% dextrose orally to the stable neonate > 34 weeks gestation with no respiratory distress. Administer 2 ml/kg of $D_{10}W$ intravenously over 1 minute for documented and symptomatic hypoglycemia.[16] Reassess

serum glucose 15 to 20 minutes after the dextrose bolus and hourly until glucose level is stable.

- If neonate is NPO, deliver maintenance intravenous (IV) fluids as indicated by patient condition. Administer $D_{10}W$ at 80 to 120 ml/kg/day via an infusion pump.[17] Fluids should be $D_{10}W$ for the first 24 hours of life and $D_{10}.2$ NaCl if over 24 hours old and voiding.

Evaluation and Ongoing Assessment

The care of the neonate is challenging and requires knowledge of transitional and immature physiology. The neonate requires meticulous and frequent reassessment. Subtle signs and symptoms of illness may be indicative of critical illness in the neonate. Ongoing evaluation of airway patency, breathing effectiveness, circulation, temperature, and urine output are essential in evaluating progress toward expected outcomes. Key to assessment is the knowledge of normal behaviors in this stage of life and an awareness of what the normal neonate should look like and do.

Table 14-4 Infant Reflexes

Reflex	Response	Duration
Sucking	Exhibits strong movements of the mouth in response to stimulation	12 months
Rooting	When cheek is touched or stroked along the side of the mouth, the infant turns head toward that side and begins to suck.	12 months
Grasp	Digits flex when palm of hand or sole of the foot are touched	3 to 8 months
Startle	With sudden loud noise, arms abduct with flexion of the elbows	4 months
Babinski	When the sole of the foot is firmly stroked in an upward direction from heel to toe, the great toe flexes toward the top of the foot and the other toes fan out.	24 months

Table 14-5 Additional Neonatal Assessments

Assessment	Normal	Cause for Concern
Muscle tone and posture	The neonate's normal posture is one of flexion with good muscle tone. The arms are flexed at the elbows, and the hands are usually clenched. The legs are flexed at the knees, the hips are flexed, and the feet are dorsiflexed.	Neonates stressed by an acute disease process may have outstretched, limp extremities.
The umbilicus	Assess the umbilicus for the presence and condition of the umbilical cord stump. The cord should completely separate in 7 to 14 days, and the cord base should be healed by the end of the first month.	Until the umbilicus is completely healed, the umbilical vessels are a potential site of entry for infection. Abnormal findings include redness, swelling, drainage, or foul odor.
The circumcision site	The site will develop a yellowish-white scab by the second day after the circumcision. If the Plastibell procedure was used, the plastic ring remains on the penis until it separates in approximately 5 to 8 days.	Abnormal findings include bleeding, swelling, exudate, foul odor, or erythema extending down the shaft of the penis.

Table 14-6 Abnormal Neonatal Assessment Findings and Potential Causes

Assessment Findings	Potential Causes

Cyanosis (mucous membranes or trunk)	• Hypoxia
	• Respiratory distress or failure
	• Congenital heart disease
	  - Congestive heart failure causing impaired alveolar ventilation
	  - Right-to-left shunting due to cardiac lesion
	• Infection/sepsis
	• Poor perfusion, shock
	• Acidosis
	• Polycythemia
	• Methemoglobinemia
	• Central nervous system (CNS) injury, malformation, or disease causing a diminished respiratory drive

Mottling of skin	• Hypothermia/cold stress (vascular instability) • Poor perfusion from hypovolemia • Infection/sepsis • Hypoxia • Congenital heart disease
Pallor–soles of feet, palms of hands, nail beds, mucous membranes	• Poor perfusion • Poor oxygenation • Low hemoglobin • Infection/sepsis • Hypothermia • Shock • Hypoxia • Congenital heart disease
Jaundice	• Hyperbilirubinemia secondary to blood group incompatibilities • Primary liver disease • Extrahepatic obstruction such as biliary atresia • Infection/sepsis • Hemolysis reaction secondary to bruising during delivery • Physiologic jaundice • Breast milk jaundice • Genetic and metabolic disorders
Lethargy, hypotonia–decreased muscle tone, poor feeding or lack of interest in feeding, difficult to arouse or elicit a response to stimuli, increased sleeping times, decreased reflexes (i.e., suck, grasp, startle, rooting)	• Sepsis • Hypoxia • Respiratory distress or failure • Dehydration • Shock • Hypoglycemia
Irritability–increased activity level, poor sleep patterns or decreased sleeping times, inconsolable	• Infection • Pain or discomfort • Colic • Withdrawal from maternal substance abuse • Hypoglycemia • Feeding intolerance • Overstimulation

Table 14-6 Abnormal Neonatal Assessment Findings and Potential Causes (cont.)

Assessment Findings	Potential Causes
Hypertonic–arms and hands tightly flexed, arching of back and neck, legs stiff and extended, startles easily	• Meningitis • Neurologic injury or dysfunction

Jittery, seizure activity–lip smacking, eye fluttering or repeated eye movements, bicycling movements of legs, shaking of one or more extremities	• Hypoglycemia
	• Hypocalcemia
	• Sepsis
	• Seizure disorder
	• Electrolyte disturbance
	  - Secondary to diarrhea and vomiting
	  - Secondary to error in formula preparation
	• Meningitis
	• Increased intracranial pressure
	• Neurologic injury or dysfunction

Hypothermia
  Axillary temperature < 36.5°C (< 97.9°F)
  Rectal temperature < 36°C (< 96.9°F)
	• Sepsis
	• Cold ambient environment
	• Neurologic dysfunction

Hyperthermia
  Axillary temperature > 37.5°C (> 99.5°F)
  Rectal temperature > 38°C (> 100.4°F)
	• Sepsis
	• Warm ambient environment
	• Bundled heavily in clothing and blankets in warm environment

Apnea	• Airway obstruction (congenital deformity, swelling, secretions, positioning) • Sepsis • Respiratory infection • Gastroesophageal reflux • Hypoglycemia • Seizures
Bradypnea	• Respiratory failure • Cardiopulmonary failure • Neurologic compromise
Tachypnea–consistent respiratory rate > 60 breaths/min after 6 to 8 hours of age	• Respiratory infection, pneumonia • Hypoxia • Sepsis • Hyperthermia • Congenital heart disease, congestive heart failure • Hypoglycemia • Acidosis • Dehydration • Shock • Pain or discomfort
Bradycardia–heart rate < 100 beats/min	• Late response to hypoxia • Late response to shock • Apnea • Sepsis • Hypothermia • Neurologic compromise

Table 14-6 Abnormal Neonatal Assessment Findings and Potential Causes (cont.)

Assessment Findings	Potential Causes
Tachycardia–sustained heart rate > 180 beats/min	• Dehydration • Shock • Hypotension • Acidosis • Sepsis • Respiratory distress • Hypoxia • Congenital heart disease • Hyperthermia • Crying
Depressed or sunken anterior fontanel	• Dehydration
Bulging anterior fontanel–assessed with infant in an upright position and quiet	• Hydrocephalus • Increased intracranial pressure
Diarrhea–an increase in the number of stools with an increased water content	• Viral infection • Bacterial infection • Toxic reaction to food or other poison • Formula intolerance • Antibiotic therapy side effect
Constipation–first newborn stool should be passed by 36 hours of age	• Infrequent passage of stool • May be accompanied by abdominal distention and discomfort • Stool may be hard • Stool may be blood streaked, formula incompatibility (change of formula) • Meconium plug • Meconium ileus (early sign of cystic fibrosis) • Congenital intestinal obstruction, atresia, or stenosis • Malrotation • Hirschsprung disease
Vomiting–a forceful ejection of the gastric contents, may be present with abdominal distention	• Infection • Pyloric stenosis • Bowel obstruction, atresia, or stenosis • Malrotation • Gastroesophageal reflux • Necrotizing enterocolitis
Hypoglycemia–symptomatic infant with blood glucose < 45 mg/dl or asymptomatic term infant with risk factors and blood glucose < 36 mg/dl[14]	• Increased glucose utilization (asphyxia, hypothermia) • Sepsis • Prolonged seizures • Elevated insulin levels (infant of diabetic mother) • Inadequate substrate supply (premature infant, intrauterine growth retardation, SGA) • Congenital defects or syndromes

Selected Emergencies

Delivery of a Baby in the Emergency Department (ED)

Although the obstetrical suite is the ideal location for delivery, many births will occur either in the ED or prior to arrival at the hospital. The ED staff must be prepared to care for both the mother and the neonate and have an understanding of the neonate's special needs in the first few minutes of life. Any neonate born prior to arrival in the ED must receive the same serial assessment and care as outlined for the neonate born in the hospital.

The assessment and resuscitation of the newly born infant should occur simultaneously.

There are many conditions that place the neonate at risk for complications at the time of or immediately following delivery. Examples of these conditions are described in **Table 14-7**.[4,18]

Additional History

Although a maternal history can alert the health care team to potential neonatal problems, it may be impractical to obtain a detailed history in the ED when delivery is imminent. Although early and thorough prenatal care is recommended, it must be remembered that the lack of prenatal care does not mean there will be problems with delivery, nor does it mean the neonate will have problems.

Should a delivery be necessary in the ED, the following may aid in preparing for the birth.

- Assess for the presence of meconium in the amniotic fluid. Ask, "What color was your water when it broke?" Meconium-stained infants who are not vigorous at the time of delivery will need immediate intubation and suctioning.

- Estimate gestational age of the fetus. Ask, "When is your baby due?" Premature infants require ventilatory support more frequently than term infants.

- Determine anticipated number of fetuses. Ask, "How many babies are there?" A multiple birth will require more personnel and equipment at the time of delivery.

Table 14-7 Conditions That Place Neonate at Risk for Complications Following Delivery[4,16]

Maternal Factors	Environmental Factors	Fetal Factors
• Maternal age < 16 or > 35 years	• Poverty (related to poor nutrition and health care)	• Multiple gestation (carrying two or more fetuses)
• Prepregnant weight < 100 lbs (45.5 kg)	• Maternal drug use (alcohol, cocaine, narcotics)	• Abnormal fetal heart rate
• Anemia	• Exposure to environmental toxins	• Meconium-stained amniotic fluid
• Cephalopelvic disproportion	• Narcotics administered to mother within 4 hours of delivery	• Prematurity
• Maternal nutritional deficiencies		• Postterm gestation
• Chronic disease (renal disease, diabetes, heart disease)		
• Hypertension		
• Infection		
• Surgery during pregnancy		
• Prolonged labor (> 24 hours)		
• Prolonged rupture of membranes (> 18 hours prior to delivery)		

Table 14-8 Equipment Specific to Delivery in the ED

- Personal protective items such as gloves, gowns, and masks with eye shield
- OB kit–usually contains items for a normal, uncomplicated delivery, such as towels, cord clamps, scalpel, bulb syringe, footprint and thumbprint kit, and ID bands
- Radiant warmer or heat lamps
- Resuscitation bag capable of delivering 90 to 100% oxygen and capable of avoiding excessive pressures—200- to 750-mL bag-the smaller bag is for preterm infants. A 450- to 500-mL bag will work for most neonates, regardless of gestational age.
- Resuscitation masks–sizes for premature to term infants
- Laryngoscope handle and blades-sizes 0 and 1
- Endotracheal tubes (sizes 2.5, 3, 3.5, and 4) with stylets
- Suction catheters–sizes 5 or 6, 8, and 10 Fr
- CO_2 detector (optional)–infant use up to 15 kg
- Meconium aspirator
- Gastric tube–8 or 10 Fr
- Medications–Epinephrine 1:10,000; sodium bicarbonate 4.2% (0.5 mEq/cc); naloxone

- Determine drug history. Ask, "Have you taken any medications or drugs in the last day?" A history of narcotic use in the 4 hours prior to delivery may result in a neonate with a depressed respiratory effort. The use of some illegal drugs may cause uterine contractions and premature labor.

Table 14-8 provides a list of the equipment needed to facilitate a delivery in the ED.

Delivery

In preparation for a delivery, it is important to remember that approximately 90% of neonates are able to make the transition from intrauterine to extrauterine life without difficulty. These infants require little or no assistance in establishing effective ventilation. About 10% of neonates require some assistance with ventilation whereas only 1% require extensive resuscitative measures.[4]

Figure 14-1 represents the relationship between resuscitative measures and the number of newly born infants who need those procedures. The top of the inverted pyramid illustrates the interventions needed by all infants; the bottom those interventions needed by only a few infants.[4]

Figure 14-2 illustrates the neonatal resuscitation process, beginning with the birth of the neonate. Based on the assessment of the newborn, resuscitation, if necessary, proceeds from one step to the next.

During and following the clamping and cutting of the umbilical cord, the initial assessment is made. If the answer to the first five questions is yes, the newly born

infant will need little intervention other than drying and keeping warm.

If the answer to any of the first five questions is no, the initial steps of resuscitation should be provided.[4]

- Dry and warm the neonate.
  - Place the neonate in a warm area and dry thoroughly.
  - A radiant warmer, heat lamps, or an exam light may be used as a heat source.

Figure 14-2 Neonatal Resuscitation Flow Diagram

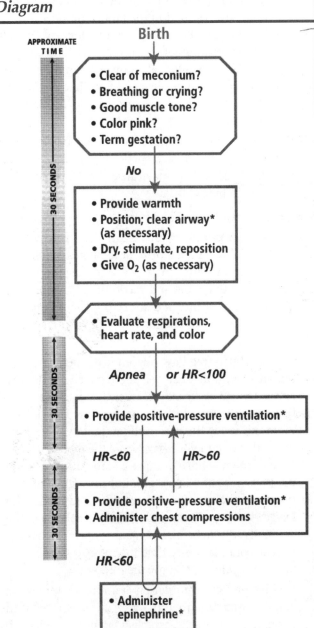

* Endotracheal intubation may be considered at several steps.

Reprinted with permission from Kattwinkel, J. (2000). Overview and principles of resuscitation. In *Neonatal resuscitation* (4th ed., pp. 1-1–1-22). Elk Grove Village, IL: American Academy of Pediatrics and American Heart Association.

Figure 14-1 Relationship of Neonatal Resuscitation Procedures to Number of Newborns who need them

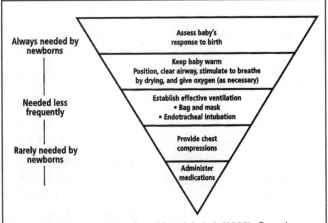

Reprinted with permission from Kattwinkel, J. (2000). Overview and principles of resuscitation. In *Neonatal resuscitation* (4th ed., pp. 1-1–1-22). Elk Grove Village, IL: American Academy of Pediatrics and American Heart Association.

- Quick removal of amniotic fluid from the head and body helps prevent evaporative heat loss.
- Remove wet towels and wrap the neonate with pre-warmed towels or blankets; cover the neonate's head with a blanket or hat.

• Maintain airway patency.
- Position the neonate in a neutral position. A rolled washcloth or cloth diaper may be used under the shoulders to facilitate maintenance of correct airway position.
- Using a bulb syringe, suction the mouth and then the nose. Always suction the mouth first because nasal suctioning may cause gasping or crying, resulting in the aspiration of oral secretions. The bulb syringe is usually adequate; however, an 8 Fr or 10 Fr suction catheter connected to mechanical suction may be used (negative pressure must not exceed -100 mm Hg).
- Repeated suctioning of the mouth may be performed as necessary. Avoid deep suctioning of the posterior pharynx because this may cause a vagal response resulting in bradycardia.

• Maintain breathing effectiveness.
- Assess the respiratory rate, effort, and effectiveness of respiration. The majority of neonates will begin effective respirations in response to the stimulation provided with drying and suctioning. Newborns may be dusky at the time of delivery but should rapidly turn pink with the establishment of effective respirations.
- Deliver 100% free flow oxygen if the newborn remains centrally dusky with effective respirations and an adequate heart rate. A simple face mask held firmly on the face with an oxygen flow rate of 5 liters/minute is the preferred method. An alternate method is to cup your hand over the mouth and nose of the newborn and place standard oxygen tubing (flow rate of 5 liters/minute) through your fingers so that your hand becomes a "reservoir" for oxygen buildup. Once the newborn's color is pink, gradually withdraw the oxygen, continually assessing the color. If at any time the newborn again becomes cyanotic, reapply the oxygen.
- Positive pressure ventilation at a rate of 40 to 60 breaths/minute with 100% oxygen is required if the neonate is not able to establish effective respirations after these interventions or if the heart rate is less than 100 beats/min. Intubation may be performed at this time.

• Maintain adequate circulation.
- Palpate central pulse (femoral or umbilical). The heart rate should be > 100 beats/minute. If the newborn's heart rate is < 100 beats/minute, initiate positive pressure ventilation with 100% oxygen.
- Begin cardiac compressions if the heart rate is below 60 beats/minute after 30 seconds of positive pressure ventilation with 100% oxygen. Use two fingers or two thumbs placed one finger breadth below the nipple line to provide compressions at a ratio of three compressions to one ventilation (approximately 120 beats/minute). Reevaluate the heart rate after 30 seconds of chest compressions, and stop compressions when the heart rate is 80 or greater but continue ventilation

• Obtain vascular access.
- The umbilical vein is the most common and accessible route for administering drugs and fluids in the neonate. Umbilical catheter insertion is a sterile procedure performed only by trained individuals.
- Veins in the scalp and extremities can be used; however, these sites can be difficult to access in the neonate with poor perfusion. Also, they are impractical if large volumes of fluid or emergent medication boluses are necessary because they cannot accommodate fast infusion rates.
- The intraosseous route can also be used in the neonate.
- Volume expanders should be given when there is evidence of hypovolemia such as profound pallor, weak pulses with a good or rapid heart rate, and a poor response to resuscitation.
  ■ Administer 10 ml/kg of a crystalloid solution, such as lactated Ringer's or 0.9% normal saline, or O-negative blood crossmatched with the mother, over 5 to 10 minutes. Warmed solutions are preferred.

• Administer medications.
- If the heart rate is < 60 beats/minute after 30 seconds of chest compressions accompanied by positive pressure ventilation with 100% oxygen, medications need to be given.
  ■ Epinephrine is the drug of choice for bradycardia or asystole.
- If positive pressure ventilation has restored good heart rate and color, but the newborn continues to have poor respiratory effort, consider the possibility of narcotic effects. Naloxone will reverse the effects of the narcotic on the neonate; however, do not give to the neonate of an addicted mother because this will result in seizure activity. Narcotic duration may exceed that of naloxone, and repeat doses may be needed; therefore, close monitoring is necessary.

Delivery of Neonate with Meconium-Stained Amniotic Fluid

Meconium is the first stool passed by the newborn. If passed by the fetus prior to delivery, meconium will appear in the amniotic fluid and can be described as thin or thick. If meconium is aspirated by the neonate, it can interfere with the normal expansion of the alveoli. This begins a cascade of events that prevents the transition from intrauterine to extrauterine ventilation and circulation.

Table 14-9 describes the additional interventions for delivering a neonate with meconium-stained amniotic fluid.

Apgar Score[4]

The Apgar score is a standardized rating system of five factors that reflect the infant's ability to adjust to extrauterine life (see **Table 14-10**). It is used to relay information about the newborn's response to the initial steps of resuscitation at birth, not to determine the need for resuscitation. The Apgar score is assigned at 1 minute and at 5 minutes of age. When the 5-minute Apgar score is less than 7, additional scores should be assigned every 5 minutes for 20 minutes.

The Premature Infant[2,4,19]

Prematurity is defined as the birth of an infant born at less than 37 weeks gestation. Premature infants will generally be discharged to home when the following criteria are met.[2]

- Weight around 1900 g with a steady weight gain of 20 to 30 g/day
- Able to maintain temperature when bundled in an open crib
- Able to tolerate feedings (either oral or tube)

Considerations in the Assessment and Care of the Premature Infant in the ED

The premature infant is

- More prone to hypothermia and cold stress
- More prone to hypoglycemia if stressed
- More prone to dehydration and shock if vomiting and diarrhea occur
- More prone to bruising (fragile skin and capillaries)
- Less able to tolerate periods without fluids and nutrients
- More prone to feeding difficulties

Delays in all areas of development may be seen in the premature infant. The delays may be secondary to the prematurity itself, to complications of prematurity, or to an extended time spent on ventilatory support and medications.[19] Development should be assessed by using the corrected age for the first 2 years. Many premature infants, although they start out slow, will exhibit normal development by their second birthday. Using a

Table 14-10 Apgar Score

Sign	0	1	2
Heart rate	Absent	< 100 beats/min	> 100 beats/min
Respiratory effort	Absent	Slow, irregular	Good, crying
Muscle tone	Limp	Some flexion	Active motion
Reflex irritability	No response	Grimace	Cough or sneeze
Color	Blue or pale	Pink body with blue extremities	All pink

Table 14-9 Additional Interventions for Delivering a Neonate with Meconium-Stained Amniotic Fluid

Meconium present in amniotic fluid	Allow the birth to continue. Do not suction until after the birth is completed.
	Bulb syringe or mechanical or wall suction with negative pressure no greater than 100 mm Hg and a 10 Fr or larger suction catheter can be used.
Assess the infant for vigor (after cord clamped and cut)	The vigorous infant will have strong respiratory efforts, good muscle tone, and a heart rate greater than 100 beats/minute.
• Infant vigorous	Proceed with the initial steps of resuscitation as outlined in Figure 14-2.
• Infant not vigorous	Suction the hypopharynx under direct vision.
	Using a meconium aspirator and an appropriately sized endotracheal tube, intubate the trachea and suction any meconium present in the lower airway as the endotracheal tube is being removed.
	Reintubation may be necessary if a large amount of meconium was obtained and the heart rate is < 100 beats/min.

corrected age helps prevent concerns in the premature infant who is not developing according to the standard charts for age.

Corrected age is the postdelivery age minus the number of weeks the infant was born prematurely. An alternative method to calculate the corrected age is by using the expected date of delivery as the birth date for the corrected age.

Neurologic abnormalities, such as abnormal posture, increased or decreased muscle tone, or increased or decreased deep tendon reflexes, may be present related to a delay in maturation of the CNS or secondary to neurological damage.

Abdominal musculature and structures close late in fetal development. Problems related to abdominal wall development, including inguinal or umbilical hernias or undescended testes, are common in premature infants.

Complications of prematurity include bronchopulmonary dysplasia; vision loss secondary to retinopathy of prematurity that occurs from the effects of hyperoxemia, hypoxemia, acidosis, and hypercarbia on the poorly vascularized retina; and hearing loss as the result of infection, ototoxic drugs, or hypoxemia causing injury to the auditory pathways of the brain.

Neonatal Sepsis

The incidence of neonatal sepsis is between 1 in 1,000 and 8 in 1,000 term births and 1 in 250 preterm births.[2] The neonate is at risk for infection and sepsis because of an immature immune system, impaired phagocytosis, and decreased complement levels. Other contributing factors include exposure to infectious agents in the birth canal and environmental exposures. Due to the infant's decreased ability to respond to pathogens, there is frequently not a localized reaction, and symptoms are vague and generalized. Common sites of infection include blood, lungs, urinary tract, and cerebrospinal fluid (CSF).[6]

Table 14-11 describes the signs and symptoms that a neonate with sepsis may exhibit.

Additional Interventions

Septic infants may present with mild symptoms or may present in shock and a prearrest state. Interventions to support airway, breathing, and circulation (ABCs), as previously listed in Chapter 4, *Initial Assessment*, should be performed.

The key intervention, after support of ABCs, is the prompt initiation of antibiotic therapy. In addition, do not administer anything by mouth if any respiratory distress is noted or if the neurologic status is depressed.

Vascular access should be obtained and maintenance IV fluids started.

The lumbar puncture should be deferred until infant is stabilized. Additional diagnostic tests that may be ordered as part of a sepsis workup include the following.

- Complete blood count with differential and platelets
- Electrolytes, including blood glucose and bedside glucose
- Prothrombin time, partial thromboplastin time
- Bilirubin
- Arterial or capillary blood gas
- Blood and/or urine cultures; surface cultures (i.e., eyes, umbilical cord, and nares); culture from any obvious infected or draining site
- CSF analysis, culture, and gram stain
- Chest radiograph

Table 14-11 Signs and Symptoms of Neonatal Sepsis

General appearance and behavior	• Change in behavior pattern, "not acting right" • Increased crying • Increased sleeping, not awakening for feeding • Temperature instability (increased or decreased core temperature)
Respiratory	• Episodes of apnea • Respiratory distress • Cyanosis • Tachypnea
Circulatory	• Central cyanosis or pallor • Tachycardia or bradycardia • Mottled extremities despite warming measures
CNS	• Seizure activity (e.g., smacking of lips, eye deviation and fluttering, bicycling) • Decreased or altered level of consciousness • Does not focus, will not track objects, does not maintain eye contact • Decreased muscle tone (decreased resistance to extension of extremities) • Posture: extremities extended, may be limp or flaccid rather than flexed • Weak or absent reflexes • Inconsolable, paradoxical irritability • Decreased or no response to procedures
Gastrointestinal	• Poor feeding–lack of interest in feeding • Feeding intolerance–gastric distention and vomiting • Hemoccult® positive stools
Hematopoietic	• Jaundice • Petechiae

Congenital Heart Disease

Congenital heart disease occurs in 8 per 1,000 live births[2] and is the major cause of death in term infants in the first year of life.[6] Some infants with congenital heart defects may exhibit signs and symptoms at birth, but others may not appear symptomatic for days, weeks, or months; however, the majority exhibit symptoms by 3 months of age. Congenital heart lesions may include a single structural anomaly or a combination of anomalies. They are classified in broad terms as either cyanotic and acyanotic, then further classified based on hemodynamics using the ratio of pulmonary to systemic blood flow and the direction of blood flow through the lesion as a descriptor. **Table 14-12** provides a summary of the major congenital cardiac defects using these classifications.

Defects that produce left-to-right shunts result in increased pulmonary blood flow. In the heart, the blood is shunted from the left (systemic) side of the heart to the right (pulmonary) side. The increased pulmonary blood flow may lead to congestive heart failure if significant. These defects are also termed acyanotic.[6, 20, 21] Cyanotic defects, or right-to-left shunts, are those in which blood is shunted from the right side of the heart to the left side, bypassing the pulmonary circulation and mixing with blood being pumped to the systemic circulation. Obstructive defects may occur on either side of the heart, and when in combination with other anomalies, shunting of blood may occur. Some obstructive and right-to-left shunt congenital heart defects would not be compatible with life except for the presence of other anomalies or a patent ductus arteriosus.

The ductus arteriosus is a fetal circulation structure connecting the pulmonary artery to the aorta. The rising arterial PaO_2 after birth stimulates constriction and closure of the ductus arteriosus. However, neonates with congenital heart disease may have a delayed closure of the ductus arteriosus, in part due to a lower PaO_2. Neonates with defects dependent on the patent ductus to maintain pulmonary blood flow will exhibit symptoms within the first weeks of life as the ductus arteriosus begins to close. Congestive heart failure, pulmonary edema, or shock occurs.[20] If the circulation to the lower extremities is dependent on the patent ductus arteriosus, the infant will show signs of profound deterioration as the ductus closes. Because Prostaglandin E1 (PGE1) has a direct dilatory effect on the ductus, it is used to reestablish the patency of the ductus arteriosus.

Infants with right-to-left shunting will exhibit a lower arterial PaO_2 and saturation in their left arm and lower extremities. Measurements that are preductal (before the patent ductus arteriosus through which blood shunts) may be higher than those that are postductal. For this reason, the pulse oximeter should be placed on the right arm. If a second pulse oximeter is available, it can be placed on a lower extremity, and concurrent readings can be recorded. Always record the location of the pulse oximeter probe along with the actual reading. An oxygen challenge test may be performed when trying to differentiate a cardiac or pulmonary origin for cyanosis in the neonate.[20]

History, Signs, and Symptoms

Neonates with congenital heart disease may exhibit any or all of the signs and symptoms listed in **Table 14-13**. Because the caregivers may not recognize all of these as a problem, specific behavioral information must be elicited.

Additional Interventions

Neonates with congenital heart disease typically present to the ED in severe distress, shock, or a prearrest state. Interventions to support airway, breathing, and circulation, as previously listed in Chapter 4, *Initial Assessment*, should be performed. In addition, the following interventions should be initiated.

Table 14-12 Summary of Congenital Cardiac Defects

Left-to-right shunts (acyanotic)
- Patent ductus arteriosus
- Atrial septal defect
- Ventricular septal defect
- Complete atrioventricular canal defect

Right-to-left shunts (cyanotic)
- Transposition of the great arteries
- Tetralogy of Fallot
- Total anomalous pulmonary venous return
- Truncus arteriosus
- Tricuspid atresia
- Hypoplastic left heart syndrome

Obstructive lesions
- Aortic stenosis
- Pulmonic stenosis
- Coarctation of the aorta

Reprinted with permission from Redfearn, S. (1998). Cardiovascular system. In T. E. Soud & J. S. Rogers (Eds.), *Manual of pediatric emergency nursing* (pp. 233-265). St. Louis, MO: Mosby.

- Administer oxygen as ordered. There are circumstances when oxygen may be ordered at a level of 30 to 40% even though the oxygen saturation is lower than normal. This is because there are some conditions in which delivering oxygen at too high a concentration can be detrimental.[6]

- Initiate monitoring of heart rate and oxygen saturation.

- Obtain vascular access for maintenance fluids and medication administration.

- Obtain appropriate laboratory work and other diagnostic studies, such as arterial blood gases, blood glucose, blood cultures, chest radiograph, and echocardiogram.

- Keep NPO.

- Administer PGE1 via continuous IV infusion to reestablish patent ductus arteriosus.[21] PGE1 also causes vasodilatation of all arterioles, inhibits platelet aggregation, and stimulates intestinal smooth muscle.
  - May be given via a peripheral IV or an umbilical arterial or venous line but must be given directly into the hub of the neonate's vascular access; cannot be piggybacked several inches up the IV tubing.
  - Maximal drug effect is usually seen within 30 minutes, but immediate effects, such as an increase in oxygen saturation and decreased cyanosis, are noted within minutes.
  - Monitor for side effects of PGE1.
    - Apnea, hypoventilation
    - Hypotension
    - Edema
    - Cutaneous vasodilatation
    - Fever
    - Hypoglycemia
    - Hemorrhage
    - Thrombocytopenia
    - Irritability

- Be prepared to intubate. If the neonate is to be transported to another facility, the neonate should be intubated due to the potential for apnea secondary to the PGE1.

Health Promotion

The first few weeks of life require major adjustments from both the neonate and the caregivers. A new mother is experiencing hormonal changes, body image changes, and sleep deprivation. Although the caregivers may have attended prenatal classes and received educational information after the birth of the child, the overwhelming responsibilities of the neonate may cause frustration and exhaustion. Information previously learned may be forgotten. The following information is a sample of what can be shared both verbally and via written materials.

Illness Prevention

- Educate caregiver concerning immunizations and immunization schedule. Provide referral to community immunization resources as needed.

- Review with caregiver the importance of well-baby checks and establishing a relationship with a primary care provider (PCP) for the infant. Provide PCP referral or resources for obtaining or selecting a PCP.

- Review with caregiver what to do in case of an emergency including
  - When to call the PCP
  - When to go to the ED

Table 14-13 Signs and Symptoms Exhibited with Congenital Heart Disease

General appearance and behavior	• Easily fatigued • Doesn't cry much or for long ("Such a good baby")
Respiratory	• Cyanosis during crying or feeding • Dyspnea during crying or feeding • Respiratory distress • Clear breath sounds in a tachypneic, cyanotic infant (highly suspicious of congenital heart disease) • Cyanosis • Dyspnea • Increased work of breathing
Circulatory	• Excessive sweating • Diminished lower extremity pulses; some cardiac defects may result in diminished pulses in the lower extremities (e.g., coarctation of the aorta) • Lower blood pressure reading in lower extremities (may be as much as 20 mm Hg difference with some defects)[20] • Murmur may or may not be present • Tachycardia • Visible precordial impulse
CNS	• Decreased level of consciousness • Poor muscle tone • Poor sucking response
Gastrointestinal	• Doesn't feed well or for as long as would be expected; falls asleep early in feeding • Poor weight gain
Hematopoietic	• Profound pallor • Polycythemia

- Advise caregiver to keep the infant's environments (home and car) smoke free.

- Teach caregiver the early signs of illness in the neonate and infant: fever, poor feeding, vomiting, diarrhea, unusual irritability, decreased activity, decreased responsiveness, or extended posture.

- Encourage caregiver to learn infant cardiopulmonary resuscitation. Provide information on hospital- or community-based classes.

- Review feeding information as appropriate.
  - Stress need for good maternal diet when breastfeeding.
  - Refer to lactation consultant if experiencing difficulties with breastfeeding.
  - Review types of formulas and preparation process.
  - Review risks associated with giving honey to an infant–associated with infant botulism.
  - Review safe bottle-feeding practices. For example, do not prop the bottle or put the infant to bed with a bottle, and do not microwave infant bottles to heat them.

Injury and Abuse Prevention

- Review use of infant car seat restraint devices. Stress the importance of using a rear-facing car seat, properly secured in the backseat, with the infant strapped into the car seat at all times.

- Discuss infant's sleeping position with caregiver. Current recommendations state that an infant should be positioned on the back or side, not prone.

- Discuss cosleeping, in which parents and infants sleep in the same bed. Although this is a common practice in some cultures, recent studies have shown that cosleeping is associated with an increased incidence of sleep-related deaths, most likely from suffocation.[6]

- Review and discuss general infant safety measures with the caregiver.
  - Set the hot water heater thermostat at less than 120°F.
  - Always test the water temperature with a bath thermometer or at your wrist to make sure it is not too hot before bathing the infant. Never leave the baby alone in a tub of water.
  - Ensure crib slats are no more than 2 3/8 inches apart with a snug-fitting mattress. Keep the sides of the crib raised.
  - Do not put the infant on soft surfaces such as a water bed, couch, or pillow.
  - Do not leave the infant on high places, such as changing tables, beds, sofas, or chairs. Always keep one hand on the infant.
  - Never leave the baby alone or with a young sibling or pet.
  - Do not drink hot liquids while holding the infant or pour hot liquids while reaching over the infant.
  - Avoid overexposure to the sun and use sunscreen.
  - Install smoke detectors if not already in place.
  - Never shake an infant.
  - Provide information on prevention of foreign body aspiration, both from improperly prepared foods and objects in the environment.
  - Do not use mobile infant walkers.

- Monitor the environment both at home and when visiting family or friends to make sure that it is child safe.

- Provide information as appropriate for community resources to assist with financial concerns, parenting skills, inadequate housing, limited food resources, lack of transportation, lack of appropriate car seat, or domestic violence and child abuse prevention.

Summary

Neonates are our smallest patients and often our scariest. They cannot speak for themselves, so we must be their advocates. Illness signs are often subtle so we are challenged to look for the pieces of the puzzle if we are to obtain the whole picture. Let us not forget the incredible miracle of this small being and what we can offer. Our ability to fine-tune our assessment, discover and treat a problem, provide educational information to the caregiver, and offer support and encouragement to the family can make a difference in the lives of the infants and their families.

References

1. Minino, A. M., & Smith, B. L. (2001). Deaths: Preliminary data for 2000. *National Vital Statistics Reports*, 49(12). Retrieved September 3, 2003 from http://www.cdc.gov/nchs/data/nvsr/nvsr49/nvsr49_12.pdf

2. Landry, N. (1999). Uncomplicated antepartum, intrapartum, and postpartum care. In J. Deacon & P. O'Neill (Eds.), *Core curriculum for neonatal intensive care nursing* (2nd ed., pp. 2–17). Philadelphia: Saunders.

3. Cloherty, J. P., & Stark, A. R. (Eds.). (1998). *Manual of neonatal care* (4th ed., p. 53). New York: Lippincott.

4. Kattwinkel, J. (2000). *Neonatal resuscitation textbook*. Elk Grove Village, IL: American Academy of Pediatrics and American Heart Association.

5. Harrell, H. A. (1999). Neonatal delivery room resuscitation. In J. Deacon & P. O'Neill (Eds.), *Core curriculum for neonatal intensive care nursing* (2nd ed., pp. 101–116). Philadelphia: Saunders.

6. Hockenberry, M. J., Wilson, D., Winkelstein, M. L., & Kline, N. E. (2003). In *Wong's nursing care of infants and children* (7th ed.). St. Louis, MO: Mosby.

7. Burke, S. S. (1998). Neonatal topics. In T. E. Soud & J. S. Rogers (Eds.), *Manual of pediatric emergency nursing* (pp. 660–685). St. Louis, MO: Mosby.

8. Hazinski, M. F. (1992). Children are different. In M.F. Hazinski (Ed.), *Nursing care of the critically ill child* (2nd ed., pp. 1–17). St. Louis, MO: Mosby.

9. Cheng, T. L., & Partridge, J. C. (1993). Effect of bundling and high environmental temperature on neonatal body temperature. *Pediatrics, 92*(2), 238–240.

10. Grover, G., Berkowitz, C. D., Lewis, R. J., Thompson, M., Berry, L., & Seidel, J. (1994). The effects of bundling on infant temperatures. *Pediatrics, 94*(5), 669–673.

11. Johnston, P. G. B. (1998). *The newborn child.* New York: Churchill Livingstone.

12. Glass, S. M. (1999). Hematologic disorders. In J. Deacon & P. O'Neill (Eds.), *Core curriculum for neonatal intensive care nursing* (2nd ed., pp. 383–412). Philadelphia: Saunders.

13. Bailey, C., Boyle, R., Kattwinkel, J., & Ferguson, J. (1997). *Outpatient perinatal education program book two: The infant at risk after discharge* (pp. 1.3). Charlottesville, VA: Division of Neonatal Medicine, University of Virginia Health Sciences Center.

14. McGowan, J., Enzman Hagedorn, M., & Ha, W. (2002). Glucose homeostasis. In G. B. Merenstein & S. L. Gardner (Eds.), *Handbook of neonatal intensive care* (5th ed., pp. 301–302). St. Louis, MO: Mosby.

15. Zupan, J., & Garner, P. (1998). *Routine topical umbilical cord care at birth (Cochrane review).* Retrieved September 3, 2003 from http://www.update-software.com/abstracts/ab001057.htm.

16. American Heart Association. (2005). Neonatal Resuscitation Guidelines. *Circulation, 112*(24)(Suppl.), IV188–IV195.

17. Berry, D., Adcock, E., & Starbuck, A. (2002). Fluid and electrolyte management. In G. B. Merenstein & S. L. Gardner (Eds.), *Handbook of neonatal intensive care* (5th ed., pp. 292). St. Louis, MO: Mosby.

18. Bailey, C., Boyle, R., Kattwinkel, J., & Ferguson, J. (1997). *Outpatient perinatal education program book one: The high risk mother and fetus* (pp. 1.14–1.23). Charlottesville, VA: Division of Neonatal Medicine, University of Virginia Health Sciences Center.

19. Louch, G. (1999). Follow-up of the preterm infant and outcome of prematurity. In J. Deacon & P. O'Neill (Eds.), *Core curriculum for neonatal intensive care nursing* (2nd ed., pp. 781–795). Philadelphia: Saunders.

20. Redfearn, S. (1998). Cardiovascular system. In T. E. Soud & J. S. Rogers (Eds.), *Manual of pediatric emergency nursing* (pp. 233–265). St. Louis, MO: Mosby.

21. Hazinski, M. F. (1992). Cardiovascular disorders. In M. F. Hazinski (Ed.), *Nursing care of the critically ill child* (2nd ed., pp. 117–394). St. Louis, MO: Mosby.

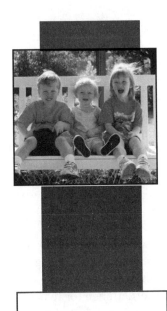

CHILDHOOD ILLNESSES

Introduction

Emergency department (ED) visits by children for illness encompass the entire spectrum of acuity. The most common chief complaints include fever, ear pain, respiratory symptoms, vomiting, diarrhea, sore throat, rash, urinary tract symptoms, and abdominal pain.[1] This chapter will provide an overview of selected childhood illnesses, including infectious diseases, neurologic, gastrointestinal, genitourinary, endocrine, hematologic, and immune system disorders.

Anatomic, Physiologic, and Developmental Characteristics as a Basis for Signs and Symptoms

Temperature Measurement

Body temperature in children can be measured by a variety of different methods with different degrees of sensitivity and specificity. The best sites for temperature measurement in children are those closest to the brain that reflect central or "core" temperature.[1] Although rectal temperatures are still recognized as being the gold standard for temperature measurement in children less than 2 years of age, recent studies suggest that rectal temperatures may be slower to change in relation to core temperature and are affected by depth of measurement, conditions affecting local blood flow, and presence of stool in the rectum.[2,3]

Due to their dependence on environmental factors, axillary temperatures are not considered to be a specific nor sensitive route of measurement. They are, however, still recommended by the American Academy of Pediatrics as a screening test for neonates due to the risk of perforation with rectal temperature measurement in this age group.[2,3,4] Tympanic membrane thermometry is considered to be a reasonable method of measurement in children, but readings may be influenced by cerumen, otitis media, tympanostomy tubes, and ear canal size.[3] Whatever the method, the accurate measurement of body temperature is a key element in the evaluation of sick pediatric patients and an important ongoing measure of response to therapy.

Fever

Fever is a nonspecific symptom of an underlying infectious or inflammatory process and is one of the most common symptoms encountered in pediatrics. The public readily recognizes fever as a symptom of illness, and approximately 20% of all ED visits by children are attributable to fever.[3]

Fever is a rise in the core body temperature that follows a resetting of the body's thermostat, which is located in the hypothalamus. A pediatric patient is generally considered febrile when the rectal temperature is at least 38°C (100.4°F).[1]

The duration and degree of fever may provide clues to the underlying illness, although the degree of fever does not reflect severity of illness. Seriously ill infants and children may be normothermic or hypothermic rather than febrile. The presence or history of fever at home may affect triage and treatment decisions in pediatric patients who are at increased risk for sepsis or other serious illness. This includes infants less than 90 days of age, immunocompromised patients, patients with chronic illnesses, and children less than 2 years of age without an identified source of infection.[3,5]

Fever in itself is not an emergency. Low-grade fevers may, in fact, enhance the immune response through mobilization of white blood cells (WBCs) and production of antigens.[1,6] However, a febrile state does affect physiologic function. Fever can contribute to increases in insensible fluid losses, metabolic rate, oxygen and calorie consumption, heart rate, and respiratory rate.[4] Control of fever with cooling measures and antipyretics often helps the child feel better but more importantly may decrease some physiologic demands in the seriously or critically ill child.

Fluid and Electrolyte Balance

Total body water is comprised of extracellular (ECF) and intracellular fluid (ICF). Extracellular fluid is composed of the interstitial fluid and the circulating blood plasma. Essential and insensible fluid losses occur through the skin, respiratory system, gastrointestinal tract, and urinary systems. The following characteristics of fluid and electrolyte balance are unique to the pediatric population.

- The child's higher metabolic rate increases heat production, which in turn increases insensible fluid losses.
- A greater body surface area to mass ratio results in a larger quantity of water loss per unit of mass, particularly through evaporation.
- The immature kidney function of neonates results in a limited ability to concentrate and dilute urine and conserve or secrete sodium resulting in a larger daily turnover of body water.[1]
- Normal urine output in well-hydrated infants is 2 ml/kg/hr and 1 ml/kg/hr in the child. The well-hydrated adolescent on average may only excrete 0.5 ml/kg/hr.[6]
- Although infants and young children have a larger ECF to ICF volume ratio, dehydration occurs more rapidly due to a large body surface area, increased metabolic rate, and a smaller absolute volume of ECF.

In the otherwise healthy pediatric patient, dehydration is most often due to gastrointestinal losses from vomiting or diarrhea coupled with inadequate fluid intake.[1,7,8] Other causes of dehydration include increased insensible fluid losses due to respiratory illness or fever, excessive renal losses (diabetes insipidus or diabetes mellitus), skin losses (burns, cystic fibrosis), third-spacing of fluids, and incorrect formula preparation.[9]

Dehydration is usually classified according to serum sodium levels because the level in dehydrated patients may be low, normal, or high. There are three types of dehydration that reflect the proportion of sodium to water losses: isotonic (serum sodium 130 to 150 mEq/L), hyponatremic (serum sodium < 130 mEq/L), and hypernatremic (serum sodium > 150 mEq/L).[8,10] By far the most common type of dehydration in children is isotonic dehydration, in which sodium and fluid losses are equal.

Hyponatremic (or hypotonic) dehydration is less common but may develop from excessive water intake (water intoxication) or excessive sodium losses. This is often the result when a pediatric patient experiencing diarrhea or vomiting at home is given free water as replacement for dehydration. Hypernatremic (or hypertonic) dehydration usually results from a deficit of free water (water is lost in excess of sodium). Improper formula dilution as well as gastrointestinal losses coupled with high fever or decreased intake can result in hypernatremic dehydration.

The degree of dehydration is described as a percentage (mild-5%, moderate-10%, or severe-15%) and is based on loss of body weight. Clinical signs and symptoms are used to correlate the degree of weight loss.[8] In moderate and severe levels of dehydration, urinary output decreases, and mental status alterations become apparent. **Table 15-1** compares the signs and symptoms with the degree of dehydration.[11]

Rashes

Rashes are one of the most common symptoms of pediatric patients presenting to the ED. The etiology of the rash can be related to acute or chronic conditions and include systemic or localized infections (bacterial, viral, fungal); hypersensitivity reactions (environmental allergens, medications, bites and stings, or products such as latex); or infestation (lice, scabies). The evaluation of the lesion must include

- Pattern of distribution
- Appearance and texture of the lesions
- Presence or absence of fever
- History related to the eruption and evolution of the rash (chronic versus acute)

Although most rashes are not life threatening, petechial and purpuric rashes may be associated with emergent conditions that require immediate intervention.[12] Appendix 15-A summarizes common infectious exanthems.

Nursing Care

Assessment

Refer to Chapter 4, *Initial Assessment*, for a review of the initial assessment of the pediatric patient. Additional assessment data, signs and symptoms, and additional interventions are discussed with each selected emergency.

Diagnostic Procedures

Monitors

The use of cardiac and pulse oximetry monitoring is based on the pediatric patient's condition. Indications for initiating monitoring are described in the selected emergencies section.

Laboratory Studies

Specific laboratory studies will be ordered, depending on the appearance of the pediatric patient; the history, signs and symptoms; and the absence of an identifiable source of infection. Specific laboratory studies are discussed in the additional interventions for each selected emergency.

Radiographs and Imaging Studies

Radiograph and imaging studies may be indicated based on clinical status and evaluation. Specific studies are discussed in the additional interventions for the selected emergency as appropriate.

Planning/Implementation

Refer to Chapter 4, *Initial Assessment*, for airway, breathing, and circulation interventions appropriate during the primary assessment as well as general interventions. Refer to Chapter 6, *Respiratory Distress and Failure*, and Chapter 7, *Shock*, for additional interventions related to respiratory compromise and shock respectively.

- Monitor vital signs including temperature.

Table 15-1 Degrees of Dehydration

Degree of Dehydration	Mild (< 5%)	Moderate (10%)	Severe (15%)
Signs and symptoms			
Dry mucous membrane	±	+	+
Reduced skin turgor (pinch retraction)	-	±	+
Depressed anterior fontanel	-	+	+
Mental status	Alert	Irritable	Lethargic
Sunken eyeballs	-	+	+
Hyperpnea	-	±	+
Hypotension (orthostatic)	-	±	+
Increased pulse	-	+	+
Capillary refill	≤ 2 sec	> 2 sec	> 2 sec
Laboratory			
Urine			
Volume	Small	Oliguria	Oliguria/anuria
Specific gravity*	≤ 1.020**	> 1.030	> 1.035
Blood			
BUN	WNL**	Elevated	Very high
pH (arterial)	7.40–7.30	7.30–7.00	< 7.10

+, Present; -, Absent; ±, Variable

* Specific gravity can provide evidence that confirms the physical assessment

** Not usually indicated in mild or moderate dehydration

Reprinted with permission from Dehydration. (1999). In R. M. Barkin & P. Rosen (Eds.), *Emergency pediatrics: A guide to ambulatory care* (5th ed., pp. 69–77). St. Louis, MO: Mosby.

- Avoid rectal temperatures and rectal suppositories in a child who is immunocompromised or has rectal pathology.
- Maintain standard precautions.
- Initiate appropriate isolation measures.
- Administer antipyretics per protocol.
- Administer fluids, medications, and blood products as indicated.

Evaluation and Ongoing Assessment

The pediatric patient with a serious or life-threatening illness requires frequent reassessment and evaluation of progress toward desired outcomes. Improvements in airway, breathing, circulation, or neurologic status may not be sustained, and additional interventions may be required. To evaluate the patient's response and progress, monitor the following.
- Airway patency
- Effectiveness of breathing
- Color, pulse rate, and quality of peripheral and central perfusion
- Level of consciousness and activity level
- Urinary output
- Level of pain
- Cardiac rhythm as indicated
- Oxygen saturation as indicated

Selected Childhood Illnesses

The following selected childhood illnesses occur primarily in the pediatric population. Additional history, signs and symptoms, and interventions specific to the selected illness are listed. Standard assessment data and interventions are outlined in Chapter 4, *Initial Assessment*, and at the beginning of this chapter; therefore are not repeated with each disorder, but should be applied as appropriate.

Infectious Disorders

Gastroenteritis

Worldwide, gastroenteritis is second only to respiratory illness as a cause of morbidity from complications of dehydration, electrolyte imbalance, and malnutrition. It is responsible for up to 10% of all hospitalizations in children less than 5 years of age.[13] Gastroenteritis is an inflammation of the gastrointestinal tract caused by bacterial, viral, or parasitic agents. Viral diarrhea is the most common and accounts for 80% of all infections in

children.[13,14] Rotavirus is the most common form, followed by adenovirus and enterovirus. Antibiotic therapy, malabsorption problems, milk allergy, diet, and infections outside of the gastrointestinal (GI) tract may also cause diarrhea.

Identification of risk factors can assist the caregiver in identifying the transmission of the causative agent. **Table 15-2** identifies risk factors and their associated pathogens.

Additional History
- Duration of associated symptoms–vomiting, fever
- Description of diarrhea stool, frequency, number, and onset
- Number of wet diapers in last 8 hours; last urination
- Use of antibiotics or other medications
- Change in diet
- Day care attendance, others ill at home, recent travel, pets in the home

Signs and Symptoms
- Vomiting
- Diarrhea (consistency, color, presence of blood)
- Fever
- Abdominal pain or cramping
- Lethargy, with or without irritability
- Signs and symptoms of dehydration: sticky or dry mucous membranes, sunken fontanelle, sunken eyes,

Table 15-2 Risk Factors and Their Associated Pathogens

RISK FACTORS	ASSOCIATED PATHOGENS
Day care centers	• Rotavirus • Giardiasis • Shigella
Household Pets Iguanas, turtles, snakes Puppies, kittens Birds, reptiles	• Salmonella • Campylobacter • Cryptosporidium
Food Raw hamburger Raw eggs, poultry	• Escherichia coli (E. coli) • Salmonella
Antibiotic Use	Clostridium difficile
Travel (international)	Enterotoxigenic E. coli

Adapted from Belamarich, P. (1997). Gastrointestinal emergencies. In E. F. Crain & J. C. Gershel (Eds.), *Clinical manual of emergency pediatrics* (3rd ed., pp. 191–248). New York: McGraw-Hill.

decreased tearing, decreased urine output, poor skin turgor, weight loss, and changes in vital signs, such as tachycardia, tachypnea, or orthostatic blood pressure changes

Additional Interventions

- Fluid replacement therapy is based on the level and type of dehydration.
- Initiate rehydration via oral or intravenous route as indicated.
  - Oral rehydration using oral replacement therapy (ORT) is usually adequate for the pediatric patient who has mild isotonic dehydration and can tolerate fluids.
  - Moderate to severe isotonic dehydration requires intravenous fluids and an initial bolus of crystalloid solution (i.e., normal saline or lactated Ringer's solution) at 10 to 20 ml/kg. For the severely dehydrated child, up to 60 ml/kg may be required.
- Fluid boluses are followed by replacement of calculated fluid losses along with maintenance fluid therapy of dextrose/saline solutions. See **Table 15-3** for one method to calculate maintenance fluid replacement.
- Accurate monitoring of fluid intake and output
- Administer antipyretics as needed. Antidiarrheal agents are rarely indicated.
- Stool for culture, ova, and parasites; rapid enzyme immunoassay for rotavirus; and hemoccult.
- Provide caregivers with proper home care instructions for oral replacement therapy and prevention of disease transmission (i.e., hand washing).

Meningitis

Meningitis is an inflammation of the meninges covering the brain and spinal cord and is identified by an abnormal number of WBCs in the cerebrospinal fluid (CSF). It is caused by a variety of bacterial and viral agents. Incidence is generally based on age. *Haemophilus influenzae* historically has been the most common organism causing bacterial meningitis in children, but it has markedly decreased following the institution of widespread immunization programs.[15] The most common bacterial organisms in newborns are *streptococcus ß-hemolytic*, Group B and *E. coli. Neisseria meningitidis* and *Streptococcus pneumoniae* are responsible for the majority of cases in children.[16]

Viral meningitis, commonly caused by enteroviruses, is generally self-limiting and associated with a lower morbidity and mortality rate. Treatment is usually symptomatic and is often limited to rest, antipyretics, and analgesia.

Meningitis results from entrance of organisms into the CSF, commonly by two routes. They may enter via direct invasion from penetrating trauma, or more commonly, organisms can enter indirectly through invasion of the upper respiratory tract, the bloodstream, or the CSF.

Complications of bacterial meningitis include cerebral edema, increased intracranial pressure (ICP), seizures, septic shock, syndrome of inappropriate antidiuretic hormone, disseminated intravascular coagulation (DIC), subdural effusions, and anemia.

Meningococcal meningitis caused by *Neisseria meningitidis* is often accompanied by high fever, changes in level of consciousness, and a petechial or purpuric rash. Because this form of meningitis can lead to profound shock, DIC, and death, the presence of these symptoms in pediatric patients is treated emergently.[15,16]

Mortality rates are as high as 30 % for bacterial meningitis.[17] The outcome varies according to the infectious organism, the child's age, and state of immune competence. Long-term effects may include deafness, epilepsy, hydrocephalus, and learning and motor disorders.[17]

Additional History

- History of vomiting, poor feeding, or decrease in appetite
- Fever
- Recent ear or upper respiratory tract infection
- Presence of ill-looking child with petechial or purpuric rash
- Seizure
- Headache, photophobia, or neck stiffness
- Decreased activity level, irritability, decreased level of consciousness

Table 15-3 Calculation of Maintenance Fluid

Body Weight (kg)	Fluid requirement per hour	Example 15 kg child
First 10 kg	4 ml/kg +	10 x 4 = 40 ml
Second 10 kg	2 ml/kg for each kg above 10 kg +	+ 5 x 2 = 10 ml
Each additional kg	1 ml/kg for each kg above 20 kg	+ 0
	Total	Total = 50 ml/hr for maintenance

Adapted from Roberts, K. (2001). Fluid and electrolyte balance. In M. A. Curley & P. A. Moloney-Harmon (Eds.), *Critical care nursing of infants and children* (2nd ed., p. 381). Philadelphia: Saunders.

Signs and Symptoms

Clinical signs and symptoms depend on the age of the child, type of organism, and underlying medical conditions. It is important to remember that infants and children in early stages of meningitis may present with subtle signs and symptoms (see **Table 15-4**). An accurate patient history and clinical assessment are key to early diagnosis, treatment, and minimization of negative outcomes.

Diagnostic Procedures

Laboratory Studies

- Complete blood count with differential
- Blood culture
- Electrolytes
- Blood glucose
- Urinalysis and culture (catheter specimen in pretoilet-trained child)
- CSF for cell count, gram stain, protein, glucose, and viral studies, if appropriate

Radiographic Studies

- Chest radiograph
- Computerized tomography (CT) scan of head which is typically completed prior to lumbar puncture if required to rule out space-occupying lesion

Monitors

- Cardiac monitor
- Pulse oximeter

Additional Interventions for Bacterial Meningitis

- Administer oxygen.
- Obtain vascular access and administer intravenous fluids judiciously. If signs and symptoms of shock exist, administer a 20 ml/kg bolus of isotonic crystalloid solution (i.e., lactated Ringer's solution or 0.9% normal saline). Repeat the bolus as necessary.
- Administer medications as ordered.
  - Intravenous antibiotic therapy. In suspected bacterial meningitis, do not delay antibiotic administration while awaiting laboratory specimen collection or results.
  - Antipyretics
  - Consider topical analgesia prior to lumbar puncture.
  - Anticipate need for inotropic agents or vasoactive therapy to support cardiac output.
  - The use of dexamethasone in reducing the complication of deafness in bacterial meningitis remains controversial and is based on individual patient evaluation.[16]
- Evaluate and trend neurologic status and vital signs for increased intracranial pressure.
  - Minimize increases in cerebral metabolic rate by controlling temperature, instituting comfort measures, and monitoring seizure activity.
  - Document serial measurements of head circumference in infants.
- Initiate respiratory isolation (Droplet Precautions) for 24 hours after the start of antibiotics.[18]
- Administer antibiotic prophylaxis for household contact or health care providers who experience intimate contact with the pediatric patient's respiratory secretions or blood.

Meningococcemia

Meningococcemia is a potentially life-threatening clinical entity in which the organism, *Neisseria meningitidis*, gains access to the bloodstream. The incubation period is 2 to 10 days, and as in meningitis, the bacterium is

Table 15-4 Signs and Symptoms of Meningitis by Age[10]		
Less than 2 Months of Age	**3 Months to 2 Years of Age**	**Greater than 2 Years of Age**
Fever	Irritability	Fever
Apnea, cyanosis	Fever	Headache
Temperature instability	High-pitched cry	Altered mental status/irritability
Altered level of consciousness	Poor feeding	Seizures
Seizures	Vomiting	Stiff neck
Vomiting/diarrhea	Ataxia	Petechiae or purpura (bacterial infection)
Bulging fontanel (may or may not be present)	Seizures	Vomiting
Jitters, irritability	Stiff neck	Photophobia
Petechiae or purpura (bacterial infection)	Altered mental status	Positive Brudzinski's sign
Poor feedings	Petechiae or purpura (bacterial infection)	Positive Kernig's sign
	Bulging fontanel (late sign)	

usually spread via oral or nasal droplet. The disease course can be fulminating with a rapid onset of symptoms, and death may occur within hours. It may exist as sepsis or as a complication of meningococcal meningitis. Most cases occur in younger children and adolescents. Survival may be determined in the first 12 hours after treatment has been initiated. With use of antibiotics and supportive measures, the fatality rate is below 10%.[19] The ultimate prognosis and outcome depends on the pediatric patient's immune status, splenic function, fulminance of the infection, and prompt medical intervention. Complications include meningitis, shock, septic arthritis, pneumonia, pericarditis, myocarditis, DIC, and death.[19]

Additional History

- Recent exposure to known infected person
- Fever
- Nausea or vomiting
- Irritability, lethargy, or poor feeding in infants
- Headache, malaise, or joint pain
- Onset of petechial or purpuric rash

Signs and Symptoms

- Fever or temperature instability
- Changes in level of consciousness, irritability
- Poor feeding, vomiting
- Petechiae (initially) then purpura
- Bleeding from puncture sites
- Tachycardia, poor perfusion, hypotension
- Gangrene and tissue necrosis (late)

Diagnostic Procedures

- Blood for septic workup
- Coagulation studies
- Fibrinogen split products
- Lumbar puncture for CSF analysis

Additional Interventions

- Initiate respiratory isolation (Droplet Precautions).[18]
- Initiate cardiorespiratory, pulse oximetry, and blood pressure monitoring.
- Monitor for signs of DIC and anticipate need for clotting factor replacement therapy.
- Anticipate the need for inotropic or vasoactive agents to support cardiac output.
- Administer antibiotic prophylaxis for household contact or health care providers who experience intimate contact with the pediatric patient's respiratory secretions or blood.

Table 15-5 Types of Seizures and Symptoms

Generalized	Partial seizures (focal, local)	Unclassified
Absence seizures–brief lapses in awareness; staring	Simple partial seizures are associated with motor, sensory or autonomic symptoms. Consciousness is not impaired.	Febrile seizures–tonic-clonic movements lasting < 15 minutes. Most are benign and self-limiting. Normally they do not lead to neurologic sequelae or seizure disorders. The peak incidence is 8 to 20 months and most resolve by 5 years of age. There is a 30% chance of reoccurrence.[20]
Myoclonic seizures–sudden brief muscle jerks occur unilaterally or bilaterally		
Tonic–means to become tense or stiff	Complex partial seizures are associated with impaired consciousness.	
Clonic–refers to rapid rhythmic jerking or flexion of extremities		
Tonic-clonic (grand mal)–tonic followed by clonic phase	Partial seizures can progress to generalized seizures.	Neonatal seizures–due to metabolic, toxic, infectious, congenital, or maternal disturbances. They include subtle behavior changes such as rhythmic eye, arm, and leg movements, chewing, swimming, and bicycling. They occur due to the immature neonatal cortex, and may be unilateral or bilateral in presentation.
Atonic seizures–abrupt loss of muscle tone usually causing the pediatric patient to collapse		
All are associated with a loss of consciousness and may be convulsive (tonic-clonic) or nonconvulsive (absence)		

Adapted from Vernon-Levett, P. (2001). Neurologic critical care problems. In M. A. Curley & P. A. Moloney-Harmon (Eds.), *Critical care nursing of infants and children* (2nd ed., pp. 695-720). Philadelphia: Saunders.

Neurologic Disorders

Seizures

Seizures are one of the most frequently encountered pediatric medical emergencies. The most common causes of seizures in children include febrile illness, infections, and metabolic disturbances, but they may also be caused by toxins, trauma, tumors, and noncompliance with seizure medications.[20,21] Approximately 5% of all children experience one or more seizures.[22] The clinical manifestations of the seizure depend on several factors, including the part of the cortex involved, the rate and direction of electrical discharge of neurons within the cortex, and the age of the child.[20] **Table 15-5** identifies types of seizures and their symptoms.

Most childhood seizures are single, generalized tonic clonic events lasting only a few minutes. A seizure lasting longer than 15 minutes is considered a prolonged seizure. Status epilepticus is defined as continuous seizure activity exceeding 30 minutes in duration or recurrent seizures without an intervening period of recovery.[21,23]

Prolonged seizure activity results in airway obstruction, hypoxia, acidosis, increased intracranial pressure, hypoglycemia, and hyperthermia. If not abated, hypotension can develop along with respiratory, cardiovascular, and renal failure. A single, brief seizure (< 30 minutes) is usually not associated with permanent sequela.[23]

Additional History

- Past history of seizures
- History of neurologic or metabolic disorder
- Family history of seizure disorder or febrile seizures
- Description of seizure activity prior to arrival to the ED including length of seizure, type of movements, color change, presence of aura
- Associated head trauma, fever, infection, or presence of ventriculoperitoneal shunt
- Possibility of toxic exposure

Signs and Symptoms

- Tonic and/or clonic muscle activity
- Dilated pupils, salivation, tachycardia, and increased blood pressure during tonic phase
- Incontinence of urine or stool
- Decreased level of consciousness during and following the seizure (postictal state) followed by lethargy, confusion, blank stare, or tremors
- Presence of pallor or cyanosis
- Headache

Additional Interventions

- Ensure patent airway.
- Provide supplemental oxygen.
- Obtain intravenous (IV) access.
- Obtain laboratory work. Consider whole blood or serum glucose (especially in infants), toxicology screen, anticonvulsant levels (if on current therapy), and electrolytes.
- Administer medications.
  - Benzodiazepines, such as lorazepam or diazepam
  - Anticonvulsant therapy as indicated, such as phenobarbital or phenytoin
  - Antipyretics as indicated
- Initiate seizure precautions to protect against self-injury according to institution-specific protocol.
- Reevaluate neurologic status and vital signs.
- Initiate cardiac or pulse oximetry monitoring for pediatric patients with status epilepticus, prolonged seizure, or as indicated by the pediatric patient's condition.
- Provide education on seizure management and fever control (if febrile seizure).

Hydrocephalus

Hydrocephalus is a condition that causes excess CSF to accumulate in the ventricular system either through obstruction, overproduction, or reduced absorption of CSF. Hydrocephalus can be communicating or noncommunicating. In communicating hydrocephalus, CSF flows freely but is not absorbed or is blocked in the subarachnoid space. In noncommunicating hydrocephalus, the normal pathway for CSF circulation is blocked at the ventricles.[15,16]

Table 15-6 Clinical Manifestations of Hydrocephalus in the Infant and Child

Infant	Child
Increased head circumference	Nausea; vomiting
Setting-sun eyes	Headache
Widening sutures	Altered LOC
Dilated scalp veins	Papilledema
Irritability, lethargy; poor feeding; high-pitched cry	Diplopia
	Seizures
Seizures	

Adapted from Vernon-Levett, P. (2001). Neurologic critical care problems. In M. A. Curley & P. A. Moloney-Harmon (Eds.), *Critical care nursing of infants and children* (2nd ed., p. 713). Philadelphia: Saunders.

Hydrocephalus is typically treated with the implantation of a valve-regulated shunt. One example is a ventriculoperitoneal shunt (V-P shunt) in which the proximal catheter is placed in the lateral ventricle and the distal end can be placed in the peritoneum.

The most common complication of valve-regulated shunts is obstruction or disconnection. When this occurs, signs and symptoms of increased ICP will develop. The second most common complication is shunt infection. The pediatric patient may present with signs and symptoms of local or systemic infection. Regardless of the cause, pediatric patients with increased ICP must be treated emergently through early identification of symptoms and prompt intervention.

Signs and Symptoms

Table 15-6 summarizes clinical manifestations of hydrocephalus in the infant and child.

Diagnostic Interventions

- CT scan or magnetic resonance imaging (MRI)
- CSF analysis, if infection suspected
- Shunt series: Series of radiographs determining position, integrity, and length of shunt[15]

Additional Interventions

- Anticipate the need for temporary removal of CSF from the shunt reservoir (usually performed by neurosurgery), and prepare for surgical intervention
- Blood, urine, and CSF analysis
- IV antibiotics (if shunt infection present)
- Ongoing evaluation of neurologic status and vital signs, and repeated measurement of head circumference in infants

Table 15-7 Comparison of Common Inflammatory and Obstructive GI Disorders

Disorder	Cause	Age of onset	Signs & Symptoms	Diagnosis	Treatment
Obstructive					
Pyloric stenosis	Hypertrophy of the circular muscle of the pylorus causing constriction & obstruction	Commonly 2 to 6 weeks	Projectile vomiting, persistent hunger, weight loss, dehydration, constipation, "olive-shaped" abdominal tumor, peristaltic waves	History and physical Ultrasound	Correct dehydration NPO Nasogastric tube Pyloromyotomy
Intussusception	Telescoping of a portion of the proximal bowel into the distal bowel	3 months to 5 years. Most common between 3 to 12 months	Colicky abdominal pain (crying, drawing up legs), currant-jelly stool, vomiting, lethargy, RUQ mass	History and physical Abd x-ray	NPO Barium or water-soluble contrast/air enema Surgical repair (late)
Hernia	Protrusion of an organ through an abnormal opening in the musculature	Usually < 1 year	May be inguinal, femoral, or umbilical. Noted by a bulging mass when the child cries. If the hernia becomes incarcerated, pain and edema will develop and the hernia will not be reducible.	Clinical evaluation	Manual reduction (if early) Surgical repair (incarcerated) No treatment for umbilical hernia unless incarcerated
Inflammatory					
Appendicitis	Inflammation and/or obstruction of the vermiform appendix	9 to 12 years most common, but may be earlier	Progressively worsening pain increasing with movement, guarding, RUQ & rebound tenderness, fever, vomiting	Clinical evaluation X-ray Ultrasound CBC, urine	NPO IV fluids Appendectomy

Reprinted with permission from Horton, M., Soud, T., Inman, C., & Standifer, P. (1998). Gastrointestinal system. In T. E. Soud, & J. S. Rogers (Eds.), *Manual of pediatric emergency nursing* (pp. 332-343). St. Louis, MO: Mosby.

Gastrointestinal and Genitourinary Disorders

Gastrointestinal (GI) Disorders

Many children present to the ED with abdominal discomfort related to a variety of origins. Although gastroenteritis is one of the most common causes of abdominal pain, there are also inflammatory and obstructive disorders that affect children of all ages. **Table 15-7** summarizes symptoms and treatment of the more common inflammatory and obstructive GI disorders in infants and children.

Genitourinary Disorders

In addition to gastrointestinal disorders, children present to the ED with a variety of genitourinary disorders. Most of these are self-limiting and easily treated; however some may be associated with long-term complications and/or underlying medical conditions.

Urinary tract infection (UTI) is defined as the presence of bacteria anywhere in the urinary tract.[24]

Up to 80% of cases of UTIs in children are caused by *E.coli* but other gram-negative enteric organisms are not uncommon.[25] The incidence is higher in males less than 3 months of age, but with growth and changes in anatomy, the incidence becomes dramatically higher in older females.[24] Factors contributing to UTI include the shorter female urethra, urinary stasis, and reflux. UTIs can be difficult to pinpoint and may present with a variety of symptoms ranging from fever, poor feeding, lethargy, and crying in infants to the more localized symptoms in older children of dysuria, frequency, and hematuria. Neonates can become septic quickly, and consideration of UTI in this population is critical to early intervention.

Urine collection methods range from clean catch to catheterization, depending on the age of the child. Bag urine specimens are considered inadequate for definitive diagnosis due to contamination from perianal and perineal flora.[24,25] Methods of urine collection in pediatric patients are summarized in **Table 15-8**.

Testicular torsion is caused by a twisting of the spermatic cord and vessels supplying the testicle.[24] Once the cord twists, it decreases blood flow, causing extreme testicular pain. Testicular torsion has a peak onset of 13 years of age but may occur at any age.[25] It should always be considered as a diagnosis for any male pediatric patient presenting to the ED with testicular pain. In addition to severe pain, nausea, and vomiting, erythema or edema of the testicle may accompany torsion. Diagnosis can often be made clinically but Doppler ultrasound may also be used. Surgery is required for detorsion, and if not treated immediately, the testicle may become ischemic and require removal.

Table 15-8 Methods of Urine Collection for Pediatric Patients

Method	Technique	Rationale/Comments
Clean catch	• Clean area with soap and water • Specimen collected midstream	Antibacterial agents may affect results of culture
Bag specimen	• Remove bag as soon as urine is present • Not reliable for culture	To reduce bacterial growth in bag
Catheterization	• Intermittent catheterization performed for urine specimen collection. • Age and size of child determine the catheter size: #5 Fr. feeding tube may be used for infants and #8 Fr. for toddler • To avoid catheter curling in bladder, use short-length tube and stop advancing when urine flow is established	Gold standard for urine culture collection
Suprapubic bladder aspiration	Needle is inserted into cleansed area above pubis symphysis and urine is aspirated using a syringe	• Ensure infant has not voided prior to procedure. • Performed by physician. • Seen less frequently. More common in neonates. • Consider topical analgesia.

Adapted from Pye, T., & Soud, T. E. (1998). Genitourinary system. In T. E. Soud & J. S. Rogers (Eds.), *Manual of pediatric emergency nursing* (p. 376). St. Louis, MO: Mosby.

Endocrine Disorders

Diabetes

Table 15-9 provides a comparison between type 1 and type 2 diabetes mellitus.

Diabetic Ketoacidosis (DKA)

DKA is a condition caused by insulin deficiency that results in hyperglycemia, mobilization of fatty acids, and excess counterregulatory hormones causing gluconeogenesis. When this occurs, body lipids and proteins are broken down and utilized for energy. Mobilization of fatty acids and the production of lactic and ketoacids results in ketoacidosis. Osmotic diuresis from profound hyperglycemia results in hyponatremia, potassium shifts, and potential dysrhythmias related to electrolyte imbalances. DKA can be life threatening and is the most common cause of death in diabetic children.[26,27] Forty percent of children with new onset of diabetes present to the ED with DKA.

Diabetic ketoacidosis is characterized by[26,28]

- Hyperglycemia
- Dehydration
- Metabolic acidosis
- Ketonemia or ketonuria

Additional History

- Frequent urination
- Excess thirst
- Fatigue
- Weight loss
- History of diabetes and/or viral illness

Signs and Symptoms

- Abdominal pain (poorly understood)
- Nausea and vomiting—related to electrolyte imbalances, acidosis, and underlying factors
- Kussmaul breathing: Hyperventilation in an effort to eliminate CO_2
- Mental status changes related to fluid shifts with correction of dehydration and degree of acidosis
- Signs and symptoms of dehydration related to osmotic diuresis
- Electrolyte imbalances related to fluid shifts and osmotic diuresis

Table 15-9 Comparison of Type 1 and Type 2 Diabetes Mellitus

Characteristic	Type 1	Type 2
Age of onset	Usually < 20 years	Usually over 30 years but there is now a recent increased incidence in children
Incidence (overall)	10%	90%
Associations:		
Family history	Possible	Probable
Genetics	HLA gene is present. Triggered by autoimmune response	No association
Ethnicity	Primarily Caucasian	Aboriginal; Hispanics; African American
Lifestyle	No association	Increased incidence with age, physical inactivity, obesity
Insulin requirement	Always	Sometimes
Oral medication	Not effective	Commonly used
Diet	Controlled balance of nutrition, activity, insulin	Weight loss encouraged through dietary interventions and physical activity then oral or insulin therapy.
Presenting symptoms	Polyuria, polydipsia, polyphagia, weight loss, fatigue	May be asymptomatic. Associated with long-term complications, fatigue, frequent infections, yeast infections
Ketoacidosis	Common	Infrequent

Adapted from Hockenberry, M. J., Wilson, D., Winkelstein, M. L., & Kline, N. L. (Eds.). (2003). *The child with endocrine dysfunction.* In *Wong's nursing care of infants and children* (7th ed., pp. 1703-1756). St. Louis, MO: Mosby.

- Cardiac dysrhythmias related to electrolyte imbalances
- Acetone or "fruity" odor on breath related to build up of ketones

Diagnostic Procedures

Laboratory Studies

- Arterial or capillary blood gas
- Serum or whole blood glucose test
- Complete blood count (CBC), electrolytes, blood urea nitrogen (BUN), creatinine, osmolality
- Urine for urinalysis, ketones, glucose
- Serum beta hydroxybutyrate
- Glycosylated hemoglobin

Additional Interventions

- Correct dehydration
  - For mild dehydration ORT may be used.
  - For moderate to severe dehydration, obtain vascular access and initiate intravenous fluids.
  - Administer a 5 to 20 ml/kg bolus of 0.9% normal saline over 1 to 2 hours. Repeat the bolus as necessary.[29]
  - Continue to replace fluid deficit as per institution-specific protocol, adding glucose to the solution once hyperglycemia corrects.
- Obtain serial laboratory specimens per institutional protocol.
- Correct acidosis through administration of continuous intravenous infusion of regular insulin as per institutional protocol.
- Replace potassium losses with IV fluids once urine output is established.
- Evaluate neurologic status and vital signs for signs of cerebral edema.
- Monitor fluid intake and output.
- Monitor ECG for dysrhythmias related to hyper- or hypokalemia.

Hematologic Disorders

Sickle Cell Crisis

Sickle cell disease (SCD) is an inherited hemoglobinopathy characterized by the presence of an abnormal type of hemoglobin (hemoglobin S) in the red blood cell. It occurs in approximately 1 out of every 500 African Americans; however, it may also be seen in individuals of Mediterranean, Middle Eastern, and Indian descent.[30] In SCD, red blood cells that are normally round assume an irregular sickle shape when deoxygenated. Once sickled, the cells become fragile, clump together, and cannot easily flow through capillaries. This causes an increase in blood viscosity that results in stasis, sludging, and further deoxygenation. Occlusion of small vessels causes tissue ischemia and infarctions resulting in painful sickle cell crisis.[31] The sites most commonly involved are the bones (joints), mesenteric vessels, liver, spleen, brain, lungs, and penis.[31] Sickle cell crisis is considered a medical emergency in pediatric patients.

Children with SCD normally have an elevated cardiac output. This allows blood to travel between the capillaries and lung more rapidly so that sickling does not occur. Any process that interferes with this compensatory mechanism can promote sickling. Common factors are hypoxia, acidosis, hypotension, vasoconstriction, and increased hematocrit. Sickle cell crisis may therefore be precipitated by infection, dehydration, fatigue, exposure to cold, emotional stress, or change in altitude.[32]

The most common manifestations of SCD are vaso-occlusive crisis, aplastic crisis, and sequestration crisis. Vaso-occlusive crisis, the most common form of crisis, is an acute, painful episode produced by stasis of red blood cells in small capillaries leading to tissue ischemia and infarction. The joints and extremities are most often affected.[33] Aplastic crisis normally follows a viral infection and presents with erythropoietic failure in the bone marrow, resulting in bone marrow suppression and anemia. Splenic sequestration crisis occurs with pooling of red blood cells in the spleen resulting in splenomegaly. It may range from mild splenomegaly to massive engorgement, severe anemia, and shock. If left untreated, organ failure and death can occur.[33,34]

Children with sickle cell disease are at higher risk for serious bacterial infections (e.g., meningitis, pneumonia, and sepsis) secondary to functional asplenia and immunosuppression.[30] Infection remains the leading cause of death in early childhood for these patients. Causative agents include *Streptococcus pneumoniae*, *hemophilus influenza*, and *Neisseria meningitidis*.[33]

Other complications of sickle cell disease include cerebral vascular accident (CVA), abdominal crisis, bony crisis, and acute chest syndrome, a painful crisis resulting from sickling in the pulmonary vasculature. It presents similarly to pneumonia with pleuritic chest pain, cough, dyspnea, fever, tachypnea, hypoxia, leukocytosis, and pleural effusions.[35]

Additional History

- Known presence of sickle cell disease or trait
- Family members with sickle cell anemia
- Frequent infections, failure to thrive, jaundice, or anemia (general)
- Pain, swelling, or warmth of joints or extremities

- Dactylitis or hand-foot syndrome (painful inflammation of the fingers or toes) in infants and toddlers[33]
- Current medications
  - Prophylactic penicillin
  - Immunizations (pneumococcal, *Haemophilus influenzae B*, and meningococcal)
  - Folic acid
  - Home pain regimes

Signs and Symptoms

- Weakness, fatigue, pallor (anemia)
- Joint or extremity soft tissue swelling and pain (vaso-occlusive crisis)
- Acute left upper quadrant pain, abdominal distention, vomiting (splenic sequestration)
- Nausea or vomiting, abdominal pain, fever, malaise (abdominal crisis)
- Headache, visual disturbances (CVA)
- Chest pain, dyspnea, fever (acute chest syndrome)
- Priapism (vaso-occlusive crisis)
- Fever (sepsis)

Additional Interventions

- Promote rest to minimize oxygen expenditure.
- Administer oxygen if evidence of hypoxia present.
- Hydration for hemodilution through oral or IV therapy.
- Anticipate the need for transfusion in severe anemia. Exchange transfusion may be required in severe cases.
- Consider need for early catheterization.
- Administer medications.
  - Analgesics (Morphine sulphate is the drug of choice; avoid meperidine[36]).
  - Antipyretics
  - Antibiotics
- Complete laboratory and radiographic studies.
  - CBC and reticulocyte count
  - Type and cross match when need for transfusion identified
  - Arterial or capillary blood gas
  - Cultures of blood, urine, and CSF if infection suspected
  - Chest radiograph for suspected pneumonia or acute chest syndrome

Disorders of Coagulation

Coagulation disorders are compared in **Table 15-10**.[24,25,33,37]

Immunological Disorders

Human Immunodeficiency Virus (HIV)/Acquired Immunodeficiency Syndrome (AIDS)

In June 1999, 8,596 cases of AIDS in children under 13 years of age (pediatric AIDS) were reported in the United States. Worldwide, there are 1.1 million children living with HIV.[38] Eighty percent of all HIV-infected children are symptomatic by 2 years of age.[39] Between 1996 and 1997, the incidence of pediatric HIV declined 40%, largely due to voluntary HIV testing and antiretroviral therapy for pregnant mothers and their infants diagnosed with HIV.[38] In addition to mother-infant transmission, infection can occur through blood and blood products, sharing of needles, contaminated blood, and unprotected sexual intercourse.

HIV disease is defined as the period of time from exposure to the virus until death. AIDS is considered to be the period between onset of symptoms until death. AIDS is a progressively debilitating, multisystem, viral infection that most commonly attacks the immune and nervous systems. The etiologic agent is the retrovirus HIV that selectively invades white blood cells, particularly T-helper lymphocytes. Because the pathology of the disease involves the immune system, children are at high risk for developing bacterial, viral, parasitic, and fungal infections, eventually leading to death.[38] Pneumonia from *Pneumocystis carinii* is the most common acquired infection. The incubation period and disease course is shorter for children than for adults.

The diagnosis of HIV may not be known when a pediatric patient presents to the ED. Testing may be completed as part of the ED workup or at an alternative site, if the child is not ill, but has risk factors for HIV.

Additional History

- If acquired in the perinatal period, history may include failure to thrive, recurrent infections, and lymphadenopathy
- Frequent or recurrent infections (e.g., Candida)
- Progressive regression from developmental achievements
- Persistent weight loss
- Mother is HIV positive or has developed AIDS
- Pediatric patient is sexually active or has been sexually abused
- History of substance abuse or sharing needles
- Maternal history of blood transfusion prior to 1985
- Current medication regime

Signs and Symptoms

Most of the presenting signs and symptoms of HIV infection are nonspecific.

- Chronic diarrhea, vomiting, anorexia, failure to thrive
- Recurrent fever or infection
- Generalized lymphadenopathy, hepatosplenomegaly
- Chronic encephalopathy (e.g., generalized weakness, ataxia)
- Other signs and symptoms may vary and are associated with opportunistic infections and organ-system related disease

Additional Interventions

- Universal precautions. Initiate protective or reverse isolation measures to protect pediatric patient from exposure to other pathogens in the ED.
- Administer antiretroviral therapy.
- Provide psychological support for family and patient.
- Give consultation or teaching regarding adequate nutrition.
- Obtain laboratory work as appropriate for patient condition.
- Obtain consent according to policy or procedure prior to drawing specimens.
- Provide referral for counseling and follow-up if HIV test obtained in the ED or if HIV suspected, and testing at an alternate site preferred.

Table 15-10 Comparison of Coagulation Disorders

Disorder	Cause	Signs & Symptoms	Treatment
Hemophilia	• Genetic disorder characterized by a deficiency or absence in one of the clotting proteins in the plasma • Deficiencies in factor VIII (hemophilia A) or factor IX (Christmas disease) are most common • X-linked recessive disorder affecting mostly males. Incidence is 1:7,500 male births. Inheritance is sex linked recessive. Up to 33% of cases occur through spontaneous gene mutation. • Classified mild to severe according to level of circulating factor. 60% to 70% considered severe.	• General–hemorrhage; easy bruising; prolonged bleeding • CNS–headache; vomiting; altered LOC; seizures related to intracranial bleed • Neck–paralysis; weakness; back pain related to spinal cord bleed • GI–hematemesis; melena; abd pain; palpable mass; rigidity • GU–scrotal bleeding; pain; hematuria • Joint–common bleeds; hemarthrosis; pain; swelling; limited range of motion • Muscle–warmth; pain; swelling. Common sites are calf, upper arm, forearm and thigh.	• Replace missing clotting factors according to protocol with antihemophilic factor (AHF) VIII or coagulation factor IX concentrate. • Aminocaproic acid (Amicar®) or tranexamic acid (Cyklokapron®) may be used to control oral bleeding • Immobilization of affected joints • Analgesia • Minimize invasive procedures-intramuscular injections, venipunctures, catheters • Avoid medications that prolong bleeding time (i.e., ASA, ibuprofen)
von Willebrand's disease	• Most common hereditary bleeding disorder • Deficiency or defect in a component of factor VIII–von Willebrand factor. • Affects both males & females	Superficial bruising; epistaxis; prolonged menses; gum bleeding; prolonged bleeding post surgery	Desmopressin acetate (DDAVP®) or plasma-derived product depending on type
Idiopathic Thrombocytopenic Purpura (ITP)	• Destruction of antibody sensitized platelets (usually by the spleen). May follow a viral illness. • Often self-limiting (4 to 6 weeks). Occasionally may be chronic.	Petechiae; purpura; bruising; thrombocytopenia; spontaneous bleeding of skin and mucous membranes (oral, GI)	• Depends on severity • May range from IgG and steroid administration to treatment of shock and replacement of RBCs

Adapted from Wulff, K., Zappa, S., & Womack, M. (Eds.). (1999). Emergency care for patients with hemophilia: An instructional manual for medical professionals (2nd ed.). The Nursing Group of Hemophilia Region VI and Manley, L., & Bechtel, N. M. (1998). Hematologic and immune systems. In T. E. Soud & J. S. Rogers (Eds.), *Manual of pediatric emergency nursing* (pp. 390-416). St. Louis, MO: Mosby.

Neutropenia

Severe neutropenia is defined as an absolute neutrophil count (ANC) of 500/mm^3 or less.[40] This may occur from a decreased production of neutrophils in the bone marrow or by the production of abnormal granulocytes that do not participate in phagocytosis. Children who receive chemotherapeutic agents or radiation therapy or have undergone transplants typically become both neutropenic and thrombocytopenic during the course of their disease or treatment. Infections, drugs, and chemical toxins may also cause neutropenia.[40,41]

Febrile neutropenia can rapidly progress to septic shock, hypotension, and cardiovascular collapse. Neutropenic children with fever require early identification and emergent intervention to prevent further complications associated with sepsis.

Additional History

- History of an immune deficiency disorder or immuno-suppression
- Fever
- Signs and symptoms of infection: irritability, lethargy, pallor, chills, and myalgia
- Presence of a central line
- Obvious infection source, such as a lesion or open wound

Additional Interventions

- Strict hand washing and aseptic technique when performing procedures
- Isolation to prevent contact with other children in waiting area
- Laboratory specimens for CBC, platelets, cross match, cultures (from central line if present)
- Calculate ANC: $\frac{(\% \text{ neutrophils } + \% \text{ bands}) \times WBC}{100}$
- Initiate IV fluid therapy
- Administer antibiotics and antipyretics as ordered
- Avoid rectal temperatures, examinations, catheterizations, enemas, and suppositories

Apparent Life-Threatening Events (ALTE)

An apparent life-threatening event is an episode that is frightening to the observer and characterized by some combination of apnea (central or occasionally obstructive), color change (usually cyanotic or pallid but occasionally erythematous or plethoric), marked change in muscle tone (usually marked limpness), choking, or gagging. In some cases, the observer fears that the infant has died. The terms aborted crib death or near-miss sudden infant death syndrome (SIDS) should be abandoned because they imply a possibly misleadingly close association between this type of spell and SIDS.[42,43] **Table 15-11** identifies the possible etiologies of ALTE.[44-46]

Additional History

- Obtain thorough history of events from the witness; it is the most valuable part of evaluation. Assume the witness's perceptions are valid. Ascertain the following information.
  - Awake or asleep state
  - Appearance
  - Color changes
  - Tone changes
  - Length of event
  - Association with feeding
  - Position and sleep surface
  - Interventions and recovery time
- Patient history: GERD, previous ALTE, normal sleep position, who does the child sleep with, breathing abnormalities, chronic illness, acute illness, medications
- Family history: GERD, previous early deaths or ALTEs, seizures, obstructive sleep apnea, asthma, hypothyroidism, medications

Diagnostic Procedures

Testing may include but is not limited to

- Infection: CBC, blood culture, urine culture, RSV antigen, viral cultures, CXR, lumbar puncture
- Gastroesophageal reflux: esophageal pH monitoring or barium swallow
- Seizure disorder: EEG

Table 15-11 ALTE Etiologies

Gastroesophageal reflux disease (GERD)	Anemia
Seizure disorder or hydrocephalus	Central hypoventilation syndrome
Infection: respiratory syncytial virus (RSV), pertussis, sepsis, meningitis	CNS tumors
Upper airway obstruction	Toxins or medications
Cardiac disease	Trauma or child abuse
Breath holding	Hypo- or hyperthermia
Endocrine or metabolic disorders	Munchausen by proxy
Neuromuscular disorders	

- Cardiac disease: ECG, echocardiogram
- Pulmonary disorders: ABG, pulse oximetry, exhaled CO_2 monitoring, CXR, sleep study, lateral airway films, plethysmography
- Metabolic disorders: CBC, electrolytes, blood sugar, calcium, phosphorus, serum ammonia, magnesium, urine toxicology
- Neuromuscular disorders: Electromyogram, CT scan, MRI, hemolytic uremic syndrome
- Child abuse: CT scan, video monitoring

Management strategies are based on underlying etiology.

Health Promotion

Prevention measures and recommendations that will have an impact on medical illness include the following.

- Educate caregivers and pediatric patient about disease processes and prevention strategies, including temperature measurement, fever control measures, and resources to obtain immunizations.
- Educate about safe practices and safe sex strategies to reduce risk of sexually transmitted diseases including HIV.
- Provide referrals to available support groups in the area for children with chronic conditions (e.g., hemophilia, HIV, diabetes).
- Educate about appropriate nutrition for healthy children and those with chronic conditions.
- Educate pediatric patient and caregivers on how to obtain a primary care provider (PCP) and the importance of care continuity. Provide referral to a PCP or referral resource and encourage the caregiver to obtain a PCP.
- Provide caregivers with written information identifying common prevention strategies for each developmental stage.

Summary

Childhood illnesses encompass a vast array of disorders. Knowledge of the unique characteristics of the pediatric patient is essential for the interpretation of assessment data, the formulation of nursing diagnoses, and the provision of interventions. Early recognition of respiratory and/or cardiovascular compromise and neurologic alterations are fundamental to identification and prompt intervention of childhood illnesses and medical emergencies. The interlocking relationship between recognition of life-threatening illness and the initiation of rapid interventions is the central piece to the puzzle of care for the pediatric patient.

References

1. Soud, T. E. (1998). The febrile child. In T. E. Soud & J. S. Rogers (Eds.), *Manual of pediatric emergency nursing* (pp. 606–621). St. Louis, MO: Mosby.
2. Hockenberry, M. J. (2003). Physical and developmental assessment of the child. In M. J. Hockenberry, D. Wilson, M. L. Winkelstein, & N. E. Kline (Eds.), *Wong's nursing care of infants and children* (7th ed., pp. 170–239). St. Louis, MO: Mosby.
3. Canadian Paediatric Society. (2002). Temperature measurement in pediatrics [Position statement]. *Paediatrics and Child Health 2000, 5*(5), 273–276.
4. Coulter, K. (1997). Temperature taking. In R. A. Deickmann, D. H. Fiser, & S. M. Selbst (Eds.), *Illustrated textbook of pediatric emergency and critical care procedures* (pp. 21–23). St. Louis, MO: Mosby.
5. Warren, D., Jarvis, A., & LeBlanc, L. (2002). The Canadian pediatric E.D. triage and acuity scale: Implementation guidelines for emergency departments. *Canadian Journal of Emergency Medicine, 3*(4), 2–27.
6. Hazinski, M. F.(1997). Anatomic and physiologic differences between children and adults. In D. Levin & F. Morriss (Eds.), *Essentials of pediatric intensive care* (2nd ed., pp. 1112–1126). New York: Churchill Livingstone.
7. Barkin, R. M., & Rosen, P. (1999). Dehydration. In R. M. Barkin & P. Rosen (Eds.), *Emergency pediatrics: A guide to ambulatory care* (5th ed., pp. 69–77) St. Louis. MO: Mosby.
8. Noble, M. N. (1998). Fluid and electrolyte imbalances. In T. E. Soud & J. S. Rogers (Eds.), *Manual of pediatric emergency nursing* (pp. 313–331). St. Louis, MO: Mosby.
9. Sacchetti, A., & Brilli, R. J. (1997). Fluid and electrolyte balance. In R. M. Barkin (Ed.), *Pediatric emergency medicine: Concepts and clinical practice* (pp. 166–189). St. Louis, MO: Mosby.
10. Watkins, S. L. (1995). The basics of fluid and electrolyte therapy. *Pediatric Annals, 24*(1), 16–22.
11. Kresch, M. J. (1984). Axillary temperature as a screening test for fever in children. *Journal of Pediatrics, 104*(4), 596–599.
12. Benjamin, V. L. (1998). Pediatric history and physical examination. In T. E. Soud & J. S. Rogers (Eds.), *Manual of pediatric emergency nursing* (pp. 70–88). St. Louis, MO: Mosby.
13. Belamarich, P. (1997). Gastrointestinal emergencies. In E. F. Crain & J. C. Gershel (Eds.), *Clinical manual of emergency pediatrics* (3rd ed., pp. 191–248). New York: McGraw-Hill.
14. Horton, M., Soud, T., Inman, C., & Standifer, P. (1998). Gastrointestinal system. In T. E. Soud & J. S. Rogers (Eds.), *Manual of pediatric emergency nursing* (pp. 332–343). St. Louis, MO: Mosby.
15. Masiulis, B., & Schultz, A. (1998). Neurologic system. In T. E. Soud & J. S. Rogers (Eds.), *Manual of pediatric emergency nursing* (pp. 266–289). St. Louis, MO: Mosby.
16. Vernon-Levett, P. (2001). Neurologic critical care problems. In M. A. Curley & P. A. Moloney-Harmon (Eds.), *Critical care nursing of infants and children* (2nd ed., pp. 695–730). Philadelphia: Saunders.

17. Strawser, R. (1997). Pediatric bacterial meningitis in the emergency department. *Journal of Emergency Nursing, 23*(4), 310–315.

18. Bank, D. E. (1997). Dermatologic emergencies. In E. F. Crain & J. C. Gershel (Eds.), *Clinical manual of emergency pediatrics* (3rd ed., pp. 69–114). New York: McGraw-Hill.

19. Felter, R. A., & Bower, J. R. (1997). Infectious disorders. In R. M. Barkin (Ed.), *Pediatric emergency medicine: Concepts and clinical practice* (2nd ed., pp. 926–971). St. Louis, MO: Mosby.

20. Fuchs, S. M. (1997). Neurologic emergencies. In R. M. Barkin (Ed.), *Pediatric emergency medicine: Concepts and clinical practice* (2nd ed., pp. 972–1024). St. Louis, MO: Mosby.

21. Dannenbery, B. W. (1996). Pediatric seizure disorders: Prompt assessment and emergency management. *Pediatric Emergency Medicine Reports, 1,* 41–52.

22. Bunch, B., & Avner, J. R. (1997). Neurologic emergencies. In E. F. Crain & J. C. Gershel (Eds.), *Clinical manual of emergency pediatrics* (3rd ed., pp. 437–476). New York: McGraw-Hill.

23. Segeleon, J. E., & Haun, S. E. (1996). Status epilepticus in children. *Pediatric Annals, 25*(7), 380–386.

24. Pye, T., & Soud, T. (1998). Genitourinary system. In T. E. Soud & J. C. Rogers (Eds.), *Manual of pediatric emergency nursing* (pp. 364–389). St. Louis, MO: Mosby.

25. Hockenberry, M. J. (2003). The child with renal dysfunction. In M. J. Hockenberry, D. Wilson, M. L. Winkelstein, & N. E. Kline (Eds.), *Wong's nursing care of infants and children* (7th ed., pp. 1255–1302). St. Louis, MO: Mosby.

26. Rosenbloom, A. L., & Hanas, R.(1996). Diabetic ketoacidosis (DKA): Treatment guidelines. *Clinical Pediatrics, 35*(5), 261–266.

27. Klekamp, J., & Churchwell, K. B. (1996). Diabetic ketoacidosis in children: Initial clinical assessment and treatment. *Pediatric Annals, 25*(7), 387–393.

28. Craig, J. (1998). Endocrine system. In American Association of Critical-Care Nurses & M. C. Slota (Eds.), *Core curriculum for pediatric critical care nursing* (pp. 410). Philadelphia: Saunders.

29. Trimarchi, T. (2001). Endocrine critical care problems. In M. A. Curley, & P. A. Moloney-Harmon (Eds.), *Critical care nursing of infants and children* (2nd ed., pp. 805–819). Philadelphia: Saunders.

30. Bachman, D. T., Barkin, R. M., Brennan, S. A., & Recht, M. (1997). Hematologic and oncologic disorders. In R. M. Barkin (Ed.), *Pediatric emergency medicine: Concepts and clinical practice* (pp. 907–911). St. Louis, MO: Mosby.

31. Lombardo, D. M. (2003). Hematologic emergencies. In L. Newberry (Ed.), *Sheehy's emergency nursing: Principles and practice* (5th ed., pp. 633–640). St. Louis, MO: Mosby.

32. Drake, E. E. (1997). Hematologic system. In J. A. Fox (Ed.), *Primary health care of children* (pp. 455–464). St. Louis, MO: Mosby.

33. Brinker, D., & Moloney-Harmon, P. A. (2001). Hematologic critical care problems. In M. A. Curley, & P. A. Moloney-Harmon (Eds.), *Critical care nursing of infants and children* (2nd ed., pp. 821–850). Philadelphia: Saunders.

34. Weinblatt, M. (1997). Hematologic emergencies. In E. F. Crain & J. C. Gershel (Eds.), *Clinical manual of emergency pediatrics* (3rd ed., pp. 314–319). New York: McGraw-Hill.

35. Raghuram, N., Pettignano, R., Gal, A. A., Harsch, A., & Adamkicwicz, T. V. (1997). Plastic bronchitis: An unusual complication associated with sickle cell disease and the acute chest syndrome. *Pediatrics, 100*(1), 139–142.

36. Soglin, D., & Kramer, J. (1996). Sickle cell disease. In G. Strange, W. Ahrens, S. Lelyveld, & R. Schafermeyer (Eds.), *Pediatric emergency medicine: A comprehensive study guide* (pp. 451). New York: McGraw-Hill.

37. Wulff, K., Zappa, S., & Womack, M. (Eds.). (1999). *Emergency care for patients with hemophilia: An instructional manual for medical professionals* (2nd ed.). The Nursing Group of Hemophilia Region VI.

38. Felter, R. A., & Bower, J. R. (1997). Infectious disorders. In R. M. Barkin (Ed.), *Pediatric emergency medicine: Concepts and clinical practice* (2nd ed., pp. 926–971). St. Louis, MO: Mosby.

39. Shea, K. A. (1997). Human immunodeficiency virus/acquired immunodeficiency syndrome. In J. A. Fox (Ed.), *Primary health care of children* (pp. 878–892). St. Louis, MO: Mosby.

40. Jenkins, T. (2001). Oncologic critical care problems. In M. A. Curley & P. A. Moloney-Harmon (Eds.), *Critical care nursing of infants and children* (2nd ed., pp. 853–873). Philadelphia: Saunders.

41. Manley, L., & Bechtel, N. M. (1998). Hematologic and immune systems. In T. E. Soud & J. S. Rogers (Eds.), *Manual of pediatric emergency nursing* (pp. 390–416). St. Louis, MO: Mosby.

42. National Institutes of Health Consensus Development Panel (1986). *Infantile apnea and home monitoring* [*Consensus statement*]. Retrieved February 24, 2003 from http://consensus.nih.gov/cons/058/058_statement.htm

43. Kahn, A., Groswasser, J., Rebuffat, E., Sottiaux, M., Blum, D., Foerster, M., et al. (1993). Sleep and cardiorespiratory characteristics of infant victims of sudden death: A prospective case-control study. *Sleep, 16*(4), 391.

44. Tirosh, E., & Jaffe, M. (1996). Apnea of infancy, seizures, and gastroesophageal reflux: An important but infrequent association. *Journal of Child Neurology, 11*(2), 98–100.

45. Samuels, M. P., McClaughlin, W., Jacobson, R. R., Poets, C. F., & Southall, D. P. (1992). Fourteen cases of imposed upper airway obstruction. *Archives of Disease in Childhood, 67*(2), 162–170.

46. Southall, D. P., Plunkett, M. C., Banks, M. W., Falkov, A. F., & Samuels, M. P. (1997). Covert video recordings of life-threatening child abuse: Lessons for child protection. *Pediatrics, 100*(5), 735–760.

Appendix 15-A Summary of Infectious Exanthems

Disease	Etiology	Period of Communicability	Mode of Transmission	Incubation	Prodrome	Clinical Presentation	Complications
Rubeola (measles)	Paramyxovirus	From prodrome until 5 days after rash begins	Respiratory-airborne droplets	10-14 days	3-4 days high fever, cough, nasal congestion, conjunctivitis; Koplik's spots appear 2 days before rash	Erythematous maculo-papular rash; begins on face and spreads downward; initial discrete lesions become confluent; after 3-4 days rash appears reddish-brown; fine desquamation occurs Photophobia; high fever; conjunctivitis; harsh cough	Otitis media; pneumonia; encephalitis
Mumps	Paramyxovirus	Immediately before and after swelling begins	Saliva of infected persons	14-21 days	Fever, headache, malaise, anorexia, earache (especially when chewing)	By day 3, parotid gland enlarges, accompanied by pain and tenderness	Deafness; arthritis; epididymoorchitis; sterility
Rubella	RNA virus; Rubivirus in the togavirus family	From 7 days before to 5 days after rash	Respiratory-airborne droplets; objects freshly contaminated with nasopharyngeal secretions	14-21 days	Absent in children; in adolescents low-grade fever, malaise, sore throat, cough, nasal congestion, lymphadenopathy	Discrete pink maculopapular rash with downward progression from face; rash disappears in same order as it began; usually gone in 3 days	Greatest danger is teratogenic effect on fetus Rare: arthritis, encephalitis, purpura
Varicella (chickenpox)	Varicella zoster	From 1 day before rash erupts until lesions have crusted (approximately 1 week after rash begins)	Direct contact with infected persons via droplet spread; objects contaminated with nasopharyngeal secretions	14-21 days	Slight fever, anorexia, malaise for 24 hr.	Pruritic rash rapidly progressing from macules to papules to thin vesicles that break and form crusts; all stages of rash occur simultaneously; begins centrally, spreads to face and proximal extremities Fever; lymphadenopathy	Secondary bacterial infections; varicella pneumonia; encephalitis
Scarlet fever	Group A Beta-hemolytic streptococci	During incubation period and clinical illness or until 24 hr after antibiotics are initiated	Close direct contact with infected person or by respiratory droplet spread; indirectly by contact with contaminated objects and food, especially dairy products	2-4 days	Acute onset of high fever, increased heart rate out of proportion to fever, headache, sore throat, stomach ache, vomiting, chills	Erythematous maculo-papular "sandpaper" rash begins on neck and skinfold areas; spreads to trunk and extremities; lasts approximately 4-5 days Petechiae in skin folds of axillae, groin, and antecubital area (Pastia's sign) Facial flush with circumoral pallor; "strawberry tongue," generalized lymphadenopathy Desquamation of skin lasts for 1-2 wk	Early: otitis, pneumonia, septicemia, osteomyelitis Late: rheumatic fever and acute glomerulonephritis

Appendix 15-A Summary of Infectious Exanthems (cont.)

Disease	Etiology	Period of Communicability	Mode of Transmission	Incubation	Prodrome	Clinical Presentation	Complications
Erythema infectiosum (fifth disease)	Human parvovirus B19	Uncertain, but before onset of rash during prodrome	Unknown; most likely via contact with respiratory droplets of infected persons	4-14 days	1-4 days mild fever, headache, pruritus (usually not noticed by parents)	Three-stage rash: 1. Bright-red "slapped" cheeks 2. Erythematous maculopapular rash primarily on extremities, but sometimes also on trunk and buttocks 3. Fine lacy rash as maculopapular rash fades; rash may fade and reappear over next 10-14 days	Self-limited arthralgia and arthritis Possible fetal death if mother is infected in pregnancy Aplastic crisis in children with hemolytic disease or immune deficiency
Roseola	Human herpes virus VI	During illness	Unknown	5-15 days	3-4 days high fever in otherwise well child	Temperature becomes normal when rash develops; rose-colored discrete macules or maculopapules, nonpruritic, lasting 1-2 days	Febrile seizures
Pityriasis rosea	Unknown; probably viral	Unknown	Unknown	Unknown	Sometimes malaise, headache, pharyngitis	"Herald patch," followed by small round papules that enlarge to form erythematous oval patches with scaly border; classic "Christmas tree pattern" peaks in 2-3 wk, fades over 6-12 wk	None
Hand-foot-and-mouth disease	Coxsackie A enteroviruses	From 2 days before to 2 days after eruption	Hand-to-mouth contact with infected person	3-6 days	1-2 days low-grade fever, malaise, vomiting, sore throat	Small oval vesicles on hands, feet, and mucous membranes of mouth	Dehydration Rare: myocarditis, pneumonia, meningoencephalitis

Reprinted with permission from Fioravanti, J. (1998). Integumentary system. In T. E. Soud & J. E. Rogers (Eds.), *Manual of pediatric emergency nursing* (pp. 417-451). St. Louis, MO: Mosby.

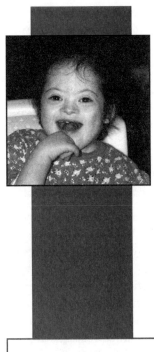

chapter 16

CHILDREN WITH SPECIAL HEALTH CARE NEEDS

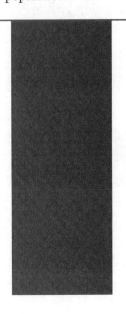

Objectives

On completion of this chapter, the learner should be able to:

1. Define the special-needs population.

2. Recognize the common causes of illness and injury in the special-needs population.

3. Describe the assessment and intervention strategies specific to the special-needs population.

Introduction

Children with special health care needs are "those who have or are at increased risk for a chronic physical, developmental, behavioral, or emotional condition and who also require health and related services of a type or amount beyond that required by children generally."[1] As medical technology continues to advance, increasing the odds of survival for children with congenital and chronic conditions, the odds of a nurse encountering one of these children in the emergency department (ED) will continue to increase.

As the definition of special health care needs indicates, there is a wide range of conditions that can qualify a child for this designation. These conditions include mental disabilities, physical disabilities, the need for technologic support, and certain chronic illnesses. **Table 16-1** outlines some of these conditions.

In 1998, approximately 18% of children in the United States under the age of 18 years had a chronic physical, developmental, behavioral, or emotional condition that met special health care needs criteria. This amounts to almost 12.6 million children annually. Among the general American population, the prevalence of special needs was higher for older children, boys, African Americans, and children from low-income and single-parent households. School-aged children were twice as likely to be classified as having an existing special need, and boys were approximately 30% more likely than girls to have special needs. Hispanic children and minorities other than African Americans were least likely to be cate-

gorized as having a special health care need under the preceding definition.[2]

It is important to keep in mind that for every anatomic part or physiologic process that exists in the human body, there can be an abnormality of that part or process. Entire textbooks are devoted to the cataloging of these anomalies, with hundreds of syndromes, associations, malformations, and defects as yet unclassified. Although it would be impossible for any one health care provider to be familiar with, yet alone an expert at, each one of these, it is not only entirely possible but also overwhelmingly likely that the child's parents or caretakers have become experts in their child's particular problem. Most families of children with special health care needs have completed training specific to their child's condition and have developed expertise in the assessment and management of their child's equipment and health-related issues. The child's family should be utilized as your most important resource in assessing and caring for a child with special health care needs.

Types of Medical Technology

Children with special health care needs often utilize some type of medical technology. Estimates from 1988 placed approximately 100,000 children in the category of dependence on medical technology.[3] Some of the more common technologies the emergency nurse is likely to encounter are reviewed following.

Tracheostomy Tubes

There are several reasons a child may require a tracheostomy tube, including nonsurgical upper airway obstruction or the need for an access port for long-term ventilation. **Table 16-2** delineates some of the tracheostomy tubes commonly used in pediatrics. **Figure 16-1** includes several types of pediatric tracheostomy tubes.

Tracheostomy tubes may be either plastic, metal, cuffed, or uncuffed.[4] Metal tubes are used infrequently and have a removable inner cannula. Plastic tubes are more commonly used in pediatrics and usually do not have an inner cannula. Plastic tracheostomy tubes may be equipped with an adaptor for easy connection to a standard manual resuscitator (Ambu® bag). Most pediatric tracheostomy tubes are cuffless.

The size of the tracheostomy tube is usually marked both on the package as well as on the flanges of each tube. The size refers to the inner diameter of the tube. Tubes are additionally marked as neonatal, pediatric, or adult. This designation refers to the length of the tube. Thus, a 3.5 neonatal tube has the same inner diameter as a 3.5 pediatric tube, but the neonatal tube is shorter.

In children who breathe spontaneously, tracheostomy tubes may have special attachments designed to protect the child's airway. A tracheostomy "nose"[4] is a filtration device that keeps particulate matter out of the airway and additionally supplies humidification because the tracheostomy bypasses the usual humidification function of the nose. Older children may have a Passy-Muir® valve (PMV) (**Figure 16-2**), which redirects the airflow and allows the child to speak. The PMV may be

Table 16-1 Descriptions of Selected Special Health Care Conditions

Body System	Description
Respiratory	*Congenital:* Laryngeal malacia; underdeveloped lungs; cystic fibrosis.
	Acquired: Pulmonary neoplasms; asthma; chronic bronchitis; bronchopulmonary dysplasia.
Cardiovascular	*Congenital:* Heart disease
	Acquired: Heart disease
Neurologic	*Congenital:* Spina bifida; Arnold-Chiari malformation; chromosomal anomalies; Dandy-Walker malformation; hydrocephalus.
	Perinatal: Infections; anoxic encephalopathy; birth trauma; cerebral palsy.
	Postnatal: Head and spinal cord trauma; neoplasms.
	Seizure disorders: Infantile spasms; Lennox-Gastaudt syndrome; epilepsy.
Immunologic	*Congenital:* Immune disorders
	Acquired: Human immunodeficiency virus; hepatitis; carcinomas.
	Induced: Immunosuppression following solid organ or bone marrow transplants and chemotherapy for cancer treatment
Mental retardation	*Physical appearance:* Well-proportioned physical features or characteristic features such as low-set ears, soft neurologic signs (e.g., microcephaly), poor fine and/or gross motor coordination
	Cognitive function: Educable or needing assistance or total care
Other	*Physical:* Limb deformities; craniofacial malformations; paralysis.
	Sensory: Alterations in hearing, vision, or tactile perceptabilities
	Cognitive: Alterations in thinking abilities

Adapted from Wertz, E. (2001). The patient with special needs. In N. E. McSwain (Ed.), *The basic EMT—comprehensive prehospital patient care* (2nd ed., p. 770). St. Louis, MO: Mosby–Year Book.

Figure 16-1 Disposable Cuffless Tracheostomy Tube and Disposable Cuffless Fenestrated Tracheostomy Tube

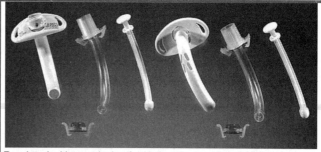

Reprinted with permission for Nellcor Puritan Bennett, Inc. Pleasanton, CA 94588.

Figure 16-2 Passy-Muir® Speaking Valves

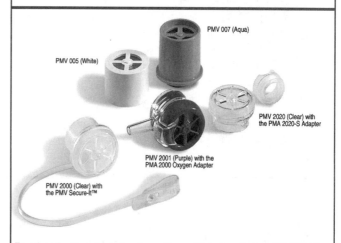

Reprinted with permission from Passy-Muir, Inc. Irvine, CA 92612

used on a tracheostomy tube and inline on the ventilator. If the child has a cuffed tracheostomy tube, the cuff must be completely deflated while using the PMV.

Oxygen

Children may be discharged home with oxygen (O_2) for a variety of reasons, including bronchopulmonary dysplasia (BPD), cystic fibrosis, and congenital cardiac disease.[5] Home O_2 may be delivered via numerous routes, including nasal cannula, tracheostomy mask, and home ventilator. The oxygen may be needed either intermittently or continuously, depending on the child's condition and the reasons for the oxygen requirement.

Apnea Monitors

Home apnea monitors are prescribed for infants who are deemed at risk for death from sudden infant death syndrome (SIDS). Risk factors for SIDS include a diagnosis of apnea of infancy (AOI), a history of apparent life-threatening events (ALTEs) or siblings with a history of AOI or ALTE.[6] Although there are many different types of home apnea monitors, all are designed to evaluate respiratory and cardiac rhythms and to alarm at predetermined levels, usually apnea of 20 seconds or greater or bradycardia. The use of home apnea monitoring is controversial because there are no studies that document a decrease in the mortality due to SIDS with their use.[11]

Ventilators

Home ventilation is most commonly used for patients who have a stable cardiopulmonary status, but are unable to provide adequate ventilatory effort on their own. It is most commonly required in children with severe BPD, neuromuscular disorders, head and spinal cord injuries, and conditions that cause chronic respiratory failure. The most common type of home ventilator is a positive-pressure ventilator.[5]

Central Venous Access Devices

Central venous catheters can be categorized into three main types: (1) short-term or nontunneled catheters, such as subclavian or jugular catheters; (2) peripherally inserted central catheters (PICC); and (3) long-term catheters, such as tunneled catheters and implanted ports.

Short-term catheters are usually used in emergency situations, such as cardiac arrests or trauma resuscitations, and are unlikely modalities to be found in the home setting.

Table 16-2 Tracheostomy Tubes Commonly Used in Pediatrics

	Single Cannula, Plastic/Silicone, Pediatric and Neonatal Tubes	Double Cannula, Plastic/Silicone Tubes
Usual age group	Premature infants, newborns, young children	Older children, adolescents, and adults
Distinguishing features	Wide variety of diameters and lengths that accommodate very small tracheas	Large outer diameter precludes use in infants, young children
	Anatomically designed to fit the curve of small children's tracheas	Available with or without fenestration (hole in outer cannula that allows for easier vocalization when inner cannula is not in use)
		Low profile cannula available (protrudes less), but does not attach to ventilator or bag-valve device
		Decannulation plugs available that occlude the trachea and allow for breathing through the upper airways
Materials	Soft, flexible materials	Made of a more rigid plastic
Cuffs	Not available with cuffs	Available with or without
Care and cleaning	Easy for home care providers to change and care for	Inner cannula may be easily removed to clean or check for mucus
	Must remove entire tube if concerned about mucus occlusion	Standard inner cannula must be in place for mechanical ventilation and ventilation with manual resuscitator

Reprinted with permission from Schultz, A., & Chalanick, K. (1998). Children with special needs. In T. Soud & J. S. Rogers (Eds.), *Manual of pediatric emergency nursing* (pp. 712–726). St. Louis, MO: Mosby.

PICC lines are used for moderate-length therapies. They are usually inserted into the antecubital area and threaded until the tip of the catheter lies within the superior vena cava or right atrium. PICC lines are used for home infusions such as parenteral nutrition[7] or for conditions requiring long-term antibiotic therapy, such as osteomyelitis.

Long-term central catheters are further categorized into either tunneled catheters or implanted infusion ports. Although tunneled catheters provide for a means of pain-free infusions, they all have some component of external tubing, which increases the likelihood of dislodgement.[7] Children, therefore, are more likely to be discharged with implanted ports and the parents given topical anesthetic cream for painless needle insertions.

Gastrostomy Tubes (G-tubes)

Gastrostomy tubes are often used for children who require long-term feeding, although they may also be employed for long-term gastric decompression.[5] Most children have indwelling tubes, of which there are several styles (see **Figure 16-3**). Button G-tubes, shown in **Figure 16-4**, are the type most commonly used in children because they sit at skin level and are less easily dislodged than those with redundant external tubing. Button G-tubes require a special adapter in order to give feedings or medications. Parents are instructed to bring this adapter with them when they visit the ED. When emergency gastric decompression is required and no

adapter is available, an intravenous (IV) extension tubing set will fit into the button.

Ventriculoperitoneal (VP) shunts

A VP shunt, surgically inserted to treat hydrocephalus, drains excess cerebrospinal fluid (CSF) from the cranial ventriculae into the peritoneal cavity. These shunts are

Figure 16-4 Button G-tube

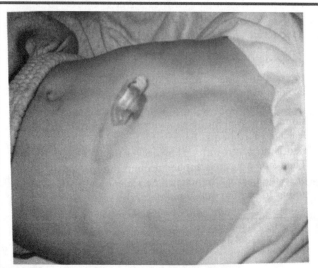

Reprinted with permission from Hockenberry, M. J., Wilson, D., Winkelstein, M. L., & Kline, N. E. (2003). Pediatric variations of nursing interventions. In *Wong's nursing care of infants and children* (7th ed., pp. 1101–1170). St. Louis, MO: Mosby.

Figure 16-3 Types of Gastrostomy Tubes

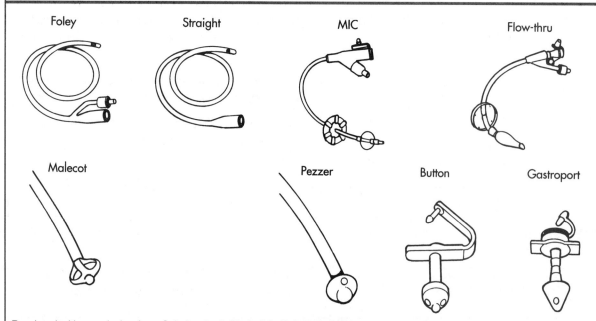

Reprinted with permission from Schultz, A., & Chalanick, K. (1998). Children with special needs. In T. Soud & J. S. Rogers (Eds.), *Manual of pediatric emergency nursing* (pp. 712–726). St. Louis, MO: Mosby.

radiopaque and usually contain both a reservoir at the cranial end to allow easy access for CSF sampling and a one-way valve to prevent backflow from the peritoneal cavity to the brain. The valve is designed to open at a predetermined intraventricular pressure and then close again when the pressure falls below that level.[7] Although the peritoneum is the most common drainage site for a CSF shunt, other sites, such as the right atrium, may be utilized.[4]

Anatomic and Physiologic Characteristics as a Basis for Signs and Symptoms

Children with special health care needs may come to the ED with illnesses and injuries related to their disabilities or with any of the complaints common to all pediatric patients. Because of their disabilities, however, they are more prone to certain problems than are other children.

Airway

Many children with special health care needs have abnormal airways. These abnormalities can occur at any level of the airway, from the oral cavity to the bronchial tree. Although the typical pediatric tongue occupies about half of the oral cavity, children with certain syndromes, such as trisomy 21 (Down syndrome), may have exceptionally large tongues, occupying even a greater proportion of their mouths. This predisposes them to airway occlusion with even a minor decrease in level of consciousness. They may also have a decreased ability to handle secretions, necessitating more frequent suctioning. Other airway anomalies can result from exceptionally small mandibles, such as in Pierre Robin's syndrome.

Abnormalities of the trachea can also occur, which include softening of the trachea (tracheomalacia), narrowing of a portion of the trachea (tracheal stenosis), an opening between the esophagus and the trachea (tracheoesophageal fistula), or incomplete formation of the trachea (tracheal atresia). These abnormalities predispose patients to obstruction by a foreign body, decreased ability to maintain a patent airway, increased risk for aspiration, and increased morbidity from common childhood illnesses such as laryngotracheobronchitis (croup).

Breathing/Ventilation/Oxygen Transport

Respiration is a complex interaction of the nervous system, respiratory muscles, the thorax, and the lungs themselves,[8] with the terminal purpose of oxygen delivery to the tissues. Children with special health care needs may have complications at any one or more of these points. Disorders of the airway, neurologic, or immunologic system or decreased activity levels may put them at higher risk for pneumonia. The pulmonary-alveolar interface itself may be altered, such as in BPD or congestive heart failure. In these children, the depth and adequacy of ventilation is offset by the inability of the oxygen to cross over from the lungs to the bloodstream.

Respiratory excursion may be limited by kyphoscoliosis or diaphragmatic hernias. The lungs themselves are normal, as is the pulmonary-alveolar interface, but lung expansion is limited by an external element. Tidal volume is subsequently decreased, leading to respiratory compromise.

Oxygen transport may be impaired by chronic anemia or by abnormal hemoglobin transport, such as in sickle cell disease. Although the respiratory system itself is anatomically normal, oxygen delivery is impaired secondary to either an inadequate amount of oxygen-carrying hemoglobin or by an altered ability of the hemoglobin to carry oxygen.

Circulation

Children with special health care needs may have circulatory abnormalities as well. These problems can occur in any of the structural entities of the circulatory system, as well as any of the homeostatic mechanisms designed to maintain a normal circulating blood volume.

Congenital adrenal hyperplasia (CAH) is a disorder of the adrenal enzymes that can result in inadequate or absent production of both mineralocorticoids and glucocorticoids. Children with CAH may present in shock resulting from intravascular volume depletion.[9]

An increasing number of children are living with congenital cardiac anomalies, ranging from relatively minor to quite severe and complex. Children with certain cardiac anomalies, such as tricuspid atresia or pulmonary stenosis, may have baseline cyanosis. Children with rhythm disorders may have implanted pacemakers or occasionally even automatic implanted cardiac defibrillators. These children need to have their presenting condition compared to their baseline, rather than to standard norms.

The peripheral circulatory system may also have anomalies. There are numerous conditions that cause anomalies of the limbs, such as CHILD syndrome (an acronym for Congenital Hemidysplasia with Ichthyosiform erythroderma and Limb Defects), or VACTERL (vertebral, anal, cardiac, tracheal, esophageal, renal, and limb defects—a group of defects that may be associated with tetralogy of Fallot and Holt-Oram syndrome).[10] Depending on the severity of malformation, these limb anomalies may be associated with peripheral vascular defects. This has implications not only for injuries to the extremities, but for vascular access as well.

There can also be anomalies in any one of the constituents of blood. Abnormalities of white cells, such as is found in leukemia, can lead to an increased susceptibility to infection. Red cell alterations can lead to vasoocclusive crises caused by sludging of the blood (sickle cell disease) and decreased oxygen-carrying capacity (thalassemia). Platelet aberrations lead to increased bleeding tendencies and easy bruising, as does a lack of any other component of the clotting cascade, such as in hemophilia. There are also numerous defects possible in the immunologic and enzymatic elements of blood. These defects may necessitate special diets (phenylketonuria), avoidance of certain medications (G-6-PD deficiency), or avoidance of common communicable diseases (severe combined immunodeficiency syndrome).

Disability

Neurologic abnormalities are found concurrently with numerous different syndromes, but may also be the child's only disability. Some syndromes cause a characteristic facial appearance, but may not cause mental disability (Nager's acrofacial dysostosis), and some mental disabilities are present in children who appear "normal" (Cohen syndrome). No assumptions should be made about the child's developmental level or level of functioning based solely on appearances. Once again, the child's parents or caretakers can provide valuable insight into whether the child's present behavior is "normal" for them.

Nursing Care of the Child with Special Health Care Needs

Assessment and Interventions

In many ways, children with special health care needs are more like their healthy, able-bodied peers than they are different;[5] however, the developmental stage, size, and language abilities of these children may vary from other children of the same age. The parents should be utilized as expert resources to determine what is normal for their child. Never hesitate to question the parents as to the presence of a chronic illness or disability, their usual complications, presenting symptoms, and treatment. As the parents have had the benefit of having received information from all of the specialists involved in their child's care, assessing the child on an everyday basis, and being involved from beginning to end in every illness that their child incurs, they are frequently the only ones with the "big picture" as it concerns their child.

In general, assessment of the child with special health care needs proceeds in the same manner as for other children. Assessment consists of three parts: (1) the pediatric assessment triangle (PAT), (2) the primary assessment, and (3) the secondary assessment.

Pediatric Assessment Triangle

The PAT is an observational assessment of the child's appearance, work of breathing, and skin parameters. In children with special health care needs, the child's developmental stage should be assessed early. This will help the emergency nurse tailor the examination to the appropriate developmental level of the child, rather than to the stated age, which may be incongruent. The child's parents can provide baseline information for the child's normal level of activity, muscle tone, level of responsiveness, and general appearance. See Chapter 3, *From the Start—Dealing with Children*, for a discussion on common developmental milestones.

Primary Assessment

Airway/Cervical Spine

Assess the airway for patency utilizing the same assessment tools used for all children. Common causes of airway obstruction in children with special health care needs include an inability to protect the airway due to altered gag reflex or other neurologic abnormality, excessive salivation, abnormally large tongue, and displacement or obstruction of the tracheostomy tube.

Observe the child to determine their ability to handle secretions, and have suction immediately available to manage these secretions. Assess the size of the child's tongue to determine their risk for airway obstruction secondary to their anatomic anomaly. Some children may require specific methods of airway positioning to facilitate breathing; check with the child's parents for optimal positioning. If abnormal airway sounds are heard, check with the parents to determine if these are new or baseline sounds. For instance, many children with tracheomalacia exhibit a stridorous sound, especially when sleeping. Potential problems with tracheostomies can be assessed by utilizing the DOPE[4] mnemonic (**Table 16-3**). This mnemonic, with modification, can be used for any tube.

Table 16-3 DOPE (for tracheostomies)	
D	Displacement of tube
O	Obstruction of tube
P	Pneumothorax
E	Equipment failure

Displacement of the tube may be assessed first by visualizing the tube. The flanges of the tracheostomy tube should be at skin level; any additional tubing that is external to the stoma indicates a displaced tube. An exhaled CO_2 detector may also be used to assess for accurate tube placement. If the tube is displaced out of the trachea, no CO_2 will be detected on exhalation. In an emergency, a standard endotracheal tube of the same inner diameter may be used instead of a tracheostomy tube.[4] For example, a 4.0 tracheostomy tube could be replaced with a 4.0 endotracheal tube, although it will need to be shortened from the distal end once proper placement is confirmed. If the tracheostomy tube needs to be replaced, have available both the size the child usually uses, as well as one size smaller. **Table 16-4** describes replacement of a tracheostomy tube.

Obstruction of the tube should be suspected when a child with a tracheostomy tube presents with fever, cough, thick secretions, decreased breath sounds bilaterally, or decreased chest rise and fall. Attempts to ventilate a child with an obstructed tube will yield minimal to no chest rise and fall, absent breath sounds, and resistance to manual ventilation. To evaluate for tube obstruction, follow these steps.[10]

1. Position the child with a rolled towel under the shoulders.

2. Consider injection of 1 to 3 ml of normal saline into the tracheostomy tube to thin the secretions

3. Select the properly sized suction catheter to fit through the tracheostomy tube. Utilize a length-based resuscitation tape to determine the correct size if the parents do not know.

4. Set the suction to 100 mm Hg or less to avoid trauma to the airway.

5. If possible, preoxygenate the child via administration of oxygen directly to the tracheal stoma or via a manual resuscitator.

6. Insert the suction catheter through the tracheostomy tube and advance until the tip of the suction catheter is even with the tip of the tracheostomy tube. If you are unsuccessful or feel that the obstruction extends beyond the end of the tube, you may gently pass the catheter beyond the tip of the tracheostomy tube.

7. Apply suction for no longer than 10 seconds. Suction should be applied on withdrawal of the catheter, while gently twisting or rolling the catheter to clear the entire inner circumference of the tracheostomy tube.

8. If the obstruction is still present, you may repeat the procedure one time after attempting ventilation between attempts. If there is still no improvement in the child's respiratory distress, the tracheostomy tube will need to be changed.

For children whose injuries or mechanism of injury suggest trauma, the cervical spine should be stabilized while the airway is assessed. Positioning the child with special needs can present distinctive challenges. Depending on the nature of the child's special needs, he or she may have concomitant cervical spine anomalies that can complicate cervical stabilization. For instance, approximately 15% of children with trisomy 21 (Down syndrome) have atlantoaxial instability.[12] Each case should be assessed individually and optimal positioning determined on a case-by-case basis. In addition, stabilization of special-needs children with developmental delays requires patience and perseverance. Having the parent at the bedside throughout the process, dimming the lights so they do not shine in the child's eyes, and speaking slowly in a calming voice can all assist in keeping the child calm until their cervical spine is cleared. Distracters such as pictures on the ceiling, playing music, or singing are also useful calming techniques.

Breathing

Certain syndromes and diseases can decrease the efficacy of the child's immunologic system, increasing their susceptibility to pneumonia. Children with limited ability to protect their airways or limited immobility are also at an increased risk for pneumonia. Although many of these children have feeding tubes or G-tubes placed to decrease the risk of aspiration pneumonia, vomiting or failure to maintain an NPO status can present significant risks. In addition, some children have baseline lung disease, poor pulmonary reserve, restrictive lung disease, or inefficient accessory muscle use. These children respond poorly to increased respiratory demands, and can progress from respiratory distress to respiratory failure more rapidly than other children.

Assessment of breathing effectiveness is accomplished by employing the same indicators used for all children; however, the results must be compared once again

---

Table 16-4 Replacement of Tracheostomy Tube[4]

Place a rolled towel under the child's shoulders to expose the stoma.

Moisten the tracheostomy tube with a sterile, water-soluble lubricant.[10]

Insert the tube using firm, gentle pressure. If the tube does not pass easily, attempt passage with a tube one size smaller.

Assess placement with two confirmatory measures, such as auscultation of bilateral breath sounds, equal rise and fall of chest, or use of an exhaled CO_2 detector. When the tube is properly placed, there should be no bleeding or subcutaneous emphysema.

against the child's own baseline. Level of consciousness, although usually an excellent indicator of end-organ perfusion, may be a misleading assessment in a child with a normally decreased or difficult-to-assess sensorium. Cyanosis, normally considered a "late" sign of respiratory distress, may be present at all times in some children, rendering this assessment tool of little use. Lung sounds may be diminished in children with restrictive lung disease; tidal volumes may be decreased in children with kyphoscoliosis; or adventitious breath sounds may be present in many children with BPD.

Children on home ventilators who develop acute respiratory distress may be evaluated using the DOPE[4] mnemonic (**Table 16-5**).

Any child who develops acute respiratory distress while on a ventilator should be removed from the ventilator and have ventilations assisted via a manual resuscitator while an assessment as to the cause of the distress ensues and reversible causes are addressed.

Children on home apnea monitors may present to the ED following activation of a monitor alarm. Home apnea monitors operate by utilizing impedance monitoring, which is subject to false alarms due to shallow breathing or normal cardiac variability.[6] Nonetheless, the activation of these alarms can cause considerable distress to parents, who are frequently not in the room with the child when the monitor alarms, and thus are unsure as to exactly what occurred. Although there are false alarms with these monitors, they may indeed detect an apneic or bradycardic episode; thus, each child must receive a complete exam to detect any life threats or underlying reasons for the alarm.

Circulation

Assessment of circulatory status in a child with special health care needs consists of the same basic assessments as that of all children, but again, the results must be compared against the child's baseline. In addition, any assistive technology the child has must be assessed.

Consideration must be given to initiation of IV access. Depending on the child's unique anatomy, certain IV sites may be less desirable or not accessible. Parents may be able to direct staff to successful IV sites. Children who require ongoing fluid or medication therapy may have some form of central line. The DOPE[4] mnemonic may again be used to guide your assessment of central lines (**Table 16-6**).

Central venous catheters can become dislodged or damaged. If the catheter is damaged, the child can be at risk for an air embolism. Although air in an IV line is never acceptable, there are some children with certain cardiac defects in whom the risk is even greater, as the air can be redirected within the heart and can embolize directly to their brain. If air is noted in the line, the catheter should not be used and should be clamped until replaced. Signs and symptoms of air embolus include respiratory distress, cyanosis, dyspnea, tachycardia, chest pain, and shock. Treatment for air embolus beyond clamping the catheter includes placing the child in a supine position left side down, head lower than the body, and administration of 100 % oxygen. If the catheter has become dislodged or disengaged, assess for bleeding, apply direct pressure over the site, and assess the child's airway, breathing, and circulation for signs of circulatory compromise.[4] Central lines may also become disconnected, with volume loss subsequent to the disconnection.

Central venous catheters can become obstructed internally from blood clots or precipitates from medications. Catheters may also be obstructed secondary to kinking of the catheter. If the medication or fluid does not infuse easily, utilize sterile technique to aspirate blood to determine patency of the catheter. With certain implanted ports, the ability to use the port is dependent on body position; the parents should be your guide to which position will yield the most success. If positioning and gentle aspiration are not successful, stop all attempts to use the catheter because further attempts to manipulate the catheter can embolize a retained clot. Signs and symptoms of embolization are dependent on the organ to which the clot embolizes. Pulmonary embolization is the most serious risk; signs and symptoms include hypoxemia, chest pain, dyspnea, or shock. Pulmonary emboli may be treated with thrombolytics or anticoagulants, oxygen, and supportive therapy.

A rare complication associated with central venous catheters is erosion or perforation of the vein in which it lies, resulting in pneumothorax or hemothorax. The

Table 16-5 DOPE (for ventilators)

D	Displacement or disconnection of the tube or ventilator circuit
O	Obstruction of airflow (i.e., kinked ventilator tubing or mucous plug in tracheostomy tube)
P	Pneumothorax or other patient-related problem
E	Equipment failure (i.e., low battery, empty oxygen supply)

Table 16-6 DOPE (for central lines)

D	Displacement, disconnection, damage
O	Obstruction
P	Pneumothorax, pericardial tamponade, pulmonary embolus
E	Equipment failure

child may require immediate pleural decompression if there is significant respiratory compromise, with subsequent placement of a chest tube as well as removal of the catheter. If the catheter tip lies within the right atrium, erosion can lead to pericardial tamponade, which may necessitate pericardiocentesis.

Equipment failure can occur with any element of the central venous catheter system. Leakage is a common problem and can occur at any one of the connections or with damage to the catheter itself. If the site of the leakage is not immediately obvious, replace all external components and attempt to flush the catheter using a small syringe.[4] This will usually either resolve the problem or reveal the location of the leak.

Children with any type of central venous catheter are at increased risk for infection. Differential diagnoses for fever in a child with a central venous catheter include catheter-related infections and fever and infection related to the underlying reason for which the catheter was placed. After stabilization of the airway, breathing, and circulation (ABCs), obtain a blood sample from the catheter for blood culture and complete blood count (CBC). Some institutions also require a peripheral blood culture as well. If the source of the infection is the catheter itself, the catheter will need to be removed.

Disability

Once the child's ABCs have been stabilized, a brief neurologic assessment is performed. In the child with special health care needs, the child's level of consciousness should be compared to their normal baseline. Another consideration in children with special health care needs is the child with a VP shunt. The most common causes of VP shunt malfunctions are shunt failure (usually due to obstruction) and shunt infection.[4] Children who present with VP shunt malfunction tend to exhibit similar symptomatology at each presentation. Often, parents will come in with a child and compare the current episode to previous episodes where the shunt was not functioning properly. Because some of the signs and symptoms of VP shunt malfunction are rather vague, the parent's perception of the episode can be a key indicator as to the etiology of the problem.

Signs and symptoms of VP shunt malfunction include headache, irritability, nausea or vomiting, bradycardia,

Table 16-7 DOPE (for VP shunts)

D	Displacement
O	Obstruction
P	Peritonitis, perforation, pseudocyst
E	Elevated temperature

ataxia, seizures, apnea, or change in mental status. In infants and young children if the rise in intracranial pressure has been gradual, the resultant increase in intracranial pressure can cause the skull sutures to expand and cause enlargement of the circumference of the head. Causes of shunt disruption can be assessed by employing the modification of the DOPE[4] mnemonic as listed in **Table 16-7**.

VP shunts may also become dislodged or fractured. Additionally, as children grow, the shunt may no longer be long enough to drain into the peritoneal cavity, thus rendering it effectively displaced. Shunts may also become obstructed from blood or protein deposits inside or around the catheter. Regardless of the etiology, the shunt is unable to drain effectively, and the child's intracranial pressure begins to rise. Suspected VP shunt malfunction is an emergency, requiring surgical repair or replacement. Temporizing measures should be taken while awaiting surgical repair if intracranial pressure is high. Furosemide, mannitol, acetazolamide, and hyperventilation are all therapies used to decrease intracranial pressure and prevent brain herniation until definitive repair can take place. In infants in whom the anterior fontanel is still open, the shunt reservoir can be tapped and CSF withdrawn to reduce intracranial pressure.[10]

Children with VP shunts can present with a perforated abdominal viscous, which occurs when the distal tip of the shunt erodes or perforates the stomach or intestinal wall.[4] When this occurs, children may present with an acute abdomen due to peritonitis, shock, and respiratory failure, requiring emergent operative repair of the damaged organ. Pseudocysts are another potential complication in children with VP shunts. A pseudocyst develops when a segment of omentum wraps around the distal tip of the shunt catheter, creating a closed sac into which the CSF drains. Accumulation of fluid within this sac leads to the development of abdominal pain and eventual shunt obstruction.[4]

VP shunts may become infected, which can lead to meningitis. These children present with elevated temperature and, occasionally, erythema, induration, and pain at the shunt site. Definitive treatment for shunt infections is antibiotic therapy and surgery to externalize the shunt.

Common diagnostics for children with VP shunts include CBC and blood cultures to investigate infective causes and computed tomography of the head to assess ventricular size and shunt function. Some institutions also recommend diagnostic radiology of the shunt itself, usually called a "shunt series." This series of three films includes a skull film, a chest film, and an abdominal film and is designed to look for integrity of the shunt catheter. In children with a suspected shunt malfunction administer oxygen, obtain vascular access, and obtain a neurosurgical consult as soon as possible.

Exposure and Environmental Control

Undress the child and examine for any unusual signs of illness or injury. Because some children may have bruising or marks associated with their condition (e.g., Henoch-Schönlein purpura or idiopathic thrombocytopenia purpura), the parents will be your best guide as to what is new or unusual for the child. Be alert to signs of maltreatment. Studies have shown that children with special health care needs are at increased risk for child maltreatment over those without disabilities.[13] See Chapter 13, *Child Maltreatment*, for additional information.

Extra care may need to be taken to maintain normothermia in some children whose underlying condition predisposes them to either cold or heat stress (Riley-Day syndrome). Frequent temperature measurement is essential in these children.

Secondary Assessment

Full Set of Vital Signs/Family Presence

All children who present with a medical illness need a baseline temperature assessment, and all critically ill children should have ongoing temperature assessments. An important point to remember is that septic children may present with a normal, below normal, or above normal temperature; therefore, absence of a fever should not be taken to mean absence of sepsis or serious illness. Temperatures should be assessed utilizing the most accurate method given the child's age and developmental level. Care should be taken to avoid rectal temperatures in children who are neutropenic, as a small laceration or tear in the rectum can lead to sepsis.

The rate and quality of pulses should be assessed, both centrally and peripherally, and compared to the child's baseline.

Assess respiratory rate and depth. If the child is on a ventilator, determine if the ventilator is set to deliver all breaths, or if the child can breathe above and beyond the ventilator settings.

Blood pressure measurement should be taken on any child with suspected fluid overload, renal or cardiac involvement, sepsis, or other significant illness. Some conditions may render a particular extremity unsuitable for blood pressure measurement (e.g., presence of a PICC line or arteriovenous fistula).

Weight is considered a vital sign in all children and is essential for proper medication and fluid dosing. A measured weight is ideal, but depending on the child's physical abilities and condition, may or may not be possible. If you are unable to directly measure a weight, you may have the parent hold the child and weigh both, then subtract the weight of the parent, use a length-based resuscitation tape, or ask the parent for the last weight (and the date of that weight).

Appropriate monitoring may be instituted at this time. If the child has an apnea or other cardiorespiratory monitor, they should be transitioned to the hospital monitor and the alarm parameters reset to the child's normal settings. Pulse oximetry may be employed, but caution should be taken as to which extremity is used, as measurement may not be accurate in an extremity with vascular malformation or compromise. Some children with underlying cardiac or respiratory diseases may have baseline oxygen saturation of 83% to 85%; for these children, it is the change in oxygenation that is significant, rather than the absolute number.

Family presence is important when caring for all children, but especially so when caring for children with special health care needs. The parent is there not only to calm the child and ease their own fears, but also as the expert in the child's illness, baseline assessments, and commonly employed interventions. Keep in mind that for some children, their needs are so extensive that the care of this child is the parent's full-time job. Their world revolves around every nuance of their child; if you can avail yourself of this expertise and allow the family to continue to participate in their child's care, many of their anxieties will be allayed, and in the end, your job will be easier and the care of the child will be optimized.

Give Comfort Measures

Regardless of a child's mental status, even children with special health care needs feel pain. Evaluation of a child's pain may be more difficult in nonverbal children, but utilization of an instrument such as the FLACC scale (see Chapter 12 for pain assessment tools), usually used for infants, can make evaluation easier. The parent can also be engaged as a pain assessment tool. Unless the child's disability involves renal or hepatic complications, medication dosing for pain is the same as for other children.

History

Additional components of the history to be obtained on a child with special health care needs vary according to the child's underlying illness or condition. Use of the Emergency Information Form (**Figure 16-5**) can be extremely useful in summarizing vital information about the child, including emergency contacts, names and doses of medications, names and phone numbers of specialists, allergies, and a list of medical

Figure 16-5 Emergency Information Form

Emergency Information Form for Children With Special Needs

American College of Emergency Physicians®

American Academy of Pediatrics

Date form completed	Revised	Initials
By Whom	Revised	Initials

Name:	Birth date:	Nickname:

Home Address:	Home/Work Phone:
Parent/Guardian:	Emergency Contact Names & Relationship:
Signature/Consent*:	
Primary Language:	Phone Number(s):

Physicians:

Primary care physician:	Emergency Phone:
	Fax:
Current Specialty physician: Specialty:	Emergency Phone:
	Fax:
Current Specialty physician: Specialty:	Emergency Phone:
	Fax:
Anticipated Primary ED:	Pharmacy:
Anticipated Tertiary Care Center:	

Diagnoses/Past Procedures/Physical Exam:

1.

Baseline physical findings:

2.

3.

Baseline vital signs:

4.

Synopsis:

Baseline neurological status:

*Consent for release of this form to health care providers

219

Figure 16-5 Emergency Information Form (cont.)

Diagnoses/Past Procedures/Physical Exam continued:

Medications:

Significant baseline ancillary findings (lab, x-ray, ECG):

1. _____
2. _____
3. _____
4. _____
5. _____
6. _____

Prostheses/Appliances/Advanced Technology Devices:

_____

Management Data:

Allergies: Medications/Foods to be avoided   **and why:**

1. _____
2. _____
3. _____

Procedures to be avoided   **and why:**

1. _____
2. _____
3. _____

Immunizations

Dates					Dates				
DPT					Hep B				
OPV					Varicella				
MMR					TB status				
HIB					Other				

Antibiotic prophylaxis: Indication: Medication and dose:

Common Presenting Problems/Findings With Specific Suggested Managements

Problem	Suggested Diagnostic Studies	Treatment Considerations

Comments on child, family, or other specific medical issues:

Physician/Provider Signature: **Print Name:**

problems/issues. It is updated with each change in medication, specialist, and so forth and is sent to hospitals and emergency medical service agencies to which the child might present. In addition, the form is kept with the child, at the child's home, at school, and with the babysitter so that the information is readily available for emergency care providers. In addition to the information provided in the Emergency Information Form, inquire about the use of assistive devices at home, sibling response to the child, and the child's normal daily activities. Regardless of their disability, do not assume that older children cannot contribute to the explanation of their history. Even when they are nonverbal or have diminished mental capacity, they frequently develop some method of communication, including nodding yes and no, use of a speech board, or hand signals. Even if you are unsure as to how much the child understands, speaking directly to them will comfort the parent by letting them know that you view their child as more than the sum of their disabilities.

Head-to-Toe Assessment

Assessment of a child with special health care needs proceeds in the same head-to-toe manner as with other children. When assessment reveals an abnormality, compare it to the child's baseline.

Children with G-tubes may present to the ED with problems related to the tube. Evaluation of potential complications related to G-tubes can be accomplished utilizing an additional modification to the DOPE[4] mnemonic (**Table 16-8**).

Although surgically implanted G-tubes contain some mechanism to maintain position in the stomach, they may still become displaced. Displacement is considered an urgent situation. For many of these children, the tube is the only means of providing nutrition and hydration to the child. In addition, once the tube is displaced from the stoma, the tract between the skin and the gastrointestinal tract begins to close. The entire ostomy can close within several hours.[4] If another G-tube is not available, a similarly sized indwelling urinary catheter may be used as a temporary substitute.

G-tubes can become obstructed by crystallization or precipitation of medications or enteral nutritional formula. Gentle attempts to alternately aspirate and irrigate with

Table 16-8 DOPE (for G-tubes)

D	Displacement
O	Obstruction
P	Peritonitis, perforation, pneumoperitoneum
E	Exudate/emesis

warm water may be attempted; if unsuccessful, the tube will need to be replaced.

Rarely, the tip of the G-tube can cause erosion or perforation of the stomach or intestine, resulting in pneumoperitoneum and acute peritonitis. Assess the abdomen for distention, rigidity, abnormal bowel sounds, and pain. Abdominal films (flat plate, upright, and lateral decubitus) can confirm the presence of pneumoperitoneum. Surgical repair of the defect is then required.

Inspect the stoma site itself for bleeding, mucus, drainage, and induration. A small amount of drainage may be normal. Any drainage beyond that may be due to blockage of the gastrostomy tube, infection of the tube tract, or erosion through an underlying structure.

Children with gastrostomy tubes who present with emesis, especially when accompanied by abdominal distention, may be exhibiting G-tube dysfunction. It is important to note for what reason the tube was placed; children who have undergone a surgical procedure called fundoplication are anatomically unable to vomit, and as such can become quite ill if their G-tube malfunctions.

Inspect Posterior Surfaces

Do not forget to assess the patient's posterior surfaces, keeping in mind the increased incidence of abuse, as well as the increased potential for pressure ulcers and other complications of immobility.

Evaluation and Ongoing Assessment

Ongoing assessment proceeds as for all children and consists of assessment of airway patency, breathing effectiveness, circulatory status, level of consciousness, vital signs, and efficacy of interventions.

Assessment can also be made at this point of family dynamics. The care of a child with special health care needs places exceptional demands on the child's primary caretaker, as well as the functioning of the entire family. A gentle discussion regarding the availability and benefits of respite care can provide relief to a family. The primary caretaker, and indeed the entire family, should be encouraged not to feel guilty about taking care of their own needs; this suggestion can sometimes be couched in terms of their increased ability to care for their child following a short respite. In addition, there are numerous family support groups available for many conditions that affect these children. Many families relay a decreased level of stress, as well as a feeling of belonging and of being understood, upon joining these groups. Information on these groups is readily available via an Internet search or from a tertiary children's hospital.

Health Promotion

Health promotion is equally, if not more, important, for children with special health care needs than for all children. Promotion strategies can include maintenance of a normal or near-normal vaccination schedule to decrease their morbidity from these common childhood illnesses. For example, children with underlying lung disease are at increased risk for serious illness from respiratory syncytial virus (RSV); as such, these families should be encouraged to investigate obtaining palivizumab (Synagis®) injections to help prevent RSV and its associated morbidity.

Families and caretakers of children with serious underlying conditions should be encouraged to complete a basic life support class. Although the need to childproof a home is usually age dependent, for children with developmental delays, this may be an ongoing need. In addition, all families of children with special health care needs should have emergency plans. The emergency plan should include a travel bag of essential equipment for trips outside the home, such as extra suction catheters, an extra battery for equipment, and extra tracheostomy tubes.

Summary

There are many more children with special health care needs in the community today than in the past. These children should in general be assessed in a similar manner to other children, though their assessment may need to be compared to their normal baseline. The child's parent or caretaker is usually the ultimate expert in the care of these children, and the nurse should not hesitate to take advantage of the parent's expertise. In addition, the children may be technology dependent, so it is essential for the emergency nurse to have a baseline familiarity with the more common technologies, such as tracheostomies, oxygen, ventilators, home apnea monitors, central lines, and G-tubes. Though in some ways these children differ from other children, they are more like their healthy, able-bodied peers than they are different, and should always be treated in a developmentally appropriate manner.

References

1. McPherson, M, Arango, P., Fox, H., Lauver, C., McManus, M., Newacheck, P. W., et al. (1998). A new definition of children with special health care needs. *Pediatrics, 102*(1 Pt 1), 137–140.
2. Newacheck, P. W., Strickland, B., Shonkoff, J. P., Perrin, J. M., McPherson, M., McManus, M., et al. (1998). An epidemiologic profile of children with special health care needs. *Pediatrics, 102*(1 Pt 1), 117–123.
3. Wallace, H. M., MacQueen, J. C., Biehl, R. F., & Blackman, J. A. (1997). *Mosby's resource guide to children with disabilities and chronic illness.* St. Louis, MO: Mosby–Year Book.
4. American Heart Association. (2002). Children with special healthcare needs. In M. F. Hazinski (Ed.), *Pediatric advanced life support* (Provider manual) (pp. 287–304). Dallas, TX: Author.
5. Schultz, A. & Chalanick, K. (1998). Children with special needs. In T. E. Soud & J. S. Rogers (Eds.), *Manual of pediatric emergency nursing* (pp. 712–726). St. Louis, MO: Mosby.
6. Letourneau, M. A., Schuh, S, & Gausche, M. (1997). Respiratory disorders. In R. M. Barkin (Ed.), *Pediatric emergency medicine: Concepts and clinical practice* (2nd ed., pp. 1056–1126). St. Louis, MO: Mosby.
7. Hockenberry, M. J., Wilson, D., Winkelstein, M. L., & Kline, N. E. (2003). Balance and imbalance of body fluids. In *Wong's nursing care of infants and children* (7th ed., pp. 1171–1206). St. Louis, MO: Mosby.
8. Helfaer, M., Nichols, D., & Rogers, M. (1996). Developmental physiology of the respiratory system. In M. Rogers and D. Nichols (Eds.), *Textbook of pediatric intensive care* (3rd ed., pp. 97–126). Baltimore, MD: Williams & Wilkins.
9. Rogers, M., & Nichols, D. (Eds.). (1996). *Textbook of pediatric intensive care* (3rd ed.). Baltimore, MD: Williams & Wilkins.
10. Lyons, K. (1997). Smith's recognizable patterns of human malformation (5th ed.). Philadelphia: Saunders.
11. American Academy of Pediatrics. (1995). *Policy statement: Atlantoaxial instability in Down syndrome: Subject review.* Retrieved November 15, 2002 from http://www.aap.org/policy/00867.html
12. American Academy of Pediatrics Committee on Child Abuse and Neglect and Committee on Children with Disabilities. (2001). Assessment of maltreatment of children with disabilities. *Pediatrics, 108*(2), 508–512.
13. Hockenberry, M. J., Wilson, D., Winkelstein, M. L., & Kline, N. E. (2003). Conditions caused by defects in physical development. In *Wong's nursing care of infants and children* (7th ed., pp. 415–492). St. Louis, MO: Mosby.

Additional Resources

Respironics Web site. Infant apnea monitor equipment. www.pedslink.com/Products/Apnea_products.htm. Retrieved 10/9/02.

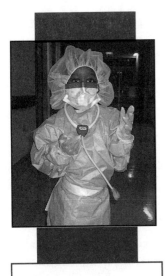

chapter 17

PROCEDURAL PREPARATION AND SEDATION

Objectives

On completion of this chapter, the learner should be able to:

1. Review developmental implications of procedural preparation.
2. Discuss techniques to facilitate procedural preparation.
3. Identify ways in which parental presence can be facilitated during therapeutic and diagnostic procedures.
4. Compare and contrast the differences between the levels of sedation.
5. Review the pharmacologic agents commonly used in sedation of pediatric patients.
6. List the equipment and preparation required to care for the sedated pediatric patient.
7. Discuss the role of the nurse in assessment and monitoring of sedated pediatric patients.

Introduction

Technologic advances and changes in health care have resulted in more pediatric procedures being performed in a variety of settings, including the emergency department (ED). Many procedures are both stressful and painful experiences for pediatric patients and their parents. To gain the cooperation of the pediatric patient and decrease his or her anxiety about a procedure or intervention, appropriate preparation is necessary that includes providing explanations and offering distractions. There are times, however, when distraction, music, and other non-pharmacologic interventions will not be effective, and sedation will need to be considered. This chapter will discuss the various elements of procedural preparation and sedation.

Procedural Preparation

When preparing the pediatric patient and family for a therapeutic or diagnostic procedure, consider the following.[3]

- Assess the pediatric patient's developmental level when determining the preparation approach and timing.
- Explain the procedure to the pediatric patient and family in a manner that is developmentally appropriate for the pediatric patient. Use age-appropriate and developmentally appropriate words and techniques and consider cultural variances.

- Provide procedural and sensory information for the child and caregiver.[1]
  - Be realistic about the time required for a procedure. Five minutes easily stretches into 15 or 20 minutes.
  - Show the pediatric patient the equipment and/or supplies that will be used. Allow the pediatric patient to touch the equipment and supplies as appropriate or have similar "play" equipment available for the pediatric patient to explore.
  - Explain any alarms that may ring; let the caregiver and pediatric patient hear what the alarm sounds like; explain why it may ring and what the staff's response will be to the alarm.
  - Provide the pediatric patients with objective information about what they may feel, hear, smell, or taste. Avoid use of words such as *hurt* or *cry*.
- Consider the pediatric patient's previous experiences. Obtaining information concerning the pediatric patient's previous experience with a procedure or painful event is useful in understanding the pediatric patient's reaction, anxiety level, and perception of the current situation.
- Be aware of cultural differences and beliefs that may affect the pediatric patient and parent's reaction to the procedure.
- Assess the pediatric patient's and parent's understanding of the information; clarify and correct any misconceptions.

- Offer the caregiver the option of staying or leaving during the procedure. Not all caregivers are comfortable being present during invasive or painful procedures. Provide adequate explanations that will allow the caregiver to make an informed decision and support the caregiver in their decision.
  - Be sure your hospital policy supports parental presence and communicate with the health care provider performing the procedure before the offer of parental presence is verbalized.
  - Clearly explain the role of the caregiver during the procedure. Give them specific directions. For example, move a chair to the side of the stretcher in a location visible to the pediatric patient and identify that the chair is the parent's chair.
  - Remind the caregiver that the pediatric patient is the staff's primary concern.
  - If the caregiver appears uncomfortable remaining present during the procedure, be supportive and "give them an out." Suggest that they have a cup of coffee or offer the use of the telephone, returning once the procedure is completed.
  - Adolescents may be uncomfortable having a caregiver present for some examinations and procedures. Ask if they prefer the caregiver to stay or leave.
- Prepare the caregiver to assume a comforting role during and after the procedure. When the caregiver understands the procedure, its sequence, and the pediatric patient's potential responses, the caregiver is better able to comfort and reassure the pediatric patient.
  - Encourage the caregiver to use comforting strategies typically used in the home environment.
  - Identify and discuss coping strategies that may be helpful for the pediatric patient.
- Provide words of encouragement during and after the procedure to promote the pediatric patient's self-esteem.

Techniques to Facilitate Coping During the Procedure

Strategies to reduce pain and distress in children undergoing painful procedures typically involve a combination of approaches. In addition to the psychological preparation, the use of specific cognitive–behavioral techniques during the procedure may assist in decreasing the pediatric patient's anxiety, distress, and pain. Nonpharmacologic interventions are discussed in Chapter 12, *Pediatric Pain Assessment and Management.*

Positioning for Comfort During Procedures

The pediatric patient should be positioned in a manner that is conducive to the procedure and comfortable for the pediatric patient. One of the developmental milestones achieved in infancy is the ability to sit unsupported. After this milestone is achieved, attempts to force an infant or child to lie down are often met with resistance, crying, and struggling. As efforts to restrain a child in the supine position increase, so do the child's resistance and attempts to get up.[2] Lying down is a significant contribution to the child's stress and anxiety during procedures.

A variety of invasive procedures commonly performed in the ED setting can be completed while the infant or child is in a sitting position. Placing children in a sitting position promotes a sense of control and decreases the stress of the event.[2] Positioning for comfort, coupled with age-appropriate preparation and other pharmacologic management techniques, improves the experience of a diagnostic or therapeutic procedure for the pediatric patient. The approach and methods advocated by Stephen and Barkey include the following.[2]

- A secure, comforting, hugging hold for the child; rocking, swaddling, or holding infants in a secure, well-supported position
- Close physical contact between the child and the caregiver
- An opportunity for the caregiver to participate in the child's care in a positive, comforting manner rather than a negative, restraining mode
- Effective immobilization of the desired body area
- Techniques to complete the procedure using fewer people

Examples of Stephen and Barkey's recommended positions are illustrated in **Figures 17-1**, **17-2** and **17-3**.[2] Creative variations to the illustrated positions accommodate the performance of many procedures. The caregiver may be positioned on the stretcher to support and hold the pediatric patient if sitting in a chair does not place the pediatric patient at a height conducive to the procedure.

Clinical Tips
- Remember that the pediatric patient's developmental level may not match their chronological age. Development may be delayed due to cognitive, emotional, and physical disabilities. These disabilities may be temporary (as with acute illness) or permanent (as with some children with chronic illnesses).[3]
- Separation from the parents or caregivers is very frightening for infants, toddlers, and preschoolers.

Try to reduce or avoid periods of separation.

- Remove the pediatric patient's shoes before starting a procedure to avoid a painful kick.[1]
- When holding the legs, position hands directly over the knee area to stabilize the extremity.
- Ensure a secure hold before starting the procedure, and utilize other staff members to assist with holding as needed.

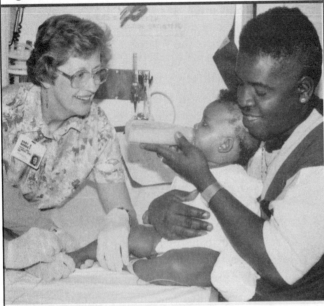

Figure 17-1 IV Placement in Foot

Reprinted with permission from Stephen, B. & Barkey, M. (1994). *Positioning for comfort.* Mt. Royal, NJ: Association for the Care of Children's Health.

- If the caregiver is assisting with holding, ensure that the caregiver is comfortable participating in holding the pediatric patient during the procedure. Give them specific directions. If the caregiver is uncomfortable or unable to hold the pediatric patient during the procedure, another staff member can hold the pediatric patient using the techniques described. The caregiver may remain involved by providing comforting measures during and/or after the procedure.
- Keep the caregiver in the pediatric patient's visual field.
- Encourage the caregiver to talk quietly to the pediatric patient and to use distraction techniques such as singing songs or telling stories.
- Keep voices at a quiet level. The louder the staff or caregiver speaks, the louder the child will scream and cry.
- Closely monitor the pediatric patient for vomiting, loss of airway patency, and respiratory compromise during the procedure.[4]

Use of Physically Restrictive Devices During Procedures

The least-restrictive methods of controlling the pediatric patient's movement should be used when possible. Preparation for the procedure and the use of pain management techniques decrease the need for restrictive devices. Assess the following when investigating the need for use of a restraint device.[5]

- The pediatric patient's developmental, cognitive, and emotional levels and coping abilities

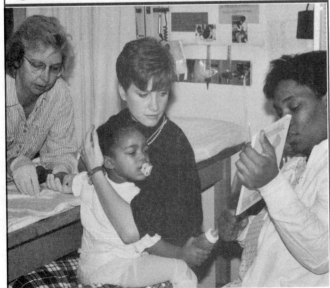

Figure 17-2 Securing child for blood draw

Reprinted with permission from Stephen, B. & Barkey, M. (1994). *Positioning for comfort.* Mt. Royal, NJ: Association for the Care of Children's Health.

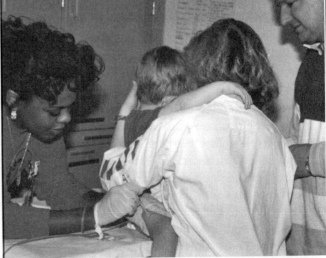

Figure 17-3 Securing child for medication injection in leg

Reprinted with permission from Stephen, B. & Barkey, M. (1994). *Positioning for comfort.* Mt. Royal, NJ: Association for the Care of Children's Health.

- The procedure to be performed (painful versus non-painful)
- The duration of the procedure
- The risk of harm to the patient if movement occurs
- Both pharmacologic and nonpharmacologic interventions already implemented and their effectiveness
- Any previous history of child maltreatment that may affect the child's response to being restrained

The following approach should be used when restrictive devices are needed.

- Explain the need for restricting the pediatric patient's movement and the method to be used to the pediatric patient and caregiver.
- Consider the length of the procedure, the pediatric patient's age, and the pediatric patient's coping abilities when choosing a securing method.
- Use the least-restrictive method or device.
- Use of the restraint device must be medically necessary and must be initiated to provide patient safety and enhance the effectiveness of the procedure.
- If the pediatric patient must not touch the sterile field or move his or her arms/or hands, one of the following three methods may be used.
  - Have the pediatric patient place his or her hands under the buttocks so that the pediatric patient is sitting or lying on his or her hands. This will remind the pediatric patient not to reach into the field.
  - Place the pediatric patient's arms in a pillowcase, pulling the pillowcase up to the pediatric patient's shoulders. Position the pediatric patient's arms at his or her side with the pillowcase across the back, so the pediatric patient lies on the pillowcase. The pediatric patient's weight on the pillowcase will keep the pediatric patient's arms in the pillowcase and restrict movement. The head of the stretcher can be raised so the patient can be in a reclined or sitting position or can lie flat. The pillowcase can be described as Superman's, Superwoman's, or Batman's cape.
  - Use a sheet to mummy the pediatric patient. Place a sheet folded into thirds on the stretcher with the length of the sheet perpendicular to the stretcher. Lay the pediatric patient on the sheet and bring one side over the same side arm and tuck the excess underneath the pediatric patient's back. Take the opposite side and repeat the process or pull across the body and tuck the excess under the pediatric patient's body. This can restrain both the upper and lower extremities.
- A child-restraint board can assist in controlling the pediatric patient's movements.
  - To avoid stress and lessen the chance that the pediatric patient will struggle, use distraction or other appropriate pain management techniques in conjunction with this method of physical immobilization.
  - Prepare the restraint board by opening the Velcro® straps on the board and placing a triangular sheet over the board (see **Figure 17-4**).
  - Place the pediatric patient supine on the board with the arms at each side. Bring the right corner of the sheet over the pediatric patient's body and tuck it under the pediatric patient's left arm; repeat on the other side.[1] Secure the Velcro® straps around the pediatric patient. If the pediatric patient is resisting the placement, open the straps and readjust the sheet.
  - Keep the caregiver in the pediatric patient's line of vision whenever possible and encourage the caregiver to talk to the pediatric patient.
  - If possible, keep one of the pediatric patient's hands free so that the caregiver can hold it. There are typically three cloth straps or sections of the device; it may not be necessary to secure all the straps to control the pediatric patient's movement.
  - Allow the pediatric patient as much control as possible (i.e., allow the pediatric patient to hold a toy or to choose their prize when the procedure is completed).
  - Monitor the pediatric patient for potential vomiting and be prepared to intervene to prevent aspiration while the pediatric patient is immobilized with this device.

Figure 17-4 Papoose Board™

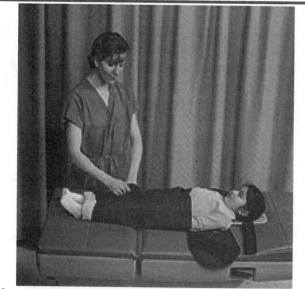

Courtesy of Olympic Medical, Seattle, Washington.

Positioning for Common Procedures

Lumbar Puncture

A lumbar puncture (LP) involves the placement of a spinal needle into the subarachnoid space of the lumbar area to obtain a cerebrospinal fluid sample, to measure pressure, or to inject medications.[4] In the ED setting, the most common rationale is for the diagnosis of an infectious or inflammatory process.[4] This diagnostic test is most often performed on pediatric patients with a suspected or potential central nervous system infection, such as meningitis. The LP is a standard component of a septic workup.

- Lateral decubitus position. Place the pediatric patient in the lateral decubitus position on the edge of the stretcher or examination table. The pediatric patient's knees are drawn up to the abdomen, and the head is flexed forward. This position curves the spine and opens the lumber vertebrae to facilitate needle insertion[7] (see **Figure 17-5**).

  - Place the pediatric patient's shoulders and hips perpendicular to the stretcher or examination table.[7]
  - Be sure that the umbilicus is pointing at an imaginary horizontal line—not pointing toward the ceiling or the floor.
  - Secure the pediatric patient throughout the procedure by placing one arm over the child's neck and the other behind the child's knees.

- Upright position (sitting). Alternatively, the health care provider performing the LP may choose to use the upright position for the infant or cooperative pediatric patient.

  - Seat the infant upright with the thighs against the abdomen and the neck flexed forward; the assistant holds the infant's arm and leg with one hand (see **Figure 17-6**).

- The upright position may also be used for pediatric patients in respiratory distress or when access to the lumbar region is difficult.[7,8] Have the pediatric patient dangle his or her legs over the side of the stretcher or examination table, bending slightly forward at the waist.[4,7]

- A pillow or rolled towel can be placed under the child's arms to facilitate a curved spine position and maintenance of a patent airway. Avoid covering the infant's mouth and nose by turning his or her head to the side.

- The infant's pliable cartilaginous airway is at great risk of collapse due to hyperflexion of the neck. Monitor carefully.[4]

- A 22-gauge, 1½-inch spinal needle may be used for neonates and young pediatric patients up to 2 years of age. For pediatric patients 2 to 12 years of age a 22-gauge, 3½-inch needle may be used. For pediatric patients over 12 years of age a 20-or 22-gauge, 3½-inch needle may be used.[8]

Clinical Tips

- If a urine specimen is needed, place a urine collection bag on the pediatric patient or perform catheterization prior to the procedure.
- Plan the use of topical anesthetic and allow adequate time for the application to take effect.
- Caution should be used with identification badges, stethoscopes, or other items that can poke and injure the child. Alternately, be aware of your body position to avoid being bitten or pinched.
- Avoid hyperflexion of the neck and vigorous holding in infants. This may lead to the loss of airway patency and respiratory compromise.

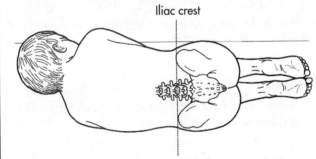

Figure 17-5 Lateral Decubitus Position for LP

Iliac crest

Reprinted with permission from Hickerson, S. L., Cross, J. T., Schutze, G. E., & Jacobs, R. F. (1997). Diagnostic procedures. In R. A. Dieckmann, D. H. Fiser, & S. M. Selbst (Eds.), *Illustrated textbook of pediatric emergency and critical care procedures* (pp. 521–537). St. Louis, MO: Mosby.

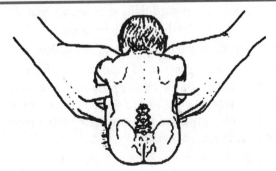

Figure 17-6 Upright Position for LP

Reprinted with permission from Hickerson, S. L., Cross, J. T., Schutze, G. E., & Jacobs, R. F. (1997). Diagnostic procedures. In R. A. Dieckmann, D. H. Fiser, & S. M. Selbst (Eds.), *Illustrated textbook of pediatric emergency and critical care procedures* (pp. 521–537). St. Louis, MO: Mosby.

- Because the procedure may be performed on acutely ill pediatric patients, observe the child's color, respiratory pattern, and muscle tone during the procedure.[4]
- Place the pediatric patient on a pulse oximeter during the procedure to monitor respiratory status.[4] Neonates are particularly at risk for cardiopulmonary changes during this procedure, regardless of the position.
- Have older children and adolescents lie flat after the procedure to avoid the risk of a post-LP headache. Younger children and infants may be held by their caregivers in a position of comfort.
- Once the LP is complete and for the pediatric patient who is taking oral fluids, offer the child a caffeine-containing fluid (such as cola) to reduce the occurrence of post-LP headache.[4]

Gastric Tube Insertion

Gastric tubes are inserted via the nasal or oral routes to decompress the stomach, perform gastric lavage, and administer medications or nutrition.

The oral route for gastric tube insertion may be used in infants less than 6 weeks of age who are obligatory nose breathers and in patients with facial trauma or suspected basilar skull fracture. The procedure for gastric tube insertion is as follows.

- Determine the appropriate-sized tube using one of the following methods.
  - The pediatric patient's age group[9]
    - Infant: 8-French
    - Toddler to preschooler: 10-French
    - School-aged: 12-French
    - Adolescent: 14-French to 16-French
  - A length-based tape, such as the Broselow™ tape
  - A larger gastric lavage tube (22-French to 36-French) may be selected when gastric lavage is needed. These larger tubes are placed orally, rather than nasally, because of their size. Airway patency must be ensured with use of these tubes.
- Determine the length of the tube to be inserted.
  - Using the appropriate-sized nasogastric tube, measure from the tip of the child's nose to the earlobe, and then from the earlobe to the tip of the xiphoid process. Mark this point on the tube with a piece of tape or permanent marker.
  - Using the appropriate-sized orogastric tube, measure from the corner of the mouth to the earlobe, and then from the earlobe to the tip of the xiphoid process. Mark the point on the tube with a piece of tape or permanent marker.
- Position the awake pediatric patient in a high-Fowler's position with the head slightly flexed.[9]

- Be prepared to suction the mouth, nose, and oropharynx with a tonsil-tip suction.
- Either hug the small child or hold the child's arms securely.
  - A caregiver may assist with the hugging hold.
  - A young infant may be swaddled and held in an upright position in the caregiver's or staff member's arms.
  - Additional staff assistance is required to assist with controlling head movement and to suction the patient if vomiting occurs or if excessive secretions are present.
- Consider placing the unresponsive pediatric patient in a head-down, decubitus position. To reduce the risk of aspiration, consider endotracheal intubation prior to gastric tube insertion.[10] Lubricate the distal end of the gastric tube with water-soluble lubricant. Topical 2% lidocaine jelly may be placed in the nares prior to insertion of the nasogastric tube.[10]
- If permitted, have an infant suck on a pacifier or a child swallow or sip water. Blowing a puff of air in the infant's face may cause reflex swallowing.
- Direct the tube straight back during insertion, not upward, along the floor of the nose. Insert the orogastric tube through the mouth following the contour of the tongue.

Never force the tube if resistance or obstruction is met.

If the pediatric patient develops signs of respiratory distress, changes in color, and/or is unable to cry or speak, remove the tube immediately.[9]

- Ensure the tube's placement by aspirating stomach contents. Then instill 3 to 10 ml of air while auscultating over the epigastric region, listening for air passage.[10] The amount of air instilled is dependent on the size of the child.
- Tape the tube securely, anchoring the tape across the bridge of the nose or upper lip area (nasogastric tube) or side of the face (orogastric tube). A clear, occlusive dressing may be used to secure the tube to the child's cheek (see **Figure 17-7**).

Clinical Tips

- Nasogastric tube placement is contraindicated in patients with major facial and/or head trauma. The oral route is used in these patients.
- Have all equipment and assistants prepared prior to beginning the procedure. Have the suction turned "ON" and a rigid tonsil tip suction ready.
- Explain the procedure using age-appropriate terms. Use age-appropriate distraction and relaxation techniques to facilitate the pediatric patient's cooperation and coping during the procedure. Encourage the care-

giver to comfort the pediatric patient and assist with distraction techniques.

- Talking or crying during the procedure is a good indication that the gastric tube has not been inadvertently placed in the trachea.

- After the procedure, protect the tube from dislogdment by applying hand mitts or soft wrist restraints, holding the pediatric patient's hands, or giving the pediatric patient something to hold, such as a security object.

- Reconfirm placement of the tube prior to instillation of any fluids or medications.

- Use universal precautions during gastric tube insertion, including goggles or face shield.

Urinary Catheterization

Urinary catheterization is performed to obtain a sterile urine specimen, relieve urinary retention, and/or monitor urine output.

The sterile procedure for urinary catheterization is the same for either an indwelling or intermittent catheter.

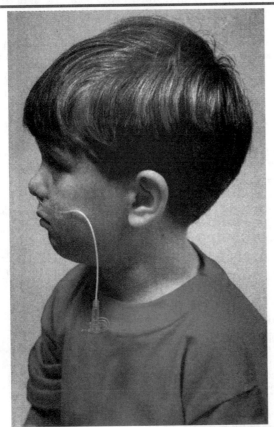

Figure 17-7 Proper method for taping NG or OG tube

Reprinted with permission from American Academy of Pediatrics. (2000). Orogastric and nasogastric intubation. In *Pediatric education for prehospital professionals* (pp. 260–262). Elk Grove Village, IL: Author.

- Position the pediatric patient. Place the female in the frog-leg position. Place the male supine, and lift the penis perpendicular to the child's body.[4]

- Assure adequate lighting and privacy.

- Select an appropriate-sized catheter.[4] The catheter size is determined by the size of the pediatric patient. A #5 French feeding tube may be used for intermittent and indwelling catheterization in young infants. A #8 feeding tube may be used for intermittent catheterization in the older infant. A #8 Foley catheter is used for indwelling catheterization in this same age group. To prevent curling in bladder, avoid using long feeding tubes and stop advancement once urine is obtained.

- If an indwelling catheter is being placed, inspect and test the balloon before insertion using sterile technique; ensure the catheter is advanced well into the bladder before the balloon is inflated to avoid urethral injury.

- Using sterile technique, lubricate and insert the catheter slowly. Never force the catheter. If resistance is felt, pull gently upward on the penis, await relaxation of the sphincter, and then continue to advance the catheter.

- If the catheter is inadvertently inserted into the vagina, obtain a new sterile catheter to insert into the bladder. Leave the first catheter in the vagina during the second attempt to assist in identifying the vaginal opening.

- Tape an indwelling catheter to the thigh in the female or the abdomen in the male

- Rinse the perineal area with warm saline or water after the procedure, ensuring povidone-iodine is removed.

Clinical Tips

- Urinary catheter insertion is contraindicated if blood is present at the urethral meatus, perineal or scrotal hematoma or ecchymosis, or there is evidence of urethral trauma.[10]

- Explain the procedure using age-appropriate terms. Use age-appropriate distraction and relaxation techniques to facilitate the pediatric patient's cooperation and coping during the procedure. Encourage the caregiver to comfort the pediatric patient and assist with distraction techniques.

- Anticipate some parent anxiety around social and psychological issues related to manipulating the pediatric patient's genitalia.

- Latex allergies are common in pediatric patients with spina bifida and should be assessed and anticipated.

- For boys that are circumcised, cleanse the glans and insert the catheter into the urethra. For uncircumcised boys, retract the foreskin only enough to visualize the urethral opening. Replace the foreskin following the procedure to prevent paraphimosis. If the foreskin is tight, aim for the center of the glans. Do not force the foreskin back.

- For girls, the meatus may be difficult to visualize. Applying gentle lateral traction to the labia with simultaneous downward traction may help with visualization. Or use the nondominant hand to pull up on the labia minora to help visualize the urinary meatus.

- For indwelling catheter insertion, encourage the child to relax and remind him or her that the catheter is in place as needed. The pediatric patient may fear wetting the bed.

Sedation

When nonpharmacologic interventions are not effective or when the procedure is lengthy in duration, sedation of the pediatric patient may be considered.

Effective and safe management of sedated pediatric patients has received significant attention in the past 10 years, particularly as the number of procedures occurring in the outpatient setting has increased. Health care providers have witnessed remarkable progress in therapeutic and procedural sedation techniques for children. Numerous articles regarding sedation medications, reversal agents, and standards of care for the sedated patient have greatly expanded our knowledge of the safety and efficacy of these medications for therapeutic and diagnostic procedures.

Sedation of the pediatric patient is different from sedation of an adult. This is primarily due to the differences in the pediatric patient's developmental stages combined with their lack of ability to cooperate, especially for pediatric patients less than 6 years of age and those with special needs due to developmental delays.[11] Pediatric patients often require additional sedation medication and deeper levels of sedation to obtain their cooperation. Furthermore, pediatric patients tend to have heightened levels of emotion due to the unfamiliar environment and health care providers (strangers), actual and anticipated pain, threatening procedures, and fear of parental separation, all of which strongly influence the need for sedation.[12]

Due to the high-risk nature of sedation, standards have been established in the United States by the Joint Commission on Accreditation of Healthcare Organizations (JCAHO) to improve the outcome of sedated patients.[13] These standards for sedation and anesthesia apply when patients receive, in any setting, for any purpose, by any route, moderate or deep as well as general, spinal, or other regional major anesthesia.[13]

These standards will be reflected in the following section covering the sedation procedure.

The goals of sedation in the pediatric patient for diagnostic or therapeutic procedures include the following.[12]

- To promote patient safety
- To encourage a calm patient and family
- To reduce physical discomfort or pain during the procedure
- To minimize patient movement
- To minimize negative psychological responses to procedures and treatments
- To increase the probability of success on first attempt for the procedure being performed
- To return the pediatric patient to their presedation state as quickly as possible

In the ED setting, pediatric patients are sedated for procedures that may necessitate cooperation and require sedation only or necessitate cooperation during a painful procedure and require both sedation and analgesia. Refer to **Table 17-1** for a listing of common procedures. There are many factors to consider when preparing for sedation of a pediatric patient that will promote a positive outcome for the pediatric patient and family as well as the health care team.

Specific factors are known to enhance the effectiveness of sedation and potentially reduce the amount of sedation medications required to complete the procedure. These include environmental factors and adjunctive pain relief.[12] The environmental factors include parental presence, use of distraction techniques, and reduction of

Table 17-1 Common ED Procedures Requiring Sedation

Sedation Alone	Analgesia Alone	Sedation/Analgesia
Neuroimaging	Wound care	Fracture reduction
Sexual assault examination	Laceration repair	Dislocation reduction
Lumbar puncture	Abscess drainage	Removal of deep foreign body
Removal of superficial foreign body	Burn care	Joint aspiration
Placement of central line	Lumbar puncture	Hernia reduction
Thoracentesis	Fracture reduction	Cardioversion
Chest tube placement		
Endotracheal intubation		

Reprinted with permission from Terndrup, T. (1999). General principles for procedural sedation and analgesia. In B. Krauss and R. M. Brustowicz (Eds.), *Pediatric procedural sedation and analgesia* (pp. 97–105). Philadelphia: Lippincott Williams & Wilkins.

Table 17-2 Examples of Topical Anesthesia

EMLA cream®	• 5% emulsion (2.5% lidocaine and 2.5% prilocaine) • Onset, depth, and duration of dermal analgesia depend primarily on duration and site of application. • A thick layer of cream is applied under an occlusive dressing for a minimum of 60 minutes. The cream is therefore of limited use when time is a factor. • Due to its vasoconstrictive properties, it may increase the difficulty of obtaining venous access.
LET	• Local anesthetic used in children 6 months and older for uncomplicated lacerations and wounds approximately 2 to 4 inches in length. • Contains lidocaine HCL, epinephrine bitartrate, and tetracaine HCL and is prepared in a KY jelly base. • Due to its epinephrine content, it should not be used on end arterioles such as fingers, toes, penis, nose, or ear cartilage. • The gel is applied to a sterile cotton or gauze, inserted into the wound, covered, and constant pressure is applied for 30 minutes. The analgesia dissipates in 15 to 30 minutes, so suturing must be done immediately after application. • Adequacy of analgesia can be assessed with skin blanching or probing of the wound edge with a needle.
Ametop gel 4%	• Effective topical local anesthetic containing tetracaine (amethocaine) • It has a minimum 30-minute onset and, like EMLA cream, is applied under occlusion. • Is safe for use in the newborn population. It is not safe for use on open wounds as is LET. It is cost effective and less vasoconstrictive than EMLA, but may have more of a local allergic component.
Buffered lidocaine	• Intradermally or subcutaneously injected • Administered quickly with minimal physiologic alterations; predictable length of efficacy • Buffered includes the addition of sodium bicarbonate to reduce discomfort • Requires needle insertion, is painful, and often requires two people for administration with younger children
Vapocoolant sprays	• Fluori-Methane®, frigiderm, ethyl chloride sprays • Instantly effective for very short periods of time • Risk of frostbite and tissue damage with inappropriate use by overspraying[12]

noise and stimulation. Pain relief may include oral systemic medications, such as ibuprofen or acetaminophen, as well as local pain relief medications, such as EMLA cream® or buffered lidocaine, which are described in **Table 17-2**.

Levels of Sedation

Sedation is currently classified into four types: (1) mild sedation, (2) moderate sedation/analgesia, (3) deep sedation/analgesia, and (4) general anesthesia (see **Table 17-3**). It is imperative to remember that these varying levels of sedation correspond to a range of responses from the medications administered. In effect, the levels of sedation are defined by the patient's level of responsiveness.

In 1998, the American College of Emergency Physicians defined procedural sedation as a technique of administering sedatives or dissociative agents with or without analgesics to induce a state that allows the patient to tolerate unpleasant procedures while maintaining car-

Table 17-3 Levels of Sedation[11,13,14]

Minimal sedation (anxiolysis)	Drug-induced state in which patients respond normally to verbal commands. Although cognitive function may be impaired, respiratory and cardiovascular functions are unaffected.
Moderate sedation/analgesia	Drug-induced state of depressed consciousness in which patients respond purposefully to verbal commands, either alone or in conjunction with light tactile stimulation. No interventions are required to maintain a patent airway or spontaneous respirations; cardiovascular function is usually maintained. This term replaces *conscious sedation*.
Deep sedation/ analgesia	Drug-induced depression of consciousness in which patients cannot be easily aroused but respond purposefully following repeated or painful stimuli. Patients may require assistance to maintain a patent airway, and ventilatory efforts may be inadequate. Cardiovascular function is usually maintained. According to the American Academy of Pediatrics, American Society of Anesthesiologists (ASA), and JCAHO, deep sedation is inseparable from general anesthesia.
Anesthesia (general, spinal, or major regional anesthesia; does not include local anesthesia)	General anesthesia is defined as a drug-induced loss of consciousness during which patients are not arousable, even by painful stimuli. Patients often require assistance in maintaining a patent airway, positive pressure ventilation may be required, and cardiovascular function may be impaired.

diorespiratory function. Procedural sedation and analgesia are intended to result in a depressed level of consciousness but one that allows the patient to maintain airway control independently and continuously. Specifically the drugs, doses, and techniques used are not likely to produce a loss of protective airway reflexes.[15, 16]

Common factors and considerations affecting sedation decisions include[12, 16]

- The pediatric patient's cardiorespiratory and neurological stability
- Presence of high-risk criteria (also known as the ASA level, which provides physical status classification for anesthesia)
- Time since last oral intake
- Extent of patient pain and anxiety
- Depth of sedation required and length of procedure
- Consent from parent or legal guardian
- Availability of equipment and sedation trained staff
- Comfort level of physician
- Increased length of stay in the ED/outpatient setting

Sedation Procedure

Policies, procedures, and practice should reflect the following standards when providing sedation to pediatric patients.[11, 13, 14]

- Preprocedure health evaluation. The pediatric patient must receive a presedation medical evaluation that should include a health history, physical assessment focused on evaluation of the pediatric patient's airway, baseline vital signs, and risk assessment.[6]
- Ideally the pediatric patient should have nothing by mouth for a designated period before the sedation

begins; however, in the ED setting sound clinical judgment should be used to identify the appropriate time interval between the last oral intake and the sedation procedure. An emergency patient may require airway protection prior to the initiation of sedation.[6]

- Consent must be obtained from the parent or legal guardian prior to the initiation of sedation. Options and risks must be discussed with the family.
- Pediatric patients receiving medications to sedate must be monitored by independently licensed sedation-qualified nursing staff. See following for further discussion on the role of nursing in sedation.
- Nursing staff monitoring these pediatric patients must be skilled in airway management and basic life support.
- The appropriate-size equipment must be in working order at the bedside, and reversal agents must be readily available should compromise occur with airway, breathing, or circulation (see **Table 17-4**).
- All sedated patients must have their cardiorespiratory status monitored by nursing staff during and after the procedure and at minimum must be continuously monitored by pulse oximetry.[6]
- Patients that are deeply sedated must be continuously assessed by nursing staff with monitoring of vital signs every 5 minutes.
- Patients must meet specific criteria before discharge;[6] criteria should be standardized for all areas of the facility to prevent complications (see **Table 17-5**).
- Documentation should include presedation assessment; medications administered with route, dose, and time indicated; status during procedure (including vitals signs); and criteria met for discharge.

Role of Nurses in Sedation

Nurses are integral members of the sedation team. Nurses are responsible for keeping the patient safe dur-

---

Table 17-4 Equipment

Minimum equipment at the bedside[13,14,17] (checked and in working order):

- Bag-mask device with appropriate-size face mask
- Supplemental oxygen source, such as nonrebreather mask
- Suction with tonsil tip
- Pulse oximetry
- Cardiorespiratory monitor
- Noninvasive blood pressure capability

Equipment that should be readily available:

- Reversal agents for sedative medication being administered
- Appropriate size intubation equipment
- Emergency equipment/code cart

Table 17-5 Sedation Discharge Criteria[6,11,14,17]

- Must exhibit stable cardiovascular and respiratory status and vital signs that are returning to baseline levels.
- Must be able to talk, sit up unaided, control his or her head and extremities, and follow commands; must be alert and oriented for age; must have returned to presedation state.
- Must be able to maintain hydration status.
- Presedation baseline returned regarding communication, mobility, and level of alertness.

NOTE: Specific discharge criteria for infants < 4 weeks of age and premature infants with postconceptual age less than 50 weeks should also be established.

ing the preprocedure, procedural, and postprocedure settings; providing emotional support and encouragement to the pediatric patient and family; ensuring that the pediatric patient has met discharge criteria; and providing discharge teaching regarding home care for the sedated pediatric patient. **Table 17-6** provides an overview of nursing roles and responsibilities in seda-tion.[18] Nurses participating in sedation must be aware of institutional policies and procedures delineating the care of patients based on various levels of sedation and the state-specific Nurse Practice Act, which dictates the level of practitioner required to monitor patients at various levels of sedation (e.g., anesthesiologist or certified registered nurse anesthetist).

Table 17-6 Nursing Roles and Responsibilities in Pediatric Sedation

Phases of Sedation	Behavioral Interventions	Monitoring Interventions	Pharmacologic Interventions
Before the procedure	Create a nonthreatening environment. Speak in a quiet, calm confident manner. Encourage family participation. Explain the sedation procedure to the family and child at the age-appropriate level. Answer questions and provide information as requested. If possible, offer the opportunity for a parent to remain in the room during the procedure. Ensure that the consent form is signed.[15]	Set up monitoring equipment; set alarms. Set up appropriate-size face mask and bag-mask device; ensure working order. Set up and check working order of tonsil tip suction. Ensure availability and location of emergency equipment/crash cart. Plan child's body position to promote airway patency and effective ventilation. Document preparation on medical record (sedation record if available).	Calculate drug doses according to weight. Verify orders. Prepare drug doses and saline flushes. Label all syringes. Calculate doses of reversal agents and have readily accessible. Establish and secure IV access.
During the procedure	Use distraction. Allow child to hold familiar object. Direct family to location to wait during procedure if family presence not an option. Involve parents. Explain progress of procedure and child's responses.	Primary responsibility to continuously monitor patient. Monitor vital signs and O_2 saturation every 5 minutes (include HR, RR).* Initiate interventions to prevent heat loss. Communicate concerns to sedating physician regarding patient status and response. Document assessments on medical record (sedation record if available).	Assess patency of IV. Administer O_2 via mask (according to hospital policy). Administer drugs, titrating to effect.
After the procedure	Maintain quiet, calm environment. Encourage parents to talk or sing soothingly to the child. Reassure parents if behavior is not the child's normal. Provide parents with individualized discharge instructions including diet, activity, sleep, when to call the doctor, and when to return to ED.	Assess child for discharge. Monitor for development of deeper levels of sedation, especially following completion of procedure and diminished stimulation. Document assessments on medical record (sedation record if available). Document discharge criteria and discharge score.	Depending upon sedative used, administer IV fluids. Discontinue IV access once child taking oral fluids well.

* If patient deeply sedated, patient must have continuous monitoring of ECG, O_2 saturation, HR/RR (with precordial stethoscope if available), capnogram if available, BP every 5 minutes, visual assessment of skin color, and airway patency.

Modified from Damian, F., & Smith, M. F. (1999). Nursing principles in the management of sedated patients. In B. Krauss & R. M. Brustowicz (Eds.), *Pediatric procedural sedation and analgesia* (pp. 108–114). Philadelphia: Lippincott Williams & Wilkins.

Medications Used for Sedation in Pediatric Patients

In the pediatric ED, the most common pharmacologic agents used for sedation include midazolam (Versed®), fentanyl (Sublimaze®), ketamine, and nitrous oxide. Longer-acting sedatives such as morphine, meperidine (Demerol®), and diazepam (Valium®) are less practical in the ED setting due to the need for lengthy postprocedural monitoring and observation. **Table 17-7** describes medications that may be used for sedation in pediatric patients.

Prevention and Management of Complications

Anticipation is the best action to prevent complications! Complications can occur at any time following medication administration. There is a higher incidence of complications with medications administered intravenously and with a rapid (versus slow) rate of administration. In pediatric patients, intravenous (IV) medication should be administered as a slow push and titrated to effect versus administering the entire dose at once.

Because a variety of medications are used to induce sedation/analgesia, staff participating in sedation must be familiar with the possible contraindications and adverse reactions with each medication being administered. In general, the most common complications include[22, 23]

- Vomiting and loss of airway patency
- Respiratory complications, such as hypoventilation, apnea, or respiratory depression
- Laryngospasm
- Cardiovascular complications, including hypotension, bradycardia, and asystole
- Emergence phenomena. Increased incidence with rapid IV administration, in children > 10 years of age, with females, and with excessive environmental stimulation during recovery.
- Anaphylactic reactions to medication or latex products
- Hypothermia

Clinical Tips

- When the noxious stimulus is decreased (e.g., fracture reduction is completed) an increased level of sedation may occur.
- It is important to remember that patients may rapidly progress from one level of sedation to another; vigilant monitoring and assessment are required to provide safe sedation.
- Infants metabolize medications, especially narcotics, differently than do older children due to decreased

---

Table 17-7 Medications Used for Sedation in Pediatric Patients[5,19,20,21]

Opioids (provide analgesia and sedation)

- Morphine sulfate
  - May be given IV, IM, SC, rectally, or PO; onset of action depends on route, with IV having the most immediate response
  - Duration of action 3 to 5 hours results in lengthy monitoring; good for longer procedures
  - Naloxone (Narcan®) will reverse effects
- Fentanyl citrate (Sublimaze)
  - May be given IV, IM, or by transmucosal route (Oralet®)
  - Rapid onset and short acting—good for brief procedures
  - Dilute IV dose with 0.9% NS to obtain 1 mg/cc concentration
  - Rapid administration can result in respiratory depression and chest wall rigidity
  - Duration of action 30 to 120 minutes
  - Naloxone will reverse effects
- Meperidine hydrochloride (Demerol) (if morphine sulfate or fentanyl citrate is not available)
  - May be given orally, IV, or IM for moderate to severe painful procedures
  - Duration of action 2 to 4 hours; results in lengthy monitoring; prolonged half-life in neonates
  - Administration of naloxone may cause normeperidine seizure

Sedatives

- Diazepam (Valium)
  - Benzodiazepine sedative may be given rectally, orally, IM, or IV
  - Long duration of action (2 to 6 hours) with half-life of 20 to 40 hours; results in lengthy monitoring
  - Flumazenil (Romazicon®) will reverse effects, but watch for resedation
- Midazolam hydrochloride (Versed)
  - Most frequently used benzodiazepine; may be given orally, rectally, IV, or sublingually
  - Rapid acting with short half-life
  - Higher doses per kg may be required for infants and toddlers to achieve desired effect
  - Flumazenil will reverse effects, but watch for resedation
- Pentobarbital sodium (Nembutal®)
  - Barbiturate may be administered orally or IV
  - Must also administer analgesic if procedure painful
  - Quick onset of action; lasting 20 to 60 minutes
  - Prolonged recovery when combined with other drugs
- Chloral hydrate
  - Most effective in children under 4 years of age
  - Delayed sedative effects can be seen up to 20 hours
  - Time is only antagonist

liver metabolism and renal excretion.[5] Delayed reactions and delays in respiratory depression may occur. Infants require extended monitoring to ensure that they return to the presedation level.

- There is no ideal drug or dosage combination. Continuous monitoring of the pediatric patient and the ability to intervene are critical to safe sedation practices.

- IV is the preferred route of administration for pediatric sedation medications.

- Avoid pushing entire dose without monitoring response. Taking a few minutes longer to administer can reduce the pediatric patient's length of recovery and reduce the occurrence of complications during the sedation procedure.

- For doses less that 1 cc, use a tuberculin syringe to make titrating easier.

- Following administration of antagonists, pediatric patients should be kept for at least 2 hours to monitor for resedation.

- Use caution in use of antagonists for patients that may be chemically dependent on opioids or for those patients taking benzodiazepines to control seizures.[6]

- REMEMBER, when an alarm sounds while monitoring a sedated patient, the first intervention is to assess the patient.

Summary

Appropriate preparation for a procedure is essential in gaining the cooperation of the pediatric patient, decreasing the pediatric patient's and the caregiver's anxiety, and helping the pediatric patient cope with the procedure. Sedation and analgesia are useful adjuncts to successfully performing diagnostic and therapeutic procedures, particularly with challenges of the pediatric population.

Sedation of patients represents a balance in that patients may easily move from lighter to deeper levels of sedation and on to unresponsiveness with a loss of the protective reflexes of the airway.[11] Continuous assessment and use of appropriate safeguards will minimize the risk of adverse events to sedative medications.

Table 17-7 Medications Used for Sedation in Pediatric Patients[5,19,20,21] (cont.)

- Ketamine
  - Produces sedation and analgesia, and is ideal for short, painful procedures with rapid onset and duration lasting 45 to 120 minutes
  - Produces a trancelike dissociative state with a disconnected stare and nystagmus being common
  - Consider giving atropine or glycopyrrolate (Robinul®) to reduce oral secretions and prevent laryngospasm

Inhaled Anesthetics

- Nitrous oxide (NO) is known for its analgesic, sedative, and amnestic effects.
  - A mixture of no greater than 50% NO with 50% O_2 is used
  - Increased complications if used in combination with other sedatives
  - Several minutes of inhaling 100% O_2 will reverse effects

Reversal Agents

- Flumazenil (Romazicon) is a benzodiazepine antagonist
  - Dose: IV: 0.01 mg/kg/dose given over 15 seconds; repeat every min to max 1 mg
  - Resedation may occur within 1 hour
- Naloxone (Narcan) is an opioid antagonist
  - Dose: IV: opioid-induced respiratory depression: 0.5 to 2 mcg/kg/dose; postoperative respiratory depression: 0.01 mg/kg/dose
  - Resedation may occur within 1 hour
  - Give in small incremental doses every 2 to 3 minutes to maximum of 2 mg

---

References

1. Bove, M. A. (1993). Positioning and securing children for procedures. In L. M.. Bernardo & M. A. Bove (Eds.), *Pediatric emergency nursing procedures* (pp. 29–34). Sudbury, MA: Jones & Bartlett.

2. Stephen, B. & Barkey, M. (1994). *Positioning for comfort.* Mt. Royal, NJ: Association for the Care of Children's Health.

3. Hazinski, M. F. (1999). Psychosocial aspects of pediatric critical care. In *Manual of pediatric critical care* (pp. 14–43). St. Louis, MO: Mosby.

4. Muscari, M. E. (2001). Laboratory and diagnostic tests. In *Advanced pediatric clinical assessment* (pp.525–543). Philadelphia: Lippincott.

5. Baker, P. (2003). Pain assessment and management. In D. O. Thomas, L. M. Bernardo, & B. Herman (Eds.), *Core curriculum for pediatric emergency nursing* (pp. 149–159). Sudbury, MA: Jones and Bartlett.

6. American Heart Association (2002). Sedation issues for the PALS provider. In *Pediatric advanced life support* (Provider Manual) (pp. 379–396). Dallas, TX: Author.

7. Cronan, K. M., & Wiley, J. F., III. (2000). Lumbar puncture. In C. King & R. M. Hentrig (Eds.), *Textbook of pediatric emergency procedures* (pp. 541–551). Philadelphia: Lippincott Williams & Wilkins.

8. King, C., & Hentrig, F. M. (2000). Lumbar puncture. In *Pocket atlas of pediatric emergency procedures* (pp.128). Philadelphia: Lippincott Williams & Wilkins.

9. King, C., & Hentrig, F. M. (2000). Gastric intubation and lavage. In *Pocket atlas of pediatric emergency procedures* (pp. 233). Philadelphia: Lippincott Williams & Wilkins.

10. King, C., & Hentrig, F. M. (2000). Bladder catheterization and suprapubic aspiration . In *Pocket atlas of pediatric emergency procedures* (pp. 258). Philadelphia: Lippincott Williams & Wilkins.

11. American Academy of Pediatrics Committee on Drugs. (2002). Guidelines for monitoring and management of pediatric patients during and after sedation for diagnostic and therapeutic procedures: Addendum (Policy statement) [Electronic version]. *Pediatrics, 110*(4), 836–838. Retrieved September 15, 2003, from http://www.aap.org/policy/0108.html

12. Nelson, D. (1999). Procedural sedation in the emergency department. In B. Krauss & R. M. Brustowicz (Eds.), *Pediatric procedural sedation and analgesia* (pp. 161–168). Philadelphia: Lippincott Williams & Wilkins.

13. Joint Commission on Accreditation of Healthcare Organization. (2002). *2002 Comprehensive Accreditation Manual for Hospitals.*

14. American Academy of Pediatrics Committee on Drugs. (1992). Guidelines for monitoring and management of pediatric patients during and after sedation for diagnostic and therapeutic procedures (Policy statement). [Electronic version]. *Pediatrics, 89*(6), 1110–1115. Retrieved September 15, 2003, from http://www.aap.org/policy/04789.html

15. American College of Emergency Physicians. (1998). Clinical policy for procedural sedation and analgesia in the emergency department. *Annals of Emergency Medicine, 31*(5), 663–677.

16. Terndrup, T. (1999). General principles for procedural sedation and analgesia. In B. Krauss & R. M. Brustowicz (Eds.), *Pediatric procedural sedation and analgesia* (pp. 97–105). Philadelphia: Lippincott Williams & Wilkins.

17. Andreoni, C. P., & Klinkhammer, B. (2000). Drugs commonly used for conscious sedation. In *Quick reference for pediatric emergency nursing* (pp. 320–323). Philadelphia: Saunders.

18. Damian, F., & Smith, M. F. (1999). Nursing principles in the management of sedated patients. In B. Krauss & R. M. Brustowicz (Eds.), *Pediatric procedural sedation and analgesia* (pp. 108–114). Philadelphia: Lippincott Williams & Wilkins.

19. Krauss, B. (1999). Practical aspects of procedural sedation and analgesia. In B. Krauss & R. M. Brustowicz (Eds.), *Pediatric procedural sedation and analgesia* (pp. 223-236). Philadelphia: Lippincott Williams & Wilkins.

20. Cote, C. J. (1994). Sedation for the pediatric patient. A review. *Pediatric Clinics of North America, 41*(1), 31–58.

21. Patterson, C. H. (2002). Sedation, anesthesia update. *Nursing Management, 33*(1), 22.

22. Bernardo, L. M., & Conway, A. E. (1998). Pain assessment and management. In T. E. Soud & J. S. Rogers (Eds.), *Manual of pediatric emergency nursing* (pp. 686–711). St. Louis, MO: Mosby.

23. Vance, C. (1999). Management of complications. In B. Krauss & R. M. Brustowicz (Eds.), *Pediatric procedural sedation and analgesia* (pp.151–159). Philadelphia: Lippincott Williams & Wilkins.

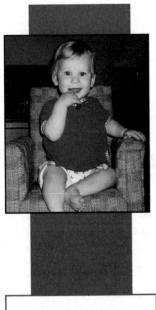

chapter 18

POISONINGS

Case Scenario: A grandmother brings her 2-year-old grandson to the emergency department. She is concerned that he has begun to exhibit signs of bizarre behavior and appears to be having hallucinations. He is flushed, his mouth is dry, and his pupils are dilated. Through history, you determine that the grandmother is on amitriptyline for neuropathic pain related to diabetes. The child has also had a viral respiratory illness and has been receiving a cough and cold preparation. What are the dangers related to the misuse of these medications in the pediatric patient? What are your immediate nursing interventions?

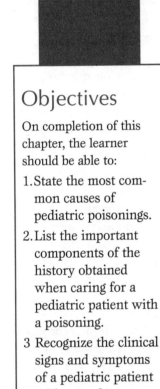

Objectives

On completion of this chapter, the learner should be able to:

1. State the most common causes of pediatric poisonings.

2. List the important components of the history obtained when caring for a pediatric patient with a poisoning.

3 Recognize the clinical signs and symptoms of a pediatric patient with an unknown or specific poisoning.

4. Discuss interventions needed to manage the pediatric patient who has suffered a poisoning.

5. Identify health promotion strategies to reduce the risk of poisoning in the pediatric population.

Introduction

In the United States, every 30 seconds a child is exposed to a potential poisoning.[1] In 2000, the American Association of Poison Control Centers (AAPCC) reported over 1.4 million exposures in children less than 19 years of age.[2] Although death due to poisoning is less common in children than in other age groups, morbidity from poisonings is significant. In 2000, the Toxic Exposure Surveillance System reported 2,526 cases of children that experienced life-threatening injury or residual disability as a result of poisoning.[2]

Poisonings may be either unintentional or intentional. The majority of poisonings in young children are unintentional and are often related to children being left unattended around open products, improper storage of poisons, and therapeutic error.[3] Almost 60 % of all exposures occur in children less than 6 years of age.[1,4,5] Males predominate in this age group but this reverses after the age of 13 years.[6] Small children are at risk for toxic exposure, particularly through ingestion, due to differences in developmental characteristics and environmental influences. Most often these are single substance ingestions, are nontoxic in nature, and are discovered soon after they occur.

There are currently 69 poison control centers located throughout the United States.[1,6] Of all pediatric poisonings reported to poison control centers in 2001, a large majority (78 %) were able to be managed at home. Of the 22 % that were referred to and treated at a health care facility, approximately 5 % were children less than 6 years of age.[6] The most common products children ingest are cosmetics and personal care products, cleaning substances, analgesics, plants, foreign bodies, topical medications, and cough and cold preparations.[6,11] Fewer than 20 types of drugs are involved in 90 % of all ingestions.[12]

Intentional poisonings as suicidal gestures are more common in the adolescent population. They are often related to academic, social, romantic, and family difficulties. Adolescent ingestions may involve more than one substance and are generally more toxic than those in younger children.[4] There may be a delay in seeking medical care after ingestion. Once medically stable, exploration of psychosocial issues is a vital part of intervention for pediatric patients presenting with intentional poisoning.

Anatomic, Physiologic, and Developmental Characteristics as a Basis for Signs and Symptoms

Anatomic and Physiologic Characteristics

A poison is any substance that can cause an unintended symptom.[1] Poisons may be solids (medication, plants, powders such as dishwasher detergent and laundry soap), liquids (furniture polish, lighter fluid, elixir medications, spray paint), or gases (carbon monoxide).[1]

The properties of a substance affect its rate of absorption, metabolism, distribution, and excretion from the body. Absorption of a substance occurs through one of five routes: (1) oral, (2) dermal, (3) ocular, (4) inhalation, and (5) parenteral. Although absorption can occur anywhere along the gastrointestinal tract, most ingested substances are absorbed by passive diffusion through the small intestine.[7] The length of the small intestine is proportionately greater in infants than in the adult, leaving a larger surface area for absorption of toxins.[8] Variability in gastric emptying, rapid peristalsis, and changes in gastric pH also influence absorption of drugs and other substances from the gastrointestinal tract in infants and younger children.[7]

Substances absorbed by a lactating mother may be excreted in breast milk and consequently ingested by the breast-fed infant. A variety of over-the-counter, illicit, and therapeutic medications as well as environmental and occupational chemicals may be excreted in breast milk at varying levels.[9] Poisoning by this route is uncommon and typically requires chronic exposure.

The epidermis of the premature infant is highly permeable, allowing the infant to absorb greater quantities of topical medication compared to the adult. The infant has a higher surface area-to-volume ratio, allowing for more efficient percutaneous drug absorption, thus the preterm infant is at risk for toxicity from topically applied medications such as cleansing solutions and topical anesthetics. Liberal use of povidone-iodine solution has been associated with high iodine levels, iodine goiter, and hypothyroidism in the newborn. Solutions containing iodine should be used with caution in the newborn and avoided in premature infants.[9]

Decreased renal clearance in infants less than 6 months of age affects the half-life of drugs and duration of effect. This is particularly concerning in the neonate whose immature renal function can lead to toxic levels of even essential medications resulting in nephrotoxicity and renal damage.[9]

Lower serum albumin concentrations in infants leave fewer binding sites for drugs that are plasma bound and increase the potential for toxicity.[8,10] With fewer available sites, these drugs are allowed to circulate freely and can rapidly build to toxic levels.

Infants and small children have low glycogen stores placing them at higher risk for hypoglycemia with ethanol or sulfonylurea ingestions.

The child's metabolic rate, ventilation, and pulmonary blood flow determine the rate of absorption of inhaled gases and fumes. Because infants and young children have higher metabolic rates, their respiratory rates are normally faster. This contributes to increased inhalation of toxic substances when exposed.

Children have a smaller airway diameter than an adult. Small amounts of airway edema can quickly lead to increased airway resistance and airway obstruction. Support and management of airway, ventilation, and oxygenation must always be considered in poisonings such as hydrocarbons and caustics that may affect airway and breathing in infants and children.

Developmental Characteristics

Young children are naturally curious, and challenges such as closed cupboards and high shelves present an opportunity to further explore their environment. Brightly colored packages and candy-coated pills make attractive items to the unknowing toddler, particularly when they are hungry. Increased oral gratification and hand-to-mouth activity in young infants increase their risk for oral ingestion. This, coupled with their increasing mobility, makes them particularly susceptible to ingestion of cleaning supplies, plants, and objects that may be on or near the floor.

Nursing Care of the Pediatric Patient with a Poisoning

Assessment

Refer to Chapter 4, *Initial Assessment*, for a review of the primary assessment. Once airway, breathing, and circulation have been established, a secondary survey is done including a full neurological assessment. In all cases, treat the patient first, not the poison. Additional assessment data related to specific poisonings are listed in the following sections.

Additional History

When obtaining a history of toxic exposure, include the following questions specific to the exposure or substance (the 5 Ws):

1. Who?
   - Other family members exposed
   - Other children exposed
2. What and how much?
   - Route(s) of exposure
   - Open bottles or containers found near the pediatric patient
   - Evidence of exposure: pills found in immediate vicinity, pill fragments in mouth, product spilled on clothing, plant leaves or pieces
   - Estimated amount of exposure: count or measure remaining pills or liquid; always assume the maximum amount has been taken
   - Treatment administered prior to arrival in the emergency department (ED)
3. When?
   - Time of exposure; time discovered
   - Estimated duration of exposure
4. Where?
   - Availability of other products in the general area where the exposure occurred
   - Location pediatric patient found (e.g., home, babysitter's, inside or outside house)
5. Why?
   - Intent of exposure (self-harm, unintentional)
   - Circumstances of exposure (error in medication administration, curiosity)

Signs and Symptoms

The symptoms, severity, and time of onset will vary, depending on the type and quantity of poison involved. Signs and symptoms of each particular exposure are listed with each poison.

Diagnostic Procedures

Laboratory studies may be indicated based on the suspected etiology of the pediatric patient's poisoning. Definitive diagnostic testing is performed while the resuscitation is in progress or after the pediatric patient is stabilized. Specific diagnostic procedures are listed under the interventions of the selected poisonings. The following general procedures and studies may be indicated for the pediatric patient with a suspected or actual poisoning.

Monitoring
- Noninvasive blood pressure monitoring and cardiorespiratory monitor
- Pulse oximeter
- Capnography (with intubated patients)

Radiographic Studies
- Chest radiograph to evaluate for infiltrate from aspiration or presence of foreign body
- Abdominal radiograph (for iron ingestion)

Laboratory Studies
- Laboratory studies may be ordered based on the suspected or known poison. The following should be considered.
  - Toxicology screens rarely lead to changes in initial patient management.[24] Treatment may be provided by obtaining an accurate history, identifying the toxin, and treating clinical symptoms.
  - Components of a toxicology screen vary among laboratories and may not be inclusive for the pediatric patient's suspected exposure. A negative toxicology screen does not indicate absence of exposure.
- Specific quantitative drug levels such as acetaminophen, methanol, ethylene glycol, iron, salicylates, carbon monoxide, anticonvulsants, and theophylline may be useful to determine appropriate ongoing management.
- Other laboratory tests may be ordered based on the potential actions of the toxin and signs and symptoms exhibited by the patient, such as arterial or capillary blood gas, electrolytes, blood urea nitrogen, creatinine, osmolality, or blood glucose.

Planning/Implementation

Refer to Chapter 4, *Initial Assessment*, for a description of the general nursing interventions for pediatric patients with alterations in airway, breathing, or circulation. After ensuring a patent airway, effective ventilation, and adequate circulation, interventions may include decontamination, administration of available antidotes, and elimination of toxins. These are initiated as appropriate for the pediatric patient's condition.

Additional Interventions

External Decontamination

Initiate external dermal decontamination for the pediatric patient with exposure to toxic or hazardous materials, as indicated by institution policies and procedures. Prompt decontamination will lessen exposure for the pediatric patient, health care providers, and treatment areas. Any clothing left on the pediatric patient should be removed. Ocular exposures should be flushed with water or normal saline for a minimum of 15 minutes and the eye further evaluated postirrigation.

Gastric Decontamination

The aim of gastric decontamination is to prevent absorption of the poison. When indicated, the recommended method is the administration of activated charcoal. The benefit from decontamination decreases as the duration of time from ingestion increases. As a rule, there is little benefit if 2 hours have elapsed.

- Syrup of ipecac is no longer recommended for the treatment of toxic ingestions.[14]

- Gastric lavage for routine gastric decontamination in poisoned patients is of unproven benefit.[13] The amount of toxin reduced with gastric lavage is limited and diminishes rapidly with time. In addition, oro- or nasogastric tubes are not often large enough to be able to retrieve pills or pill particles in the pediatric patient. The American Academy of Clinical Toxicology/European Association of Poisons Centers and Clinical Toxicologists' position statement concludes that gastric lavage "should not be considered unless a patient has ingested a potentially life-threatening amount of a poison and the procedure can be undertaken within 60 minutes of ingestion."[13,14,15] Gastric lavage is associated with a higher prevalence of aspiration pneumonia, esophageal and gastric injury, dysrhythmias, changes in oxygenation, and laryngospasm.[14,15,16]

- Activated charcoal reduces absorption of a toxin by binding with it in the gastrointestinal tract. It is derived from organic material and exposed to agents that make it extremely porous and absorbent. It can bind with up to 37% of a charcoal-absorbent toxin if given within 60 minutes of the ingestion.[14,17] As with all methods of gastric decontamination, the efficacy of activated charcoal diminishes with time, and it is of most value if given within 1 hour of ingestion. Due to its poor palatability and gritty texture, it is often given via nasogastric tube to small children. The recommended dose of charcoal is 1.0 gm/kg.

  - The addition of sorbitol to activated charcoal or the use of other cathartics is controversial in the pediatric patient.[4,14] There is no evidence demonstrating their effectiveness, and their repeated administration can lead to severe diarrhea, fluid shifts, and electrolyte complications associated with dehydration in the pediatric patient such as hypernatremia and seizures.[4,14,18]

  - Charcoal is not effective with alcohols, hydrocarbons, caustics, and heavy metals such as iron, lead, mercury, lithium, and arsenic.

Whole Bowel Irrigation

Another intervention that may be implemented for intestinal decontamination in a poisoned pediatric patient is whole bowel irrigation (WBI). This therapy was introduced during the 1980s and is useful for ingestion of toxins such as iron, lithium, or sustained-release and enteric-coated preparations, that cannot effectively be absorbed by activated charcoal.[19]

- WBI is accomplished by the administration, through a gastric tube, of a polyethylene glycol electrolyte solution (i.e., GoLYTELY®, NuLYTELY®, or Colyte®), at a rate of 25–40 ml/kg and is continued until the rectal effluent is clear.[5] This solution is designed to pass through the intestinal tract without being absorbed, thereby avoiding shifts in fluids and electrolytes.

Table 18-1 Common Toxins and Related Antidotes

Toxin	Antidote
Acetaminophen	M-acetylcysteine
Anticholinergics	Physostigmine*
Anticholinesterases (organophosphates and carbamates)	Atropine, pralidoxime
Benzodiazepines	Flumazenil*
Botulism	Botulinum antitoxin
Beta blockers	Glucagon
Calcium channel blockers	Calcium
Carbon monoxide	Oxygen, hyperbaric oxygen
Cyanide	Nitrites, sodium thiosulfate
Digoxin	Digoxin Fab antibodies
Heparin	Protamine
Iron	Deferoxamine
Isoniazid	Pyridoxine
Lead	BAL, EDTA, DMSA
Methemoglobinemia	Methylene blue
Opioids	Naloxone
Toxic alcohols (methanol and ethylene glycol)	Ethanol, fomepizole, hemodialysis
Tricyclic antidepressants	Sodium bicarbonate
Warfarin (and superwarfarins)	Vitamin K

*Use of flumazenil/physostigmine contraindicated in many situations. This is useful as an educational tool but might not represent standard of care everywhere. Please consult a poison control center in case of emergency.

Reprinted with permission from Abbruzzi, G., & Stork, C. M. (2002). Pediatric toxicologic concerns. *Emergency Medicine Clinics of North America, 20*(1), 234.

- Vomiting may occur. Intravenous (IV) medications to increase gastric motility (i.e., metoclopramide) and provide antiemetic relief (i.e., ondansetron) may be used to reduce emesis.
- WBI is contraindicated in patients with suspected paralytic ileus, bowel obstruction, or perforation.[4,19]

Antidotes

Although there are few antidotes, the administration of an antidote can be life saving or, at minimum, decrease the severity of toxic effects in instances where they are useful. The use of antidotes is reviewed with the specific poisonings where appropriate. **Table 18-1** lists common antidotes and the toxins for which they are used.

Elimination of Toxins

Once a toxin has been absorbed it is free to act systemically. Certain properties of a drug can make it more amenable for enhanced elimination from the system. Some of these methods include hemodialysis, urine alkalization, and charcoal hemoperfusion. Methods appropriate to the poison are mentioned as part of specific poison management.

Evaluation and Ongoing Assessment

Children who have been exposed to a toxic substance require meticulous and frequent reassessment of airway patency, breathing effectiveness, perfusion, and mental status. Initial improvements may not be sustained, and additional interventions may be needed. Monitoring of drug levels may be needed to achieve desired outcomes.

Selected Poisonings

The following selected emergencies are common pediatric exposures; however, the frequency and type of poisoning may vary by region. Consultation with regional poison experts to identify appropriate and current treatment modalities is an essential component of emergency care, planning, and interventions. Additional history, signs and symptoms, and interventions specific to the selected poisoning are described.

Unknown Poison or Overdose

Occasionally a pediatric patient who is unconscious or nonverbal will be seen in the ED for an exposure to an unknown poison. In these cases, the pediatric patient's clinical presentation may provide clues toward identifying the poisoning agent.

Additional History

- Unconscious
- Abnormal behavior for age
- Pediatric patient exhibiting symptoms of an unknown etiology
- History of ingestion confirmed but amount and type unknown

Signs and Symptoms

- Central nervous system (CNS) findings such as altered mentation, absence of cough or gag reflex
- Changes in color or integrity of skin and/or oral mucosa
- Odors
- Toxidromes: A toxidrome is a group of signs and

Table 18-2 Toxidromes[4,5]

Toxidrome	Signs and Symptoms	Possible Poison
Sympathomimetic	Tachycardia, hypertension, hyperthermia, mydriasis, restlessness, agitation, hyperactivity, diaphoresis, tremors, cardiac dysrhythmias	Amphetamines; cocaine; phencyclidine (PCP); Ecstasy
Anticholinergic	Flushing, hallucinations, dry mouth, tachycardia, urinary retention, mydriasis, decreased bowel sounds, seizures, coma, cardiac dysrhythmias	Cyclic antidepressants; antihistamines; atropinics; over-the-counter sleep preparations
Cholinergic	Salivation, lacrimation, urination, defecation, emesis, bronchoconstriction, muscle fasciculations, seizures	Organophosphates and carbamate insecticides; some mushrooms; severe black widow spider bites
Opiate/opioid	Altered mental status, unresponsiveness, miosis, respiratory depression, bradycardia, hypothermia, hypotension	Opioids; heroin; clonidine
Sedative hypnotics	Sedation, confusion, hallucinations, coma, diplopia, blurred vision, slurred speech, ataxia, nystagmus, respiratory depression, hypotension	Benzodiazepines; barbiturates
Salicylates	Hyperthermia, tachypnea, altered mental status, tinnitus, vomiting, acidosis, shock	Aspirin

symptoms that help identify an unknown poison. **Table 18-2** provides an overview of signs and symptoms associated with specific poison exposures. Consultation with a poison control center or toxicology expert is recommended to assist in identification of specific toxins.

Additional Interventions

- The acronym SIREN (see **Box 18-1**) may be applied to cases of unknown poisoning to assist with recalling the sequence of general interventions.
- Position the pediatric patient. Elevation of the head of the bed may help to reduce the risk of aspiration.[4]
- Suction as needed.
- Provide supplemental oxygen for lethargic, obtunded, or respiratory-depressed patients.
- Provide ventilatory assistance with a bag-mask as required.
- Consider the need for an oropharnygeal airway (if gag absent).
- Consider the need for intubation.
- Establish IV access and replace fluids as necessary.
- Consider medications, such as inotropic support, antidotes (i.e., naloxone, flumazenil), or dextrose

Acetaminophen (Paracetamol)

Acetaminophen (paracetamol) is an analgesic and antipyretic commonly found in many over-the-counter and prescription preparations. It is one of the five most common drugs ingested by children and one of the ten most common drugs used by adolescents and adults in intentional self-poisonings.[6] There are several commercially available concentrations of acetaminophen-containing products, such as infant drops, pediatric elixir, children's chewables, and junior tablets. Risk of improper dosing is increased due to a lack of understanding of the various concentrations and packaging.

Overdose of acetaminophen may lead to hepatic failure

and death. Toxicity can occur with a single large exposure or multiple exposures over time (hours or days). The onset of symptoms is dependent on the total amount ingested per kg of body weight. Children who ingest more than 150 mg/kg are at risk for hepatotoxicity. Young children tend to develop less hepatic toxicity than adults because they rarely ingest large enough doses.

Acetaminophen levels assist in assessing the severity and treatment needs of a child with potential toxicity. A level drawn at least 4 hours following a single acute ingestion should be plotted on the Rumack-Matthew nomogram (see **Figure 18-1**). The nomogram is used to determine the risk of hepatotoxicity and the need for the antidote, N-acetylcysteine (Mucomyst®). N-acetylcysteine acts as a chemical replacement for glutathione,

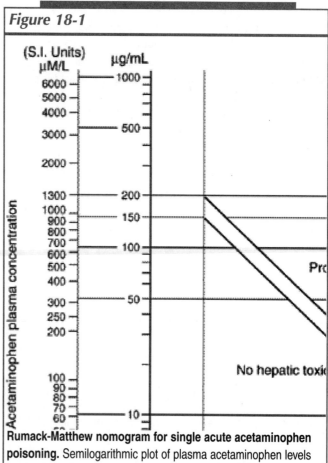

Figure 18-1

Rumack-Matthew nomogram for single acute acetaminophen poisoning. Semilogarithmic plot of plasma acetaminophen levels versus time. *Cautions for use of this chart:* (1) The time coordinates refer to time of ingestion. (2) Serum levels drawn before 4 h may not represent peak levels. (3) The graph should be used only in relation to a single acute ingestion. (4) The lower solid line 25% below the standard nomogram is included to allow for possible errors in acetaminophen plasma assays and estimated time from ingestion of an overdose.

Adapted from Rumack, B. H., & Matthew, H. (1975). Acetaminophen poisoning and toxicity. *Pediatrics, 55*(6), 871–876.

Box 18-1 SIREN

S—Stabilize the child's condition

I —Identify the poison

R—Reverse its effect; reduce absorption

E—Eliminate toxin

N—Need for consultation with poison control, ongoing physical care, and psychiatric consultation

Adapted from Ball, J., & Bindler, R. (2003). *Pediatric nursing: Caring for children* (p. 535). Upper Saddle River, NJ: Pearson Education, Inc.

the naturally occurring substance that protects against hepatocellular damage. It is optimally administered within 12 hours of ingestion and may be effective up to 24 hours after ingestion. Each case should be considered individually. Consultation with a poison control center should be made to assist with the analysis of toxicity whenever appropriate.

Signs and Symptoms of Toxicity

Acetaminophen-induced injury occurs in stages, with the first phase beginning shortly after ingestion. Symptoms progress at a variable rate depending on the dose and time of ingestion. In Phase 1 the child may either be asymptomatic or have signs of gastrointestinal (GI) irritation including anorexia, nausea and vomiting, decreased appetite, and general malaise. Phase two consists of signs of hepatic damage including elevation in liver enzymes (AST, ALT, bilirubin), prothrombin time, partial thromboplastin time, and presence of right upper quadrant (RUQ) pain. By the third phase (72 to 96 hours), the patient may have signs of hepatic failure, hepatic necrosis, and encephalopathy, including RUQ pain, altered mental status, jaundice, renal failure, and coagulation defects. Death due to hepatic failure may occur during this phase. Resolution may occur by 4 days or take up to 2 weeks if the damage done is not irreversible.

Additional Interventions

- Obtain appropriate lab work.
  - Acetaminophen level at least 4 hours postingestion
- Administer activated charcoal 1g/kg if within 1 to 2 hours of ingestion.
- Anticipate and prepare for administration of antidote.
  - N-acetylcysteine loading dose followed by maintenance. Administration is based on serum acetaminophen levels. Follow institution-specific protocol for method and route of administration. It can be administered intravenously or orally, with the former route having many advantages. When administering orally, the unpleasant taste and "rotten egg" smell may be masked somewhat if diluted in juice, poured over ice, placed in a covered cup, and sipped through a straw. Vomiting is very common after oral N-acetylcysteine.

Alcohols

For a pediatric patient, an alcohol ingestion can be a serious, life-threatening emergency. Depending on the type of alcohol, toxicity can occur with ingestion of very small amounts. Though certain alcohols such as methanol and ethylene glycol themselves are not poisonous, the metabolites they form produce toxicity.[14] **Table 18-3** outlines examples of several types of alcohols.

Signs and Symptoms

Methanol

Methanol produces a triad of clinical symptoms including GI, CNS, and ocular symptoms. If consumed with ethanol, there may be a latent period of 24 to 72 hours postingestion where the patient is asymptomatic. Organ damage occurs from its metabolite, formic acid.

- Headache, lethargy, dizziness, nausea, and vomiting
- Visual disturbances; metabolites may deposit in the retina causing permanent blindness
- Presence of elevated osmolality and anion gaps
- Metabolic acidosis
- Deterioration in mental status progressing to lethargy, seizures, and coma

Ethylene Glycol

Ethylene glycol is rapidly absorbed within 1 to 4 hours of ingestion. Ethylene glycol that is not eliminated may cause renal toxicity.

- Signs of intoxication without ethanol odor including slurred speech, confusion, nystagmus, seizures
- Nausea, vomiting
- Metabolic acidosis
- Renal failure
- Production of calcium oxylate crystals in the urine

Isopropyl Alcohol

Isopropyl alcohol is rapidly absorbed by the GI tract and excreted via the kidney. The remainder is metabolized by the liver, producing acetone.

- Sign of intoxication without ethanol odor. Will present with fruity acetone smell on breath.
- CNS depression
- GI irritation

Ethanol

Ethanol is rapidly absorbed by the GI tract, and 90% is metabolized by the liver. The remainder is excreted in the kidney.

Table 18-3 Types and Examples of Alcohols

Types	Examples of Products
Ethanol	Alcoholic beverages, perfumes, and mouthwash
Isopropyl alcohol	Rubbing alcohol and solvents
Ethylene glycol	Radiator antifreeze and deicer
Methanol	Windshield washer fluid, solvents, antifreeze, and gasoline

- Signs of intoxication include cognitive impairment, slurred speech and ataxia, and progression to lethargy, stupor, depression, and coma.
- Visual disturbances.
- Impaired gluconeogenesis causing hypoglycemia. This can result in seizures and coma in young children.

Additional Interventions

- Support airway and breathing through positioning, insertion of an oral airway (if protective reflexes are absent), suctioning, monitoring, supplemental O_2, and possible intubation.
- Obtain the following lab specimens:
  - Whole blood or serum glucose
  - Specific alcohol (ethanol, methanol, ethylene glycol) level
  - Electrolytes
  - Arterial blood gas
- Treatment varies and ranges from simple oral dilution measures to administration of ethanol or fomepizole, an antidote for methanol and ethylene glycol poisoning, by continuous infusion. Consult a poison control center for treatment recommendations.
- Administer glucose as indicated if documented hypoglycemia is present. Monitor serum glucose levels closely. Consider IV fluids with glucose for continuous or maintenance infusion.
- Anticipate and prepare for correction of metabolic acidosis through administration of sodium bicarbonate infusion.
- Anticipate the need to support cardiac output through the administration of fluids and vasopressors.
- Prepare for hemodialysis in severe ethylene glycol or methanol ingestion.

Cocaine

As a CNS and sympathetic nervous system stimulant, cocaine primarily affects the brain and heart. It can be used therapeutically as a potent vasoconstrictor or illicitly as a CNS stimulant. Cocaine may be taken intranasally, intravenously, topically, or inhaled as freebased, or "crack," cocaine. Children who intentionally or unintentionally ingest cocaine can present with altered sensorium, seizures, tachycardia, shock, and cardiovascular collapse.

Signs and Symptoms

- Altered level of consciousness; at low doses, will exhibit euphoria, hyperalertness, and talkativeness; at high doses may present with agitation, paranoia, delusions, tremor, seizures, or coma

- Tachycardia, hypertension, ventricular dysrhythmias, acute chest pain, cardiopulmonary arrest (high dose)
- Dyspnea, respiratory depression
- Mydriasis, diaphoresis, hyperthermia
- Cerebral vascular accidents, subarachnoid hemorrhage, cerebral infarction

Additional Interventions

- Support airway, ventilation, and oxygenation.
- Initiate electrocardiogram, oxygen saturation, temperature, and neurological monitoring.
- Consider gastric decontamination measures.
  - Activated charcoal for oral ingestion within the appropriate time frame.
  - WBI if drug-containing packets are present.
- Administer medications.
  - Consider benzodiazepines to treat seizures, tachycardia, hypertension, and depress CNS activity.
  - Administer IV sodium bicarbonate, amiodarone, or lidocaine for treatment of ventricular dysrhythmias.
  - Nitroglycerin and aspirin may be considered for acute chest pain.
- Treat hyperthermia with cooling measures.

Cardiac Medications

Pediatric patients are not routinely prescribed cardiac medications, but they are commonly prescribed for

Table 18-4 Cardiovascular and Neurologic Signs and Symptoms of Toxicity

Cardiovascular Signs and Symptoms of Toxicity	
Beta-blockers & calcium channel blockers	Digitalis
Bradydysrhythmias	Bradycardia
Hypotension	First-, second-, and third-degree heart blocks
AV block	Prolonged PR interval, inverted P waves
	Accelerated junctional tachycardia
	Ventricular dysrhythmias, premature atrial contractions (PAC), and premature ventricular contractions (PVC)
	Hypotension

Neurologic Signs and Symptoms of Toxicity	
Beta-blockers & calcium channel blockers	Digitalis
Syncope	Lethargy
Seizures	Seizures
Coma	Coma
	Color vision disturbances

adults. When left within reach, children may ingest these potentially lethal medications. Of the 8,844 exposures to calcium channel blockers that were reported to the AAPCC in 1999, 26% of these occurred in children less than 6 years of age.[2] Common cardiac medication poisonings seen in the ED are beta-adrenergic blockers, calcium channel blockers, and digitalis.[19] Even though beta-adrenergic blockers and calcium channel blockers act on different receptors in the cardiovascular system, the signs and symptoms of toxic ingestion have a similar presentation. Digoxin, a cardiac inotrope, is prescribed for young infants with congenital cardiac anomalies and for pediatric patients with heart failure. Digoxin toxicity may be either acute or chronic.

Signs and Symptoms

- Cardiovascular and neurologic signs and symptoms are listed in **Table 18-4**.
- Hypoglycemia and bronchospasm with beta blockers
- Hypercalcemia and metabolic acidosis with calcium channel blockers
- Hyperkalemia
- Nausea, vomiting, constipation, and decreased bowel sounds with calcium channel blockers

Diagnostic Procedures

Monitoring

- Noninvasive blood pressure, oxygen saturation, and ECG
- 12-lead ECG

Laboratory Studies

- Serum electrolytes, especially potassium and calcium
- Serum or whole blood glucose test

Additional Interventions

- Support airway, ventilation, and oxygenation.
- Establish vascular access.
- Anticipate the need for WBI if the pediatric patient has ingested a sustained-release beta blocker or calcium channel blocker.
- Anticipate the need for administration of specific antidotes or pharmacologic agents.
  - Calcium infusion in an attempt to overcome the calcium channel blockade in calcium channel blocker toxicity[2,12]
  - IV glucagon therapy for both calcium channel and beta blocker toxicity for its positive inotropic effect[12]
  - Digoxin-specific antibody fragments for digitalis toxicity[12]
  - Vasopressor therapy (norepinephrine or epinephrine) infusion to treat bradycardia and hypotension

- Prepare for and assist with external cardiac pacing or placement of a transvenous pacemaker to maintain cardiac output during initial resuscitation as indicated.

Cough and Cold Preparations

In 1998, over 64,000 cases of exposure to cough and cold preparations were reported in children less than 6 years of age.[6] These preparations are commonly found in the home, and new methods to make them flavorful and more palatable to children increase the potential for unintentional ingestion.

Cough and cold preparations may contain a variety of substances, including antihistamines (i.e., diphenhydramine, chlorpheniramine), decongestants (i.e., phenylephrine, pseudoephedrine), ethanol, and acetaminophen.

Signs and Symptoms

- Antihistamines—sedative effects. May see CNS stimulation in older children.
- Decongestants—sympathomimetic effects including anxiety, agitation, dry mouth, tachycardia, and hypertension
- Combination—hyperactivity, tachycardia, ataxia, disorientation, hallucinations, seizures, or respiratory depression
- Ethanol—CNS depression, hypoglycemia

Additional Interventions

- Close monitoring of respiratory, neurologic, and cardiovascular status.
- Administration of activated charcoal if within appropriate time frame.
- Serum or whole blood glucose.

Hydrocarbons

Hydrocarbons refer to organic compounds composed of hydrogen and carbon. There are four groups of hydrocarbons, including

1. Petroleum distillates—lighter fluid, propane, furniture polish, lamp oil
2. Aromatic—glue, nail polish, paints, paint remover
3. Aliphatics—turpentine
4. Halogenated—carbon tetrachloride, chloroform, Freon[4]

Hydrocarbons primarily affect the respiratory system. Once aspirated, direct injury to the epithelium and pulmonary capillaries causes pulmonary edema and bronchospasm to occur. The development of a chemical pneumonitis depends on the properties of the product. Those with higher viscosity such as oils tend to be less irritating to the mucosa than those with low viscosity such as gasoline or solvents.

Additional History

- Coughing and choking with initial ingestion
- Gradual increase in work of breathing
- Odor of hydrocarbon on breath

Signs and Symptoms

Hydrocarbons can also affect the CNS, GI, integumentary and cardiac systems. Some agents can cause serious systemic effects, such as hepatic failure or CNS depression. Other signs and symptoms include

- Tachypnea, dyspnea, cyanosis
- Dry, persistent cough (several hours postingestion)
- Crackles, wheezes, and diminished breath sounds
- Nausea and vomiting, irritation to the oral or nasal mucosa
- Altered mental status: headache, lethargy, agitation, confusion, ataxia, seizures, coma
- Dizziness, dysrhythmias (less common in children)
- Hepatic or renal dysfunction (halogenated hydrocarbons)

Additional Interventions

- Trend respiratory assessment. The asymptomatic patient may develop respiratory symptoms that progress to distress within hours after ingestion. Anticipate the need for intubation with worsening respiratory symptoms.
- Decontaminate skin by washing with soap and water. With prolonged contact, hydrocarbons may defat the skin and result in surface burns or continued exposure.
- Provide gastric decontamination only as recommended by the poison control center.
  - Gastric decontamination methods are controversial and depend on the type of product ingested.
  - Vomiting should be avoided to lessen the risk of aspiration. Therefore, syrup of ipecac and gastric lavage are contraindicated. Avoid the administration of activated charcoal.

Household Cleaning Agents

Most caustic injuries in children occur in the home and are caused by exposure to an acid or alkali. Integumentary injury results from neutralization of the substance in the tissue, releasing heat, and causing burns. The initial presentation and method of treatment are similar, regardless of the pH of the substance. Esophageal burns by caustic agents can result in varying degrees of damage to tissue that can occur in a number of different locations along the GI tract.

Commonly ingested acid products are toilet bowl and pool cleaners. Those containing sulfuric, hydrochloric, or phosphoric acid burn on contact, causing damage to the oral mucosa. Sources of alkali products include drain cleaners, oven cleaners, concentrated liquid alkali cleaners, dishwasher detergents, and permanent hair dye. Alkali agents usually affect the mouth, esophagus, and stomach.

Regardless of the mechanism, unless decontamination is performed, the end result will be direct tissue injury and cellular death. When caustics are ingested, it is difficult to determine if esophageal or stomach burns are present based on the presence or absence of oral burns. Therefore, recommendations from the poison control center are a vital part of management.

Additional History

- Open container of household products
- Unusual odor, stain on skin or clothing, spill in immediate area

Signs and Symptoms

- Drooling or dysphagia
- Burns in or around the mouth
- Vomiting
- Stridor, hoarseness
- Soft tissue swelling
- Respiratory distress

Additional Interventions

- Monitor respiratory status. Airway edema may continue to develop postexposure.
- Prevent vomiting.
  - Keep the pediatric patient calm and do not administer anything by mouth to avoid emesis.
  - Syrup of ipecac, gastric lavage, and activated charcoal are contraindicated.
  - Initial dilution with small amounts of water may be considered for alkali or acid ingestions.[4]
- If exposure to the skin or eye has occurred, flush with copious amounts of water for 10 to 15 minutes.
- Keep the pediatric patient NPO (nothing by mouth) and maintain hydration through IV fluids.

Iron

In 2001, over 39,000 children less than 6 years of age were reported to have unintentional exposure to vitamins.[6] Although the majority of these ingestions were nontoxic, many vitamin preparations contain iron. Prenatal vitamins, which contain greater amounts of iron, may be life threatening if a small child ingests as few as 10 tablets.

The severity of iron poisoning is directly related to the amount of elemental iron ingested. Prediction of toxicity can be determined if the number of ingested tablets is known. A serum iron concentration greater than 300 mcg/dl has been associated with vomiting. A serum iron concentration of greater than 350 mcg/dl has been associated with moderate to severe toxicity.[4]

Signs and Symptoms

Symptoms of toxicity can occur as early as 30 minutes after ingestion. Symptoms of iron toxicity are divided into four stages.

Stage 1: Approximately one half to six hours after ingestion, gastrointestinal symptoms occur. These include vomiting, diarrhea, hematemesis, and abdominal pain.

Stage 2: Six to 12 hours after ingestion, the pediatric patient may experience temporary improvement of symptoms. There is often a rapid progression from Stage 1 to Stage 3, and this stage may not occur.

Stage 3: Over 12 hours after ingestion, metabolic acidosis, circulatory failure, CNS depression leading to coma, and hepatic failure occur.

Stage 4: One to two months after ingestion, gastric scarring and strictures develop.

Additional Interventions

- Lab work including iron levels, complete blood count (CBC), liver function tests, coagulation studies, electrolytes, glucose, type and cross match.
- Abdominal radiograph is very important and used to determine the presence and number of iron tablets in the gastrointestinal tract.
- Anticipate WBI with positive radiographic findings.
- Prepare for IV administration of the antidote deferoxamine in acute iron intoxication. Deferoxamine is an iron chelation agent that removes iron from the tissues and free iron from the plasma. Following its administration, the pediatric patient's urine may turn a pink salmon or rose color indicating that the iron is binding with the antidote.

Lead

Although there has been a recent dramatic reduction in lead poisoning, there still remain a number of children with worrisome blood lead levels. Many children go undiagnosed and untreated because they have no obvious symptoms, but the detrimental effects of lead on a child's brain has lifelong implications including decreased IQ scores, cognitive defects, impaired hearing, and growth delays. Children are at greater risk for lead poisoning because they absorb and retain more lead in proportion to their weight than adults do. Lead is absorbed by the blood, tissues, bones, and teeth and is of particular harm to children less than 7 years of age. Lead absorbed by the bones and teeth is slowly released, therefore, exposure to even small amounts over time can result in toxicity. Lead-based paint and lead-contaminated dust and soils remain the primary sources of exposure in children. Children are also exposed through caregivers' occupations, hobbies, air, water, and food. Abatement of lead paint in housing is a critical measure in lead poisoning prevention.[22]

Additional History

- Exposure to lead paint
  - Living in a home painted before 1978 when lead content was not limited in residential paint
  - Playground and nursery equipment painted with lead paint
  - Recent renovation of an older home
- Caregiver with hobby (e.g., pottery glaze, lead fishing sinkers, exposure to caregivers' clothing after using indoor firing ranges)
- Use of "traditional" medicine containing lead
- Exposure to drinking water with high lead levels (e.g., cisterns with lead liners, water systems with lead soldered joints, and water systems standing on lead surfaces)
- Eating from improperly fired pottery

Signs and Symptoms

- Although now uncommon, acute lead encephalopathy may present with
  - Altered level of consciousness, apathy, bizarre behavior, seizures, coma
  - Ataxia, incoordination, myalgia, muscular exhaustion
  - Vomiting, severe abdominal pain, colic
  - Loss of recently acquired skills
- Symptomatic lead poisoning without encephalopathy may include
  - Lethargy, decrease in play activity, irritability, fatigue, difficulty concentrating
  - Anorexia, sporadic vomiting, abdominal pain, weight loss, constipation
  - Headache, anemia

Additional Interventions

- Obtain appropriate laboratory studies.
  - Blood lead level
  - Free erythrocyte protoporphyrin (FEP)
- Consider abdominal radiograph, which may show

radiopaque foreign materials that were ingested during the preceding 24 to 36 hours.

- Anticipate need for chelation therapy in symptomatic children with toxic lead levels. Calcium disodium ethylenediaminetetraacetate (CaNa$_2$EDTA), dimercaprol (BAL), d-Penicillamine, or succimer (DMSA) may be used.[20] Prepare for transport to pediatric center to provide chelation and supportive interventions.
- Refer to appropriate agencies for follow-up and environmental evaluation.

Sulfonylureas

Sulfonylureas stimulate the secretion of insulin and are used in the treatment of Type 2 diabetes. Sulfonylureas have a low threshold for toxicity, and even one tablet can cause hypoglycemia in a young child.[21] Because infants and small children have limited glucose stores, ingestion of this type of medication can cause profound and prolonged hypoglycemia.

Signs and Symptoms

- Consistent with those of hypoglycemia
- Dizziness, pallor, diaphoresis, tachycardia
- Restlessness, agitation, lethargy, seizures, coma

Additional Interventions

- Close monitoring of neurological status
- Serum or whole blood glucose levels
- Encourage feeding.
- Administer medications.
  - Consider activated charcoal.
  - Parenteral dextrose replacement for hypoglycemia.
  - Octreotide, which suppresses insulin release, may be used if dextrose and feeding ineffective for hypoglycemia. Consult a poison control center for administration.

Tricyclic Antidepressants (TCA)

Despite the increased use of newer medications to treat depression, TCAs continues to be a cause of both morbidity and mortality in children. Amitriptyline (Elavil®), imipramine (Tofranil®), amoxapine (Asendin®), and desipramine (Norpramin®) are commonly ingested TCA drugs. Although still widely used for the treatment of depression, tricyclics are often prescribed as adjuvant therapy for neuropathic pain, nocturnal enuresis, migraine headaches, and sleep disorders.[2]

Toxicity is manifested in a variety of neurologic and cardiovascular signs and symptoms. These are related to the anticholinergic activity, blockade of norepinephrine reuptake, and quinidine-like effects of the drug.

Significant complications including wide complex dysrhythmias, hypotension, seizures, or coma typically occur within 1 to 6 hours after the ingestion of a toxic amount.[4,6] Due to the drug properties of protein binding and volume distribution, the amount of TCA in the serum bears little correlation with toxicity, making serum levels of little value.[19]

The lethal cardiac effects of TCA overdose are related to the quinidine-like effects of the drug causing myocardial depression and prolongation of the PR and QRS intervals. They are responsible for intraventricular conduction delays, ventricular dysrhythmias, decreased cardiac output, and hypotension.[18] The widened QRS interval is an indicator of toxicity in overdose.

Alkalinization of the plasma with IV sodium bicarbonate is the treatment of choice to alter pH and reduce toxicity. Mild metabolic alkalosis helps to narrow the QRS, correct hypotension, and reduce the incidence of cardiac dysrhythmias.[4]

Emesis is contraindicated due to the potential for rapid deterioration in neurologic status. Gastric lavage may be initiated for gastric decontamination if the ingestion has occurred within the hour and the airway is secure.

Signs and Symptoms

- Altered level of consciousness: drowsiness, sedation, confusion, agitation, hallucinations, coma
- Seizures
- Decreased respirations
- Cardiovascular effects
  - Dysrhythmias (widened QRS, ventricular dysrhythmias)
  - Hypotension secondary to myocardial depression and norepinephrine depletion
  - Tachycardia
- Peripheral anticholinergic-related symptoms
  - Flushing, dry mouth, and dilated pupils
  - Hypertension
  - Urinary retention
  - Decreased bowel sounds
  - Hyperthermia

Additional Interventions

- Ensure adequate ventilation, monitor oxygen saturation.
- Monitor electrolytes, obtain arterial blood gas.
- Obtain 12-lead ECG.
- Continuous cardiac monitoring
- Treat hypotension with fluid bolus initially.
  - Administer medications as indicated

- IV sodium bicarbonate for signs of cardiac toxicity (i.e., widened QRS, ventricular dysrhythmias, hypotension, and seizures)
- Hypotension may be treated with dopamine or norepinephrine if blood pressure remains low following fluid administration.[4]
- Benzodiazepines for seizures
- Treat urinary retention.

Animal Bites

Animal bites to children can occur from a variety of mammals including dogs, cats, and humans. Dog bites account for 80% of bite injuries, with the majority of those being children.[6, 20] Bite injuries are frequently associated with crush injuries to the extremity and wounds can be contaminated with multiple organisms (see **Table 18-5**). Rabies is the most significant concern from animal bites. Skunks, bats, raccoons, and foxes as well as unvaccinated dogs and cats are the animals commonly associated with the spread of rabies to humans. An accurate history and clinical assessment of the wound is necessary to evaluate the risk for rabies transmission.

Envenomation

Each year, thousands of children are treated in the ED for various types of bites and stings. Although most of the creatures that inhabit the world around us are not harmful to humans, some can cause significant illness, injury, and even death. Approximately 50 to 100 people die each year as a result of insect stings.[6] It is important for emergency nurses to be familiar with their local environment and aware of local inhabitants that may

Table 18-5 Organisms That May Contaminate a Bite Wound

Aerobic Bacteria
- *Staphylococcus aureus*
- *Streptococcus*
- *Eikenella corrodens*
- *Pasteurella*

Anaerobic Bacteria
- *Bacteroides*
- *Enterobacter cloacae*
- *Proteus mirabilis*

Other Pathogens
- Hepatitis virus
- *Clostridium tetani*
- Herpesvirus
- Rabies virus

result in envenomation.

Insect Bites and Stings

Reactions to bites and stings are dependent on the individual sensitivity of the pediatric patient and the number of stings that occur. Reactions can range from local irritation to anaphylaxis. Although initial reactions may only produce local symptoms, subsequent stings may cause increasingly serious reactions due to the development of antibodies that are produced when bitten.

Additional Interventions
- Antihistamine therapy for mild cases of insect bites or stings
- Epinephrine administered subcutaneously, intramuscularly, or intravenously for signs of respiratory distress or anaphylaxis related to an insect bite or sting

Snakebites

Venomous snakes are found worldwide. Envenomation from snakebites carries with it a higher morbidity or mortality rate if left untreated due to the pediatric patient's increased metabolic rate and large body surface area to weight ratio. In addition to these physiological considerations, reactions to envenomation are based on pertinent history and presenting signs and symptoms.[22] The presence of bite or fang marks may not exist with some types of venomous snakes such as the coral snake. These snakes have rather small, nonretractable fangs that tend to scratch the skin without leaving the puncture marks characteristic of a snakebite.

All children coming to the ED with a history of a bite from a poisonous snake must be treated emergently.

Additional History
- Prehospital care and time elapsed from incident to definitive care
- Species of animal, insect, or reptile
- Amount of exertion that occurred after the envenomation
  - Since venom is transported through the lymphatics, not the bloodstream, physical exertion will assist in the rapid spread of venom throughout the pediatric patient's body.
- Type of bite or venom
  - Amount of venom injected is not always proportional to the systemic effect
  - Small amounts of venom from some creatures can result in serious anaphylactic reactions
- Known allergies or asthma
- Previous administration of antivenin

Signs and Symptoms

- Altered mental status
- Respiratory distress: airway edema, dyspnea, wheezes
- Altered skin integrity: color, fang marks, bite marks, vesicles, edema, ulcerations, hives, wounds
- Signs of neurotoxicity: paresthesia, muscle fasiculations, flaccid paralysis
- Massive tissue edema and shock due to intravascular volume depletion
- Disseminated intravascular coagulopathy, thrombocytopenia, uncontrollable hemorrhage

Additional Interventions

- Initiate IV access if signs of anaphylaxis, history of potential poisonous bite, or need for extensive wound repair are present.
- Immobilize and elevate the affected limb with a splint or sling and remove any constricting clothing or jewelry around the bite.
- Provide wound care (see **Table 18-6**).
- Provide discharge teaching regarding wound care and prevention of reoccurrence.

Additional Interventions for Venomous Snakebites

- Keep the extremity at or below the level of the heart. Do not elevate the limb.
- Apply a pressure bandage starting at the bite site. First progress distally to the end of the limb (fingers or toes) and then proximally toward the shoulder or groin. Ensure the bandage only blocks lymphatic flow and does not occlude arterial blood flow.
- Assess perfusion distal to the site.
- Observe for the development of compartment syndrome, which is compromised circulation and tissue function from increased pressure within a closed compartment. It can occur secondary to an accumulation of blood, edema, or muscle hypertrophy or from an external pressure source. Early indicators include increased

Table 18-6 Wound Care

- Inspect the wound for the presence of stingers or teeth.
- Gently remove any remaining pieces of the stinger or teeth.
- Cleanse the wound with mild soap and water.
- Irrigate potentially contaminated wounds with normal saline.
- Apply cool compresses for comfort.
- Administer tetanus prophylaxis as indicated.
- Administer antibiotics as indicated.
- Instruct the pediatric patient and caregiver regarding the following.
  - Signs and symptoms of infection
  - Proper wound care
  - When they should return to the ED or contact their physician

pain, tense or swollen extremity, and deceased sensation. Weakened or absent pulse may or may not be present and is often a late sign along with paralysis.[5]

- Do not remove the bandage until antivenin is administered.
- Apply direct continuous pressure to bites to the torso or head until definitive treatment is started.
- Determine need for and administer specific antivenin as indicated and directed by the poison control center or protocol (see Appendix A)
- Administer prophylactic antibiotics; snakebites are often complicated by staphylococcal infection.
- Obtain laboratory studies including CBC, serum electrolytes, creatine kinase (CPK), and coagulation studies.

Health Promotion

Poisoning prevention must focus on interventions that are directed at reducing toxic exposures. The following safety measures and family education should be stressed.

- Store poisons and medication in appropriately marked containers, well out of reach, and locked in a cabinet.
- Discard old medications.
- Avoid combining medications in one bottle.
- Store cleaning products and chemicals in their original containers.
- Provide the phone number of a poison control center. Instruct parents to post the number by their telephone. The number of the nearest poison control center may be found in the telephone directory or online at the American Association of Poison Control Centers, www.aapcc.org, which includes listings for centers in various states as well as countries including Australia, Canada, Brazil, and New Zealand.[16]
- Encourage caregivers to
  - Install special locks for cabinets
  - Teach child safety habits
  - Never refer to medication as "candy"
  - Remember that caps are only child resistant not "childproof"
- Refer the family to appropriate resources for information and prevention concerning
  - Childproofing the home
  - Appropriate storage of household products and cleaning chemicals
  - Initial treatment of a toxic ingestion
- Educate caregivers about reducing blood lead levels. Poison control centers can provide resources for prevention literature and additional prevention measures.
  - Instruct caregivers to make sure that the child does

not have access to peeling paint or chewable surfaces painted with lead.

- Wash the child's hands and face before they eat.
- Wash toys and pacifiers frequently.

• Prevention of bites and stings
- Become familiar with the insects, spiders, and snakes that populate your local environment or those that may be present when planning a hike or trip.
- Cover exposed areas with light, fitted clothing when working, walking, or hiking in an environment that may contain insects.
- Shake out clothing, sleeping bags, and boots before putting them on when camping or hiking.
- Use an insect repellent or natural repellent to keep insects away. Be sure it is safe for the child's age.

Summary

A pediatric patient who has been exposed to a toxic substance may be at risk for physical injury related to the direct effects of the poison or its by-products. Decreasing the risk includes knowing how to access and use the poison control center, public service agencies, and communities for education about prevention. Being aware of the dangers associated with poisons, becoming an advocate to ensure that medications and products are packaged safely, and ensuring caregivers receive age-appropriate education for their children is a responsibility we all share.

Case Scenario Answers

Dangers related to the misuse of these medications:

An overdose of tricyclic antidepressants (TCA) can produce a variety of adverse reactions including dry mouth, flushing, dilated pupils, changes in LOC including hallucinations, confusion and agitation as well as lethal cardiac effects such as intraventricular delays and ventricular dysrhythmias. Therefore, a suspected ingestion of TCA is considered a medical emergency.

Cough and cold preparations contain a variety of substances, including antihistamines and decongestants, that can cause similar symptoms as TCA ingestions.

Immediate nursing interventions:

Because of the inability to determine the nature of the ingestion, this child should be immediately placed in a room where cardiac monitoring is available. He will require close observation of his neurological status, respiratory status including rate, effort, and oxygen saturation as well as his circulatory status including color, capillary refill, blood pressure, and cardiac rate and rhythm.

Explanations of the plan and need for monitoring will need to be shared with the caregiver.

Attempts should be made to determine the origin of the ingestion (bottles retrieved from home) and the type, amount, and time of ingestion ascertained in order to provide further treatment.

References

1. American Association of Poison Control Centers. (2001). *A profile of U.S. poison centers in 2000: A survey conducted by the American Association of Poison Control Centers.* Retrieved November 11, 2002 from http://www.aapcc.org

2. Hazinski, M. F. (Ed.). (2002). Toxicology. In *Pediatric advanced life support* (Provider manual) (pp. 305–331). Dallas, TX: American Heart Association.

3. Ozanne-Smith, J., Day, L., Parsons, B., Tibballs, J., & Dobbin, M. (2001). Childhood poisoning: Access and prevention. *Journal of Paediatric Child Health, 37*(3), 262–265.

4. Madden, M. (2001). Toxic ingestions. In M. A. Curley & P. A. Moloney-Harmon (Eds.), *Critical care nursing of infants and children* (pp. 999–1023). Philadelphia: Saunders.

5. Tucker, C., & Schauben, J. (1998). Environmental and toxicologic emergencies. In T. E. Soud & J. S. Rogers (Eds.), *Manual of pediatric emergency nursing* (pp. 622–650). St. Louis. MO: Mosby.

6. Litovitz, T. L., Klein-Schwartz, W., Rodgers, G. C., Jr., Cobaugh, D. J., Youniss, J., Omslaer, J. C., et al. (2002). 2001 Annual report of the American Association of Poison Control Centers toxic exposure surveillance system. *American Journal of Emergency Medicine, 20*(5), 391–452.

7. Weisman, R. S., Howlan, M. A., Reynolds, J. R., & Smith, C. (1994). Pharmacokinetic and toxicokinetic principles. In L. R. Goldfrank, N. E. Flomenbaum, N. A. Lewin, R. S. Weiseman, M. A. Howland, & R. S. Hoffman (Eds.), *Toxicologic emergencies* (5th ed., pp. 85–98). Norwalk, CT: Appleton & Lange.

8. Smith, J. (1998). Big differences in little people. *American Journal of Nursing, 88*(4), 458–462.

9. McManus Kuller, J., & Houska Lund, C. (1998). Assessment and management of integumentary dysfunction. In C. Kenner, J. Wright Lott, & A. Applewhite Flandermeyer (Eds.), *Comprehensive neonatal nursing: A physiologic perspective* (pp. 648–681). Philadelphia: Saunders.

10. Bruckner, J. M. (1996). Pediatric pharmacology and intravenous therapy. In J. M. Bruckner & K. D. Wallin (Eds.), *Manual of pediatric nursing* (pp. 33–44). Boston: Little, Brown and Company.

11. Melini, L. V. (1991). Poisoning: An overview. In D. O. Thomas (Ed.), *Quick reference to pediatric nursing* (pp. 231). Gaithersburg, MD: Aspen Publishers.

12. Henretig, F. M., & Shannon, M. (1996). Toxicologic emergencies. In G. R. Fleisher & S. Ludwig (Eds.), *Synopsis of pediatric emergency medicine* (pp. 405–446). Baltimore: Williams and Wilkins.

13. Clinical policy for the initial approach to patients presenting with acute toxic ingestion or dermal or inhalation exposure. (1999). *Annals of Emergency Medicine, 33*(6), 735–761.

14. Tenenbein, M. (1999). Recent advancements in pediatric toxicology. *Pediatric Clinics of North America, 46*(6), 1179–1188.

15. Bond, G. R. (2002). The role of activated charcoal and gastric emptying in gastrointestinal decontamination: A state of the art review. *Annals of Emergency Medicine, 39*(3), 273–286.

16. Hayes, L. (2000). What's your gut reaction to a poison emergency? *Nursing, 30*(9), 34–39.

17. Green, R., Grierson, R., Sitar, D. S., & Tenenbein, M. (2001). How long after drug ingestion is activated charcoal still effective? *Journal of Toxicology (Clinical Toxicology), 39*(6), 601–605.

18. Liebelt, E. L., & DeAngelis, C. D. (1999). Evolving trends and treatment advances in pediatric poisoning. *Journal of the American Medical Association, 282*(12), 1113–1115.

19. Yeh, J. (2002). Poisonings. In V. L. Gunn & C. Nechyba (Eds.), *The Harriet Lane handbook* (16th ed., pp. 19–50) St. Louis, MO: Mosby.

20. Ball, J., & Bindler, R. (2003). *Pediatric nursing caring for children* (pp. 639–641). Upper Saddle River, NJ: Pearson Education Inc.

21. Abbruzzi, G. & Stork, C. M. (2002). Pediatric toxicologic concerns. *Emergency Medicine Clinics of North America, 20*(1), 223–247.

22 Hodge, D., & Trecklenberg, F. (1996). Bites and stings. In G. R. Fleisher & S. Ludwig (Eds.), *Synopsis of pediatric emergency medicine* (pp. 463–476). Baltimore: Williams and Wilkins.

23. Pharmacy Network Group. (n.d.). *Rattlesnake antivenin dosage and indications/antivenin (Crotalidae) polyvalent.* Retrieved August 8, 2003 from http://www.pharmacynetworkgroup.com/i/rattlesnake-antivenin-indications-dosage.htm

Appendix 18-A

General Indications for Antivenin Administration for Venomous Snakebites

Indications for Antivenin

- Muscle weakness
  - Respiratory and ocular muscles are particularly sensitive to snake neurotoxins.
  - Generalized muscle weakness may result in poor respiratory effort.
  - Changes in predicted peak flow measurement can be an early indicator of envenomation.
- Presence of coagulation disturbance
- Headache (early sign)
- Evidence of systemic involvement
- Tender or enlarged lymph nodes (not conclusive)

Administration of Antivenin

The use of antivenin carries a high risk of anaphylaxis and serum sickness. Treatment for anaphylaxis is discussed in Chapter 7, *Shock*. Pediatric patients who have received antivenin for previous bites have a greater risk for anaphylaxis with subsequent doses; therefore, previous administration of antivenin must be determined.

Antivenin Administration

- Ensure emergency equipment and medications to treat anaphylaxis are available.
- Assure correct antivenin is used.
  - If the snake cannot be positively identified, then polyvalent antivenin is appropriate.
  - Wound swabs as well as a urine sample can assist in the identification process with the use of a venom detection kit.
- Dosage for children and adults is the same. The amount required is the amount of antivenin necessary to relieve the presenting signs and symptoms and alleviate pain.
- Perform skin testing according to package instructions.
- The intravenous route of administration is preferred.
  - To be most effective, antivenin should be administered within 4 hours of the bite; it is less effective when given after 8 hours and may be of questionable value after 12 hours. However, it is recommended that antivenin therapy be given in severe poisonings, even if 24 hours have elapsed since the time of the bite.[23]
  - Allow the initial 5 to 10 ml to infuse over a 3- to 5-minute period, with careful observation of the patient for evidence of untoward reaction. If no symptoms or signs of an immediate systemic reaction appear, continue the infusion with delivery at the maximum safe rate for intravenous fluid administration.[23]
  - The dilution of antivenin to be used, the type of electrolyte solution used for dilution, and the rate of intravenous delivery of the diluted antivenin must take into consideration the age, weight, and cardiac status of the patient; the severity of envenomation; the total amount and type of parenteral fluids it is anticipated will be given or are needed; and the interval between bite and initiation of specific therapy.[23]
- Observe closely throughout infusion.
- Serum sickness may be prevented with a short follow-up course of oral steroids.

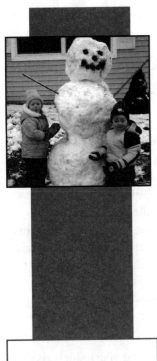

chapter 19

PSYCHIATRIC EMERGENCIES

Introduction

Psychiatric emergencies involving children and adolescents present a unique challenge to emergency department (ED) staff.[1] The primary goal for the pediatric patient brought to the ED in crisis is to keep the child safe from harm. It is important that a psychiatric consultation be obtained to make an assessment of the degree of dangerousness to self or others.

This chapter on psychiatric emergencies in pediatric patients will focus on the following.

- Suicidal behavior and ideation
- Aggressive/out-of-control behavior
- Psychosis
- Substance abuse
- Adverse psychotropic medication effects

Suicidal Behavior and Ideation

Suicidal behavior and ideation are the most frequent psychiatric emergencies for pediatric patients.[2] It is estimated that in the United States nearly 2 million adolescents attempt suicide, almost 700,000 receive medical attention for their attempt, and 2,000 adolescents commit suicide per year.[3] Overall, the most common and lethal suicide method involves the use of a firearm; however, adolescents attempt suicide most commonly with medication ingestion.[4]

Suicidal behavior and ideation must always be taken seriously, regardless of a pediatric patient's age and develop-

mental level. Pediatric patients that threaten or attempt suicide do so as a means to remove themselves from a difficult or stressful situation at home or school, to gain the love or attention of a parent, or as an act of despair in an attempt to join a significant family member who is deceased. Young children may express suicidal ideation and act in a dangerous manner that puts their safety at risk; yet developmentally they do not have a true understanding of the permanence of death.[5]

Therefore, it is important to identify those children or adolescents at greatest risk for suicidal ideation and/or behavior. These children and adolescents may present with the following.[3]

- An underlying psychiatric disorder (attention deficit hyperactivity disorder [ADHD], depression, psychosis, mania, hypomania)
- A very lethal attempt
- History of previous suicide attempts
- History of neglect and/or physical or sexual abuse
- History of drug or alcohol abuse
- Medical illness
- Exposure to family or peer suicide
- Feelings of depression and hopelessness
- Poor academic performance at school
- Parental psychopathology (depression, substance abuse)

Stressful events may precede a suicide attempt by the child or adolescent such as

- Loss of boyfriend or girlfriend
- Disciplinary action in school

- Conflicts with authorities (legal crisis)
- Family stress (illnesses or losses)

Signs and Symptoms of Depression

Table 19-1 lists signs and symptoms of depression.

Disposition of a Suicidal Pediatric Patient

The primary concern of the ED nurse is to maintain the safety of the pediatric patient. Following the assessment of the pediatric patient, a decision must be made as to whether or not the pediatric patient is safe to go home or whether psychiatric hospitalization is indicated to maintain the safety of the pediatric patient. Psychiatric hospitalization allows for additional assessment and treatment planning.

Discharge home following an assessment can be considered if the family can provide the supervision and support necessary to keep the pediatric patient safe at home and agree on a safety plan. A safety plan includes the following.

- Lock away all medications.
- Remove firearms/weapons.
- Lock away sharp objects (knives and razors).
- Develop "No Suicide" contract.
- Parent/caregiver AND pediatric patient sign safety plan contract.
- Agree to participate in outpatient appointments (provide appointment card with name, date, and time).
- Clinician witness.

An outpatient appointment should be scheduled with the family and a phone number given to a family member for emergency contact in the event the pediatric patient's safety cannot be maintained at home. Compliance with treatment depends on the development of a therapeutic alliance and relationship, and this begins with the initial session. In addition, for children and adolescents, it is important for parents to be actively involved in the therapeutic process from the beginning.

Aggressive/Out-of-Control Behavior

Pediatric patients brought to the ED for aggressive or out-of-control behavior present a frightening and overwhelming situation for all involved. Assessment of the out-of-control pediatric patient can be difficult; however, it is important to determine the reason for the aggressive/out-of-control behavior, such as whether this is an exacerbation of a chronic pattern for the pediatric patient or whether this is an acute change in behavior reflecting a psychiatric condition, physical illness, or intoxication. Listed in **Table 19-2** are potential symptoms or diagnoses that may lead to aggressive/out-of-control behavior.

Children and adolescents are at particularly high risk related to poor impulse control, poor judgment, or impaired insight.[5] Children and adolescents presenting with a developmental disability, mental retardation, or impairment in speech and/or language often communicate stress through aggressive/out-of-control behavior. Attempts should be made to understand the reason for this behavior. Precipitating events may include a change in the following areas.

- Daily routines at home or school
- Caregiver
- Medications
- Medical illness (ear infection, sinus infection, or dental caries/abscess)

Table 19-1 Signs and Symptoms of Depression

- Feeling sad or depressed most of the time
- Loss of interest or pleasure in usual activities
- Weight gain or loss
- Cannot sleep or sleeps too much
- Fatigue, loss of energy
- Feeling worthless or guilty
- Low self-esteem
- Decompensation in self-care
- Feeling hopeless about his or her future
- Cannot concentrate
- Irritable, upset by little things
- Recurring thoughts of death

Table 19-2 Symptoms or Diagnoses That May Lead to Aggressive/Out-of-Control Behavior

- Anxiety or panic attacks
- Hallucinations or paranoia
- Severe temper tantrums
- Fever, with or without electrolyte imbalance
- Seizure disorder
- Meningitis
- Encephalitis
- Brain tumor (primary or metastatic)
- Thyroid dysfunction
- Hypoxia caused by respiratory distress
- Hypo- or hyperglycemia
- Adverse reaction to medications (prescribed or over the counter)
- Overdose of medication

In addition to determining the reason for the behavior, one must obtain a history related to the aggressive/out-of-control behavior. It is imperative to determine the following.[3]

- Type of behavior exhibited (i.e., hitting, biting, spitting, throwing objects, kicking)
- Severity of behavior
- Frequency of behavior
- Targets (focused on someone or something)
- Precipitating factors (triggers)
- Destruction of property

Whatever the reason for the behavior, the priority for the ED nursing staff must be to ensure the safety of the pediatric patient and others. Initial interventions to help the pediatric patient gain control may include

- Informing the pediatric patient in a calm yet firm manner that aggressive/destructive behavior will not be tolerated
- Asking the pediatric patient to let the staff know when they feel they are losing control
- Having a caregiver or other adult remain in the exam room; the child should not be left unattended
- Providing a relatively quiet and low-stimulating exam room in the ED
- Giving one-step directions, one at a time
- Using clear verbal redirection as needed
- Recognizing and verbally praising the pediatric patient for maintaining control
- Providing support with the presence of hospital security staff
- Medication may be considered; however, a thorough medical history must be completed prior to administration
- Mechanical or physical restraint or seclusion if the pediatric patient continues to present as a danger to self and others and less restrictive interventions are not successful in helping the pediatric patient gain control of their behavior

Disposition of the Aggressive/Out-of-Control Pediatric Patient

Prior to discharge from the ED, the safety of the pediatric patient and others in the home, as well as the ability of the adults in the home to provide supervision, must be determined. Even though the behavior may resolve in the ED, a referral for outpatient treatment is made to provide more extensive follow-up care. Many pediatric patients need additional psychiatric services beyond the scope of the ED, such as individual and family therapy, anger management groups, and social skills groups.[4]

Psychiatric hospitalization must be considered if there is any concern that the pediatric patient presents a danger to self and others if discharged from the ED. The inpatient psychiatric setting provides a safe and secure environment wherein there can be further evaluation of dangerousness and initiation of treatment.

Psychosis

Children and adolescents presenting with a decompensation in behavior due to psychotic symptoms are often a danger to themselves and others and in need of emergency treatment. They may present to the ED with a history of gradual decompensation in behavior, suicidal ideation or behavior, increased agitation, aggression, or extreme anxiety.[4] In these instances the pediatric patient may exhibit characteristic signs of psychosis such as hallucinations, delusions, and unusual or bizarre behavior. In addition, they may be agitated, disorganized, and disorientated.

Physical examination, medical history, and medical workup are essential in the care of these pediatric patients in determining the reason for the psychotic symptomology. **Table 19-3** lists a number of neurologic and medical problems that may produce behavioral changes presenting as psychotic symptoms.[2,4]

Disposition of the Pediatric Patient with Psychotic Symptomology

The primary concern is the safety of the pediatric patient when considering the most appropriate treatment setting. Hospitalization is the initial treatment indicated for pediatric patients that present with the following.[2]

- Major change in behavior or personality
- Extreme distress or anxiety
- Active hallucinations (auditory, visual, or tactile)

Table 19-3 Neurological and Medical Problems That May Produce Behavior Changes

- Meningitis
- Encephalitis
- Seizures
- Brain tumors
- Subdural hematoma
- Cerebral vascular complications related to leukemia or congenital heart disease
- Hypo- or hyperglycemia
- Thyroid dysfunction
- Hypoxia related to respiratory illness
- Alcohol or drug intoxication
- Adverse medication reaction (prescription or over the counter)

Table 19-4 Physical Signs and Psychiatric Symptoms of Various Illegal Substances

Illegal Substance	Physical Signs	Psychiatric Symptoms
Amphetamines	Dilated pupils (responsive to light) Tachycardia or bradycardia Perspiration or chills Tremulousness Hyperreflexia Nausea or vomiting If severe: hypertension, hyperpyrexia, cardiac dysrhythmias	Talkativeness Restlessness Anxiety Agitation Euphoria Visual or tactile hallucinations Paranoid ideation Impaired judgment Confusion
Cannabis	Increased appetite Dry mouth Tachycardia Conjunctival injection	Impaired motor coordination Euphoria Anxiety Sensation of slowed time Impaired judgment
Cocaine	Tachycardia or bradycardia Pupillary dilation Elevated or lower blood pressure Perspiration or chills Nausea or vomiting Muscular weakness Respiratory depression Chest pain or cardiac dysrhythmias	Euphoria Confusion Hypervigilance Anxiety Tension or anger Impaired judgment
LSD (and mescaline)	Pupillary dilation Tachycardia Sweating Palpitations Blurred vision Tremors Incoordination	Apprehension Panic Perceptual distortion Depersonalization Derealization Auditory or visual hallucinations Impaired judgment
Inhalants	Dizziness Nystagmus Incoordination Slurred speech Unsteady gait Lethargy Depressed reflexes Tremor Generalized muscle weakness Blurred vision or diplopia	Euphoria Apathy Belligerence Assaultiveness Impaired judgment
PCP (and ketamine)	Pupils normal or small Nystagmus (vertical or horizontal) Muscular rigidity Grimacing Numbness or decreased perception of pain Hypertension Tachycardia Ataxia	Anxiety Euphoria Disorientation Hallucinations; suicidal behavior is not uncommon Impulsive Unpredictable Agitated Belligerent Assaultiveness

- Delusional thoughts
- Active suicidal ideation or behavior
- Extreme aggression

Inpatient psychiatric hospitalization provides a safe, secure setting that offers consistency and support for pediatric patients exhibiting psychotic characteristics.

Substance Abuse

The use of alcohol and illegal substances is occurring more frequently in children and adolescents. Oftentimes, these children and adolescents have a pre-existing psychiatric disorder.[4] The primary goal is to maintain the safety and medical stability of pediatric patients brought to the ED with acute intoxication related to substance use. Pediatric patients presenting with respiratory depression, neurologic or cardiac abnormalities, or agitation are rapidly assessed and treated.

A serum and urine toxicology screen and blood alcohol level may be helpful in determining what substance has been taken in addition to the physical exam and medical history.[2] It is important to be familiar with the physical signs and psychiatric symptoms associated with intoxication with various illegal substances.[2,6] **Table 19-4** provides an overview of various substances.

Disposition of the Pediatric Patient after Acute Intoxication

Treatment recommendations are considered once the pediatric patient is medically stable and a safe environment maintained. Recommendations may include inpatient psychiatric hospitalization, referral to a drug treatment program, or outpatient treatment.

Adverse Effects of Psychotropic Medications

Any medication can have an adverse reaction that can be a complication during treatment. Adverse reactions that need immediate medical attention include severe muscle spasms, difficulty breathing, difficulty swallowing, dysrhythmias, hyperthermia, or an abrupt change in behavior in which the pediatric patient is a danger to self or others.

Adverse effects from psychotropic medication that require immediate emergency care include lithium toxicity, extrapyramidal symptoms associated with antipsychotic medications, and bipolar switching associated with the treatment with selective serotonin reuptake inhibitors (SSRIs).

Lithium Toxicity

Serum lithium levels can markedly increase related to dehydration caused by nausea, vomiting, diarrhea, fever, exercise, hot weather, or large oral intake of salt. Concomitant use of lithium with thiazide diuretics, nonsteroidal anti-inflammatory drugs, carbamazepine, and some antibiotics may increase lithium levels.[7]

The recommended therapeutic serum level ranges from 0.6 to 1.2 mEq/L.[7] Toxic effects from lithium may be associated with therapeutic levels greater than 2.5 mEq/L.[7] Signs and symptoms of lithium toxicity are listed in **Table 19-5**.

Extrapyramidal Symptoms

Antipsychotic medications have many serious side effects, including extrapyramidal symptoms. The period of maximum risk is within hours to several days after initiation of the medication, and there may also be increased risk following increases in dosage. Symptoms may last from a few minutes to several hours, and the

Table 19-5 Signs and Symptoms of Lithium Toxicity

• Persistent vomiting or diarrhea	• Cardiac dysrhythmias
• Hypotension	• Fainting
• Staggering	• Blurred vision
• Nystagmus	• Tinnitus
• Inability to urinate	• Muscle twitches
• Hyperthermia	• Seizures
• Impaired level of consciousness	• Coma
• Death	

Table 19-6 Extrapyramidal Symptoms

Acute Dystonic Reactions	Neuroleptic Malignant Syndrome
• Muscular hypertonicity: Tonic contractions (spasms) of the neck, mouth, and tongue, which may make speaking or breathing difficult	• Life-threatening condition; can occur with a single dose but most frequently occurs within 2 weeks of initiation of antipsychotic medication or with an increase in dosage
• Oculogyric crisis: Eyes roll upward and remain in that position	• Severe muscular rigidity (hypertonicity)
• Opisthotonos: Involuntary arching of the neck and back	• Altered consciousness
	• Stupor
• Dysphagia	• Catatonia
• Laryngeal spasm	• Hyperthermia
	• Labile pulse and blood pressure
	• Incontinence
	• Pulmonary congestion

experience may be painful and frightening, particularly if the pediatric patient does not understand what is happening. Extrapyramidal symptoms are outlined in **Table 19-6**.

Bipolar Switching (Manic Reaction)

This adverse reaction includes a notable change in the pediatric patient's mood, behavior, level of activity, and impulsivity.[8] Parents will frequently present to the ED reporting that the child has never behaved in this manner and presents a danger to self or others. A manic reaction is characterized by the following symptoms.[7]

- Distinctly elevated mood, euphoria
- Grandiose behaviors
- Decreased need for sleep
- More talkative than usual or pressured speech
- Flight of ideas or feeling that thoughts are racing
- Highly distractible
- Increase in impulsivity
- Increase in psychomotor agitation

A manic reaction can occur after the pediatric patient has been on a SSRI for a period of time and has been experiencing clinical benefit.[8] Discontinuation of the medication does not ensure that the manic reaction will resolve without the use of additional medications such as mood stabilizers.[8]

Disposition of a Pediatric Patient Experiencing an Adverse Effect from a Psychotropic Medication

It is important for the ED nurse to remain with the pediatric patient and their family members to explain what is happening and to maintain a safe environment for the pediatric patient. Pediatric patients presenting to the ED experiencing an adverse medication reaction require a physical examination and may need a neurologic evaluation. In addition, laboratory tests may be indicated based on the pediatric patient's medical history and clinical findings from the physical examination.

Summary

The primary goal for the pediatric patient presenting to the ED with a psychiatric emergency is safety. The interventions that ensure a pediatric patient's safety include but are not limited to the following.

- Provide a safe environment; remove potentially unsafe objects from the treatment room to prevent harm to self and others.
- Create a calm environment by minimizing unnecessary noise and clutter.
- Maintain a calm presence.
- Use clear, direct verbal communication rather than unclear or nonverbal gestures.
- Speak slowly and clearly; avoid multiple directions and give one-step directions one at a time.
- Use verbal praise when the pediatric patient is able to follow directions.
- Explain safety precautions to family members and ED staff.

The focus of care in any psychiatric emergency in the pediatric population is maintaining the safety of the patient and those around him or her. Family members and ED staff are keys to the successful outcome of any treatment plan.

References

1. Falsafi, N. (2001). Pediatric psychiatric emergencies. *Journal of Child and Adolescent Psychiatric Nursing, 14*(2), 81–88.

2. Robinson, J. (1986). Emergencies I. In K. S. Robson (Ed.), *Manual of clinical child psychiatry* (pp. 185–211). Washington, DC: American Psychiatric Press.

3. American Academy of Child and Adolescent Psychiatry. (2001). Practice parameter for the assessment and treatment of children and adolescents with suicidal behavior. *Journal of the American Academy of Child and Adolescent Psychiatry, 40*(7 Suppl), 24S–28S.

4. Halamandaris, P. V., & Anderson, T. R. (1999). Children and adolescents in the psychiatric emergency setting. *Psychiatric Clinics of North America, 22*(4), 865–874.

5. King, R. A. (1997). Practice parameters for the psychiatric assessment of children and adolescents. *Journal of the American Academy of Child and Adolescent Psychiatry, 36*(10 Suppl), 4S–20S.

6. American Psychiatric Association. (1994). *Diagnostic and Statistical Manual of Mental Disorders (DSM-IV)* (4th ed.). Washington, DC: Author.

7. McClellan, J., & Werry, J. (2001). Practice parameters for the assessment and treatment of children and adolescents with bipolar disorder. *Journal of the American Academy of Child and Adolescent Psychiatry, 36*(10 Suppl), 157S–176S.

8. Walkup, J., & Labellarte, M. (2001). Complications of SSRI treatment. *Journal of Child and Adolescent Psychopharmacology, 11*(1), 1–4.

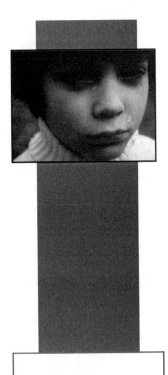

chapter 20

CRISIS INTERVENTION

Objectives

On completion of this chapter, the learner should be able to:

1. Identify factors likely to precipitate, exacerbate, and mitigate the severity of traumatic response in the pediatric patient.

2. Identify somatic signs and symptoms related to traumatic response.

3. Plan appropriate interventions for the traumatized pediatric patient for each stage of traumatic response and special situations.

4. Identify prevention strategies for vicarious traumatization.

Introduction

Illness and injury are always stressful for children and families and may precipitate crises in coping or functioning for the pediatric patient or family. Children may become ill or injured during the experience of trauma. Events that may provoke a psychological traumatic response include severe motor vehicle crashes (MVCs), natural disasters (i.e., tornados, floods), man-made disasters (i.e., explosions, war), community violence, and child abuse. The experience of traumatic stress or trauma is distinct from the experience of stress and is associated with long-term adverse consequences and with neurobiological changes. Adults may not realize the extent to which children are distressed and may underestimate their problems.

Definitions

Trauma has been referred to as "a jarring awareness of the fact of death."[1] Events universally considered traumatic have the following characteristics.

- Come from outside the person
- Pose a threat to existence
- Disrupt integrity and function
- Are outside the range of usual experience
- Overwhelm usual coping and adaptation strategies

The experience of trauma can be divided into phases that may be associated with different types of reactions, including[2]

- Preimpact—the period before the event
- Impact—when the event occurs
- Recoil—immediately after the event

- Postimpact—days to weeks after the event
- Recovery and reconstruction—months or years after the event

Identification of Traumatized Pediatric Patients

Most health care providers will interact with the pediatric patient during the recoil and postimpact period. What is done or said during that time influences the trajectory of recovery. Emergency medical treatment itself is stressful, and nurses may inaccurately presume that the pediatric patient's emotions and behaviors are due to the health care environment. In the emergency department (ED), formal mental health assessment for victims of trauma is neither practical nor necessary as a precursor to intervention. The extent to which the experience of a traumatic event has detrimental impact on the pediatric patient's well-being has consistently been found to be related to event characteristics, preexisting characteristics of the pediatric patient, and the experiences of the pediatric patient in the immediate postevent period.[3] All pediatric patients who might conceivably be experiencing trauma based on history should be treated as such.

Event Characteristics

It is particularly important to evaluate and intervene for a traumatic response when a pediatric patient has been exposed to an event in which any of the following has occurred.

- There is perception of, potential for, or actual life threat. Pediatric patients may also perceive a life threat when it did not exist.

- Death of others known to the pediatric patient occurred during the event. Grief dramatically worsens a traumatic response.
- The pediatric patient was in close proximity to the event (i.e., observed or was a victim).
- The pediatric patient had prolonged duration and intensity of exposure to event, such as prolonged extrication from a motor vehicle, prolonged pain associated with the traumatic event, or multiple exposures to traumatic events.
- Significant disruption of "normal" was caused by the event. The pediatric patient is maimed, grieving, or displaced from home or community as a result of the event.

Preexisting Characteristics

The following child and family characteristics have been found to be associated with vulnerability to long-term detrimental impact of trauma.

- Prior exposure to community violence
- Preexisting symptoms of anxiety
- Academic and attention problems
- Unstable or limited social support from significant others
- Parents with poor psychosocial functioning or impaired coping

Experiences of the Pediatric Patient in the Immediate Postevent Period

Factors that increase distress and decrease adaptive coping include

- Severe untreated pain
- Ongoing exposure to stimuli linked to the trauma (i.e., images, sounds, smells, objects, conversations)
- Lack of age-appropriate information and reassurance
- Inadequate social support

Medical and Emotional Consequences of the Experience of Trauma for the Pediatric Patient

Exposure to trauma may affect the pediatric patient's perception of, communication about, and coping with bodily sensations including pain. Immediate and long-term consequences of trauma include the development of acute stress and posttraumatic stress disorders. These problems involve distress and profound disruptions of the pediatric patient's physiological response to situations and reactions to people.

Although caring for the physiologic needs of the ill or injured child is the primary focus of the emergency care team, attention to the trauma-related emotional needs of the pediatric patient is also important. Emergency medical care teams can reasonably expect to be able to affect the pediatric patient's response by

- Minimizing exposure to trauma-related stimuli (including pain)
- Providing support and reassurance about safety
- Helping the pediatric patient access other sources of support and comfort

Initial Approach to Care of the Traumatized Pediatric Patient and Family During Recoil Period

As with all psychosocial interventions there are multiple ways to impact distress in a pediatric patient or family. The following guiding principles should be kept in mind while interacting with the pediatric patient exposed to a traumatic event.

- The experience of trauma and the awareness of threat to life. Not all pediatric patients will perceive a threat to life accurately. Communication about the event should flow from the pediatric patient's understanding, with efforts made to answer questions accurately without unnecessarily frightening the pediatric patient. It is never necessary to help the pediatric patient understand the horror of an event if the pediatric patient is not displaying symptoms of trauma. Pediatric patients may perceive medical intervention as life threatening if they do not understand what is occurring.
- Individual responses to trauma. Intense fear, helplessness, and horror are universal responses to trauma. For some pediatric patients and adults, a period of blunted response (numbing) may occur. This may be adaptive if it helps the individual function to escape danger or cope with overwhelming physical or emotional pain. Prolonged numbing signals profound distress. It is important to distinguish between active and useful coping and blunted response. The pediatric patient's pretrauma emotional style (i.e., expression or withdrawal) will influence their response to trauma.
- Developmental considerations. It is common for pediatric patients to show regressive behavior when distressed. Regression may include speaking, behaving, or coping like a much younger child. Loss of bladder control may occur. Adolescents also may show regressive behavior. Separation worries are normal. Communication to the pediatric patient should be in the simplest, most concrete language possible, regardless of age. Prolonged and severe regression reflects profound distress and failure of coping, which may require clinical attention.

- Even though infants and very young children may not understand what has occurred, they may experience long-term consequences of exposure to trauma. Infants and children respond to chaos and noise around them by becoming hypervigilant or withdrawn. Shielding them from overstimulation, giving a reassuring touch, and providing familiar distractions are useful interventions. Infants and young children are highly responsive to caregiver emotions. Attention to the state of the parent is an intervention for the child. Signs of pain should not be overlooked especially when the child appears withdrawn.

- For school-age children, the focus should be on safety and concrete images and actions that occurred during the event. Statements that address the specific things they saw and heard comfort them. Children use play to deal with distress, and opportunities for this should be provided if possible. Children may become agitated (misbehave) or withdrawn. Evaluation of the child should include questions such as "Are you afraid?" and "What questions do you have about what happened?"

- Adolescents grasp the horror of what has occurred but may lack life skills and perspective to mobilize adaptive coping. Regression, or pseudoadult behavior, may occur in response to distress. Adolescents benefit from clear, honest information and support from adults and peers who shared the experience. Adolescents previously traumatized may have engaged in risk-taking behavior that resulted in further exposure to trauma. Adults may hold unhelpful presumptions about the adolescents' own responsibility for the traumatic event (e.g., rape, assault, MVC) that interfere with assessment of traumatic response. Evaluation of adolescents should include questions such as "How are you feeling about what happened?" "What do you think will happen after you leave the hospital?" and "Do you worry about what is going to happen to you in the future?"

• Somatic manifestations of trauma response. The experience of trauma triggers predictable changes in the body that are associated with the stress response. In the immediate posttrauma period, pediatric patients will show evidence of current or recent sympathetic nervous system responses such as tachycardia, sweaty palms, dry mouth, and hyperventilation. Pediatric patients experiencing flashbacks of the trauma (intrusive reexperiencing) may report physical signs and symptoms that they experienced during the event. These are experienced as real and are not hallucinations. The pediatric patient may be experiencing a physical sensation (e.g., pain) that triggered the flashback. Helpful interventions during flashbacks focus the pediatric patient on the reality and safety of their body and environment and address autonomic arousal. Hypervigilance and continuous autonomic arousal that are associated with trauma may cause gastrointestinal discomfort, hypersensitivity to pain, sleep disruption, and changes in breathing. Distractions and relaxation techniques are extremely useful in decreasing autonomic arousal and distress. Pediatric patients who are still "in shock" or "numb" may still be able to follow instructions for deep breathing. Even pediatric patients who are unable to verbally respond due to their medical condition (e.g., intubation) benefit from brief coaching in relaxation and visualization techniques (see Chapter 12, *Pediatric Pain Assessment and Management*).

• Family and cultural considerations. Cultures and communities differ in the types of behaviors and expressions of emotion that are considered acceptable. In the aftermath of trauma, the support and acceptance of the family and community are more essential to healing than abstract conceptualizations of "proper" or "healthy" behaviors as judged by the health care team. Health care providers should be aware of the variety of cultural traditions for the expression of fear and horror. In many cultures, emotional distress may be communicated through culture-specific physical symptoms. Refugees and displaced individuals are at higher risk for traumatic response due to prior traumatization.[4] Pediatric patients' exposure to very frightening or uncontrolled emotional responses (especially from significant adults) in the immediate posttrauma period should be limited. These behaviors rarely, if ever, reflect essential cultural or community traditions, and exposure causes unhelpful autonomic arousal in the pediatric patient. Interventions and support for severely distressed family members improves outcomes for the pediatric patient. Families should be told about the importance of calmness and reassurance in helping the pediatric patient recover. The following statement is an example of what to communicate to family members. "We will help you and your child through this. Your child needs you to stay calm when you are with him. We know this is hard but it is VERY important so that your child can get better faster. Saying things like 'It will be OK' and 'The doctors and nurses can help you feel better' will help your child a lot." Tell all family members about the importance of calmness. Encourage family self-care so that exhaustion and hunger do not cause unnecessary declines in coping. Monitor the family closely and offer concrete suggestions such as "Go in the hallway to calm down if you feel too upset" or

"Take three deep breaths before speaking to your child."

Interventions During the Recoil Phase

The longer and more intensely the pediatric patient and family are exposed to the event, the greater the likelihood of developing significant posttraumatic emotional impairment. Emergency personnel can help the pediatric patient when they limit exposure to trauma-related stimuli, communicate information and reassurance, and provide a comforting environment.[3]

- Remove the pediatric patient from exposure to sights, sounds, smells, and sensations related to the trauma as soon as safely possible. The more sensory associations that the pediatric patient has to the event during the acute fear response and immediate aftermath (impact and recoil), the more likely it is to have a lasting impact.

- Sedate/distract/provide pain control. Provide the pediatric patient with all possible measures for minimizing physical discomfort, pain, and fear. Untreated pain is a potent psychological and physiological stress on the pediatric patient that interferes with recovery.

- Provide the pediatric patient with a comforting environment. Make familiar social supports available to the pediatric patient as soon as possible. If family members are critically injured but able to communicate, that should be facilitated. If parents are unable to provide even minimal reassurance due to their own distress or injury, other familiar people should be sought. Encourage use of comfort items such as a piece of clothing from a parent or a stuffed animal.

- Reassure/explain in terms the pediatric patient will understand. The focus of communication must be on the pediatric patient's need to regain a sense of safety, control, and predictability. Helpful communications include the following.
  - Realistic reassurances about the safety of the pediatric patient and their loved ones
  - Simple and honest explanations of what the pediatric patient has experienced or is experiencing
  - Preparation for what they will experience
  - Frequent messages about safety and support

- Family intervention. Providing appropriate support to the families of the traumatized pediatric patient is an intervention that will help the pediatric patient. In all cases, parents should be given information about how to help their child. Express confidence that the parent will be able to successfully do the following to help the child.
  - Provide reassurance about safety.
  - Answer questions honestly without providing extra information.
  - Acknowledge the fear and difficulty in coping that they are experiencing but express hope and a belief it will get easier.
  - Take time out for self-care.
  - Provide reassuring physical contact.

The Family in Crisis

Crisis is a state of disequilibrium that occurs when usual coping strategies are inadequate to the demands of the situation. Emotional response, problem solving, and decision making are all affected by crisis. Individuals in crisis have a wide range of responses, including

- Demanding, loud behavior or hostility
- Physical displays of anger
- Loud crying
- Withdrawal
- Blaming
- Forgetfulness
- Grief
- Agitation

Exposure to these emotional displays and behaviors are unhelpful to the traumatized pediatric patient. If a pediatric patient's support persons are in active crisis, they require intervention to regain a sense of control so that they can help the pediatric patient. Minimizing the pediatric patient's exposure to agitated worrisome adult behavior is important. Families can benefit from psychological first aid, which includes

- Direct assistance for problem solving and practical needs (i.e., housing, food)
- Assistance in evaluating information and developing a plan for the immediate future
- Activation of social support and community resources
- Factual information about the event and typical reactions of adults and children who have experienced similar circumstances

The Family Experiencing Grief from the Death of a Child

The sudden death of a child is among the most profoundly traumatic events a family can experience. Like other traumatic exposures the ability to resolve grief is affected by what families experience in the recoil phase. When a child has died or death is imminent, the family, including surviving siblings, benefit from the following.

- Timely, accurate, and clear information. Explain to the family the medical status of their child and what to expect, what they will see, hear, and smell when in the resuscitation room. Use concrete words such as *dead* and *dying* rather than *passed away* or *expired*. Children should be provided with information in developmentally appropriate but accurate language.

- The time and space to say good-bye. Facilitate family presence in the resuscitation area while the child is alive if at all possible. Provide family members the opportunity to view, hold, and touch the child. Explain the nature of what they will see regarding the child's present condition. If there are jurisdictional requirements to leave in tubes and lines, review this with the family. Facilitate baptism or other religious rites if the parents request them. Families differ in how much time they need, and space outside the ED may need to be arranged. A family member as well as a staff member should be present with the sibling who is saying good-bye.

- Validation and support during a time of overwhelming feelings. Avoid statements minimizing or negating thoughts or feelings. For example, do not say things such as "It's all for the best" or "She is your little angel." Let your concern and caring show by saying "I'm sorry." Provide support and decision-making assistance with issues such as organ donation, autopsy, and disposition of the body. Help the family contact other family members and community resources. Mobilize hospital resources such as pastoral care and social work if available.

- Support after leaving the hospital. Provide families with contact numbers for questions about the child's death. Provide written bereavement information including community resources for themselves and surviving siblings. These should also be provided to family support persons because parents may understandably not be processing the information provided. Provide bereavement follow-up over the next weeks or months through phone calls or written communication if possible. Encourage families to include children in family rituals related to death and to avoid hiding their own grief with the mistaken belief that this will "protect" the siblings from pain.

- Additional interventions in support of surviving siblings. Reassure siblings that the adults are not mad at them but are sad and may be acting in a confusing manner because of the death. Reassure them that the death was not the result of anything they said, did, or thought. Support age-appropriate responses to death, which may include playing, talking openly about the deceased, and not crying. Let families know that this is to be expected and does not mean that the child is not sad.

Care of the Pediatric Patient and Family During the Postimpact Period

Children, like adults, attempt to gain mastery over their thoughts and feelings. This begins to occur in the hours and days after trauma. Pediatric patients who appear to be coping well initially may have a different reaction later after the initial shock has subsided. There is no one "right way" to respond to a traumatic exposure. Recovery takes place over a long period of time and involves making meaning of the event, reestablishment of function, and reconnecting to or building community and personal resources.

Children differ in how they move through initial shock to disorganized coping to stabilization of coping. As soon as possible, and when developmentally appropriate, children should be offered the following options for increasing their coping capacity.

Intervention Strategies

- Choices should be offered whenever practical and possible to increase feelings of control. Nonchoices should be explained directly and nonapologetically.

- Children should be encouraged to engage in normalizing activities. For young children this includes playing, drawing, and imaginary play.

- When it is safe to do so, children are reassured by engaging in normal physical activity. This is also an adaptive way of dealing with tension.

- After the initial shock of the event, children may begin to have more questions or may express misperceptions. Communicate accurate information without frightening elaboration. Older children attempt to understand the larger picture of what has occurred. Children should be shielded from repeated and frightening media portrayals of the event. Adult conversations about what occurred should be done out of the child's earshot because children may misunderstand what is said and become unnecessarily alarmed.

  - Key points to communicate include
    - "It is normal to feel confused, scared, angry, and worried."
    - "It can be good to talk about it even though it is upsetting."
    - "Some parts might be confusing, and there may be more information you need to understand what happened and feel safe."
    - "What happened is upsetting to adults, too. They can still help you."

Discharge Issues

Discharge from emergency or hospital care may herald the beginning of recovery from the trauma or may provoke dormant fears and worries. Children whose homes, families, or bodies have been maimed will confront particularly difficult challenges. Pediatric patients and families should be provided with instructions that include the possibility that the pediatric patient may have a delayed response to the event. They can be reassured that this can be a normal part of healing and that resources for coping are available. Specific community and health system resources should be provided. It is important to reiterate the "normalness" of distress following trauma and the importance of emotional care within the family and community. Care should be taken to avoid labeling a traumatic response as a "mental illness" because such a stigma may lead some families to avoid needed support.

Special Situations

Children Traumatized During the Course of a Crime

Children who are victims of or witnesses to crimes not only become fearful due to the event but are also thrust into the confusing arena of the criminal justice system. Even young children can be reliable eyewitnesses, and their account may be important to the investigation. When children are victims or witnesses to crimes, it is most often in their homes and communities by people they know. Children may have close, dependent, and/or fearful relationships with the perpetrators of the crime. Some children have been told that they, or those they love, will be harmed if they tell someone about the crime. Emergency medical providers can assist the child and the needs of justice by staying aware of the multiple and conflicting demands on the child in the aftermath of a crime.

In addition to providing trauma interventions, the nurse must protect the pediatric patient's privacy and safety during a time when many people have an interest in knowing what the pediatric patient has seen.

- Ensure that the pediatric patient is cared for in a protected location.
- Evaluate pediatric victims or witnesses out of eyesight or earshot of perpetrators or other witnesses to the crime.
- Avoid asking unnecessary leading questions of the pediatric patient, and prevent other health care staff from doing so.

- Document direct statements made by the pediatric patient related to the crime. Document any attempts by others to influence the child's account.
- Ensure that a neutral adult is present with the pediatric patient at all times during the immediate posttraumatic period, especially prior to arrival of law enforcement personnel.
- Communicate confidence in the pediatric patients' ability to describe what they saw.
- Do not label the perpetrator as a "monster" or a "bad person" to the child.
- Consider all aspects of medical care as having possible forensic value. Follow appropriate chain-of-custody evidence procedures.
- Direct media away from the child.

The Abused Child

The abused child is a crime victim. Intentional assault of a child is among the most emotionally difficult situations that the nurse encounters. Many hospitals and communities have protocols that enhance protection and justice for the child that guide what the nurse should do and say. These protocols outline by who and when the child will be interviewed and the type of medical forensic information that should be gathered. In all cases, high-quality photographs and detailed documentation of injuries using a body chart can be invaluable in documenting the crime and ultimately protecting the child from further harm (see Chapter 13, *Child Maltreatment*, for more details). Children may have disturbing responses to and disclose disturbing information during the exam. Statements and reactions should be recorded verbatim and behaviors specifically described.

Large-Scale Tragedy of Human Design

These types of events include acts of war, terrorist attacks, sniper attacks, bombings, arson, and public transportation crashes (i.e., airplanes, trains, boats). Everyday places and situations such as schools, gas stations, and markets may become feared because of the seeming randomness and unpredictability of harm. Even if the child was not directly injured, the sounds, images, and the sense of danger in the community may provoke a traumatic response. Like victims of crimes, the experience of a traumatic event that was under the control of an individual or group of people shakes a child's trust in adults. Children may question whether parents or other trusted adults are safe and can protect them. Older children may ask "why" questions that do not have simple or knowable answers. Often "why" questions are really "will this happen again" questions.

Adults need to reassure children to the extent possible using specific examples of what is being done to protect them and to prevent the event from happening again.

Adults, including health care staff, are also profoundly affected by these same events and may have the same questions and fears as the child. In these types of situations, it is particularly important that adults take time to reassure themselves and decide on an honest and hopeful response to the child. Saying, "I don't know right now but I will let you know when I find out" is better than a reactive dishonest or anxiety-provoking response. Acute separation anxiety may be particularly prominent if there was mass confusion and separation of the child from the caregiver during the event.

Given the unpredictability and randomness of this type of trauma, the following types of messages and interventions are particularly helpful to children who are experiencing a traumatic response to a large-scale tragedy of human design.

- Provide reassurance that the child is safe and when possible that the people in charge are doing everything possible to keep or make things safe.
- Identify people that the child can talk to about worries.
- Encourage child to "face fears" in a gradual, safe, and protected way.
- Reward the child for facing fears.
- Develop a plan of action or alternative activities the child can do when worried or afraid.

Natural Disasters

Natural disasters affect all regions of the world, causing economic loss and disruption of education, government, and business. In addition to the risks or reality of injury and death, this disruption of the social fabric leads to higher risk for psychological distress. The sudden, unpredictable, and devastating nature of earthquakes, hurricanes, fires, floods, and tornados challenges the emotional resources of even the most stable adults, including health care teams. Reassurance of personal safety and immediate linkage to community-based social service resources is of paramount importance. Community-focused interventions including small-group activities for children and adults have been linked to better outcome. Regular (two times per week) massage of children in the month after a disaster has been found to diminish anxiety and depression in severely affected children.[5] As affected members of the community, personal self-care for the health care team in the aftermath of the disaster may be very challenging but necessary to sustain the long-term effort needed to restore the social fabric.

Vicarious Traumatization of the Health Care Team

Health care providers for children witness the worst of the world—the harm caused to children by people and fate. They take care of and bear witness to that which could have been prevented and that which should never happen to children. Professionals respond to constant exposure to unbearable and unspeakable tragedies in identifiable ways. Like the patients for whom they care, professionals benefit from simple environmental interventions to decrease the impact of exposure to traumatic stress in the workplace.

A critical incident is a traumatic event of sufficient magnitude to overwhelm the usually effective coping skills of health care or emergency services personnel. Critical incidents are typically sudden, powerful events that fit outside the range of normal human experience.

Reactions to these incidents may include temporary manifestations of the cognitive, physical, emotional, and behavioral signs and symptoms of trauma. Critical incident stress debriefing (CISD) is a structured intervention for professionals that is used in some settings. There is disagreement as to whether the use of CISD is helpful for all people or whether it can make symptoms worse. Important aspects of CISD that parallel the approach to the traumatized pediatric patient include access to accurate information, social support, and reassurance of personal safety and control. Some professionals prefer to get this needed support from colleagues and community rather than from a specific intervention sequence.[6]

Repeated exposure to critical incidents over time can contribute to the phenomenon of vicarious traumatization.[7] The concept of vicarious traumatization can help explain how dramatic and/or cumulative exposure to the trauma of patients can negatively affect nurses. Vicarious traumatization is a transformation that occurs within the trauma worker as a result of their empathetic engagement with the patient who has experienced trauma.

Vicarious traumatization leads to changes in cognitive and emotional functioning that affect both personal well-being and the quality of nursing care. It is associated with "burnout," substance misuse, health problems related to stress and poor sleep, and family problems. Nurses may experience flashbacks of patient care episodes or vivid images of scenes described to them. More subtle signs include a gradual numbing of emotional responses and a pervasive cynical attitude towards others.

Key Points Regarding Vicarious Traumatization[8]

- Accumulates over time and across patients
- Is different from effect of emergency nursing in general
- Can produce symptoms of posttraumatic stress such as generalized anxiety and/or irrational fears; numbing or dissociative reactions; feelings of being overwhelmed; intrusive thoughts, images, and/or nightmares; anger and poor coping; and sleep disturbances
- Can produce changes in view of self and the world, including loss of sense of safety or control, loss of trust, loss of connection with others, despair and/or cynicism, disillusionment, reduced capacity for intimacy, and poor self-image
- Is affected by situational factors such as working in isolation; lack of recognition of the real impact of trauma work, workplaces that inadequately provide for or discourage appropriate self-care, and unhelpful support systems
- Impacts the workplace environment by increasing negativity, blaming, victimhood, and turnover

Table 20-1 lists strategies for combating vicarious traumatization.[7]

Table 20-1 Strategies to Combat Vicarious Traumatization

Workplace Strategies	• Recognize vicarious traumatization as an occupational hazard of trauma work • Accept your reactions as normal responses to specialized work • Limit exposure to trauma material (e.g., books, conferences, discussions, movies) • Develop a supportive environment for discussing own reactions to work • Balance your workload as to types of patient care • Have a basic plan for care of yourself and family during a community trauma • Build a network of professional connections • Develop a balance of professional skills (e.g., trauma & nontrauma work) • Work within a supportive organizational context
Essential Personal Strategies	• Take time to laugh, have fun, socialize with coworkers (but not about work) • Seek spiritual renewal in your life however you define that • Emphasize self-care & self-nurturing activities • Take sabbaticals from trauma work • Take mental health breaks purposefully • Guard against addictive behaviors • Be rested, be fit, eat well • Seek out experiences that instill comfort & hope • Set clear boundaries between home & work. Use clothing or other rituals to mark change from work to leisure.

Reprinted with permission from McCann, I., & Pearlman, L. (1990). Vicarious traumatization: A framework for understanding the psychological effects of working with victims. *Journal of Traumatic Stress, 3*(1), 131–149.

Summary

The extent to which the experience of trauma has a detrimental impact on the child's well-being has been found to be related to preincident characteristics of the child, the quality of the response of the child's primary caregivers, the characteristics of the traumatic event, and the experiences of the child in the immediate postevent period. Although caring for the physiologic needs of the ill or injured child is the primary focus of the emergency care team, attention to the trauma-related emotional needs of the child and family may mitigate long-term traumatic responses. The principles of care for the person experiencing trauma include management of exposure, management of meaning, and control and management of comfort. Emergency medical care teams can reasonably expect to be able to affect the child's response by minimizing exposure to trauma-related stimuli (including pain), providing age-appropriate support and reassurance about safety, and helping the child access other sources of support and comfort. The health care team may also experience vicarious traumatization when caring for trauma victims, and this posttraumatic response must be addressed with strategies to mitigate its detrimental impact on work life and personal well-being.

References

1. Janoff-Bulman, R. (1992). *Shattered assumptions: Towards a new psychology of trauma.* New York: Basic Books.

2. Valent, P. (2000). Disaster syndrome. In G. Fink (Ed.), *Encyclopedia of stress* (Vol. 1) (pp. 706–709). San Diego, CA: Academic Press.

3. La Greca, A., Silverman, W., Vernberg, E., & Roberts, M. (Eds.). (2002). *Helping children cope with disasters and terrorism.* Washington, DC: American Psychological Association.

4. Marsella, A., Bornemann, T., Ekblad, S., & Orley, J. (1994). *Amidst pain and peril: The mental health and well-being of the world's refugees.* Washington, DC: American Psychological Association.

5. Field, T., Seligman, S., Scafidi, F., & Schanberg, S. (1996). Alleviating post traumatic stress in children following Hurricane Andrew. *Journal of Applied Developmental Psychology, 17,* 37–50.

6. Kenardy, J. A., & Carr, V. (1996). Imbalance in the debriefing debate: What we don't know far outweighs what we do. *The Bulletin of the Australian Psychological Society, 18*(1), 4–6.

7. McCann, I., & Pearlman, L. (1990). Vicarious traumatization: A framework for understanding the psychological effects of working with victims. *Journal of Traumatic Stress, 3*(1), 131–49.

8. Clements, K., Robinson, R., & Panteluk, L. (1998). *Annotated bibliography on vicarious traumatization and forms of traumatic stress in the workplace of psychiatric nurses.* RPNAM 2nd Annual Poster Session Competition, Selkirk, Manitoba, Canada.

Internet Resources

Comprehensive site for trauma-related information:
www.trauma-pages.com/pg5.htm

American Psychological Association:
http://helping.apa.org/therapy/traumaticstress.html

American Academy of Pediatrics:
www.aap.org/terrorism/index.html

Center for Mental Health Services:
www.mentalhealth.org/schoolviolence/parents.htm

National Association of School Psychologists:
www.nasponline.org/NEAT/crisis0911.html.

National Institute of Mental Health Web site:
www.nimh.nih.gov/publicat/violence.cfm.

Vicarious traumatization and nursing information:
http://www.psychiatricnurse.mb.ca/vt.html

Printable self-help workbooks for children and families:
www.7-dippity.com/other/op_freedownloads.html

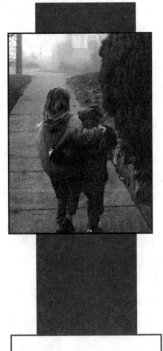

chapter 21

STABILIZATION AND TRANSPORT (OPTIONAL)

Introduction

Competent care of pediatric patients requires specialized skills, equipment, and personnel. If these components of care are unavailable, the pediatric patient must be transferred to a facility specializing in the care of children. Indications for transport include the need for pediatric expertise, the need for a diagnostic procedure, potential for deterioration because of the pediatric patient's illness or injury, and a request for transfer.[1] Although optional, this chapter will cover risks, benefits, and legalities of the transfer and transportation processes.

Rules and Regulations

Consolidated Omnibus Budget Reconciliation Act (COBRA)

Prior to 1986, there were many accounts of emergency departments (EDs) refusing to care for indigent patients.[2] In 1986, COBRA, which addresses issues related to transfer and refusal of treatment, was passed.[2] Since then there have been several additions and modifications of the COBRA provisions. General provisions include the following.[2]

- COBRA covers any individual who comes to an ED that participates in Medicare for examination of a medical condition. The hospital is obligated to provide a medical screening examination. If the patient has an emergency medical condition, the hospital must provide one of the following.

- Stabilization of a patient within the skill and capability of the hospital resources.
- Transfer of the patient to another medical facility with additional care resources. The patient cannot be transferred unless the patient or his or her guardian requests the change. A physician must sign a certificate that the medical benefits of the transfer outweigh the risks of the transfer to the patient (must have evidence that the patient received and understood the risks and benefits associated with the transfer).

- In 1994, one section of the COBRA legislation, the Emergency Medical Treatment and Active Labor Act (EMTALA), was further clarified to state that there are two circumstances when the unstable patient may be transferred:[3] (1) the patient or their family requests transfer or (2) the physician or referring personnel determine that the benefits of transfer outweigh the risks of not transferring the child.

Indications for Transport

When determining whether transfer of a pediatric patient is necessary, the following questions are essential to answer.

- Do we have the necessary resources to care for this pediatric patient?
  - Physician and/or specialist skill level
  - Nursing resource and skill level
  - Ancillary staff resources, such as radiology, respiratory therapy, physical therapy, nutrition

Objectives

On completion of this chapter, the learner should be able to:

1. Recognize indications in the pediatric patient that require transportation to a tertiary facility.
2. Identify the risks involved with transporting the pediatric patient.
3. Recognize the needed qualifications of the transporting personnel and the mode of transportation.

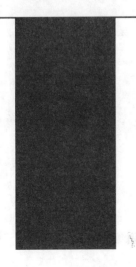

- Appropriately sized equipment—from ultrasound machines to routine supplies
- Is this pediatric patient likely to deteriorate and require emergency transport?

If the necessary resources are not available or the pediatric patient is likely to deteriorate and require emergent transport, then the child must be transferred to an appropriate facility.

Transfer Requirements

Once the decision to transfer has been made and the provisions regarding consent have been met, additional transfer requirements must also be met. These include the following.

- A physician at the receiving hospital must agree to accept the patient.
- The receiving facility must have adequate space and personnel to care for the individual.
- Medical records related to the emergency medical condition must accompany the pediatric patient to the receiving facility.
- The transfer must utilize qualified personnel and adequate equipment, as determined by the sending physician.

The following additional questions need to be addressed.

- What are the established transfer agreements?
- What is the training of the staff transporting the pediatric patient?
- What is the capability of the mode of transportation?
- Is this a medical or trauma transport?
- What is the weather like? Road conditions? Either of these can impact the choice of transport.

Table 21-1 provides comparisons between types of transport personnel and modes of transport.

Table 21-1 Comparison of Types of Personnel and Modes of Transport

Personnel	Advantage	Disadvantage
Local EMS	Readily available	Limited training experience with pediatrics
BLS crew	Direct transport to another facility	Minimal medical care capabilities; basic measures only
ALS crew	Direct transport to another facility	Increased medical training; limited pediatric expertise; limited resources
Critical care crew —adult	Critical care experience	Limited or no pediatric experience; usually trained by a pediatric team
Pediatric critical care team	Pediatric intensive care experience, initiate pediatric critical care while en route	May not be readily available; may take one hour to get to transferring facility

Mode of Transport	Advantage	Disadvantage
Ground Transport	• Availability • Space in the vehicle • Can travel in any weather conditions • Ability to carry several prehospital personnel • Ability to carry more equipment • Family may accompany child in vehicle	• Transport can take up to three times longer by ground than by air • Traffic and road conditions can interfere with transport • Loss of vehicle to the community
Air Transport	• Saves time • Improved communication ability • Heightened emergency response at receiving facility because of experience with helicopter transport patients • Continued availability of ground emergency medical services resources within the referral area	• Weather restrictions • Lack of availability • Cost • Physiologic impact • Noise • Vibrations • Temperature changes • Gas expansion with altitude • Fear of flying • Space and weight restrictions

Stabilization Prior to Transfer

Stabilization of the pediatric patient prior to transfer involves meeting the immediate needs and anticipating any change of condition that may occur during transport. The priorities of stabilization are described in **Table 21-2**.

Table 21-2 Priorities of Stabilization

Airway	• Maintain a patent airway.
	• Maintain stabilization of the cervical spine if trauma is suspected.
	• Continue the delivery of supplemental oxygen, as indicated.
	• If the pediatric patient is intubated, reconfirm endotracheal tube placement each time the patient is moved and ensure the following documentation is completed.
	- Time of intubation
	- Endotracheal tube size, cuffed versus uncuffed
	- Depth of endotracheal tube placement (location of tube at lip, teeth, or gum line)
	- Medications administered for intubation procedure and continued sedation
	- Provide copy of chest radiograph verifying tube placement
	• Insert gastric tube to decompress stomach if the pediatric patient is intubated.
Breathing	• Reassess the pediatric patient's respiratory status before transport (e.g., breath sounds, work of breathing, oxygen saturation).
	• For pediatric patients being transported by air, anticipate and prepare for additional interventions based on air physiology (e.g., placement of chest tube for a small pneumothorax).
Circulation	• Secure intravenous (IV) lines in preparation for transport.
	• Calculate intake and output; document total IV fluid and blood product administration.
Disability	• Document neurologic assessment.
Other	• Monitor and maintain temperature.
	• Apply sterile dressings to all open soft tissue injuries.
	• Splint all suspected fractures prior to transport; document neurovascular assessment of all splinted or injured extremities.
	• Facilitate family presence; allow visitation prior to transfer; never let the family leave before the child.
	• Assess pain and administer medication as needed.
	• Determine whether the pediatric patient requires isolation.

Summary

Transfer of the pediatric patient must be an organized procedure that includes prearranged agreements between referring and receiving facilities, transfer policies and protocols, standards of care for stabilization and transport, appropriate equipment, and consideration of the emotional needs of the pediatric patient and family.

References

1. American College of Emergency Physicians. (1990). Principles of appropriate transfer. *Annals of Emergency Medicine, 19*(3), 337–338.
2. Wood, J. (2002). COBRA laws. Retrieved September 10, 2003 from http://www.emedicine.com/emerg/topic737.htm
3. EMTALA. (1996). Retrieved September 10, 2003 from http://www.uplaw.net/statute.txt

North American Nursing Diagnosis Association (NANDA) Accepted Nursing Diagnoses

Activity Intolerance

Activity Intolerance, Risk for

Adjustment, Impaired

Airway Clearance, Ineffective

Anxiety

Aspiration, Risk for

Body Image Disturbance

Body Temperature, Risk for Imbalanced

Breastfeeding, Effective

Breastfeeding, Ineffective

Breastfeeding, Interrupted

Breathing Pattern, Ineffective

Cardiac Output, Decreased

Caregiver Role Strain

Caregiver Role Strain, Risk for

Communication, Impaired Verbal

Confusion, Acute

Confusion, Chronic

Constipation

Constipation, Perceived

Constipation, Risk for

Coping, Defensive

Coping, Ineffective Individual

Coping, Ineffective Community

Coping, Readiness for Enhanced Community

Coping, Compromised Ineffective Family

Coping, Disabling Ineffective Family

Coping, Readiness for Enhanced Family

Death Anxiety

Decisional Conflict

Delayed Development, Risk for

Denial, Ineffective

Dentition, Impaired

Diarrhea

Disuse Syndrome, Risk for

Diversional Activity, Deficit

Dysreflexia

Dysreflexia, Risk for Autonomic

Energy Fluid Disturbance

Effective Management of Therapeutic Regimen: Individual

Environmental Interpretation Syndrome, Impaired

Failure to Thrive, Adult

Falls, Risk for

Family Processes Dysfunctional: Alcoholism

Family Processes, Interrupted

Fatigue

Fear

Fluid Volume, Deficient

Fluid Volume, Excess

Fluid Volume, Risk for Deficient

Fluid Volume, Risk for Imbalance

Gas Exchange, Impaired

Grieving, Anticipatory

Grieving, Dysfunctional

Growth and Development, Delayed

Growth, Risk for Disproportionate

Health Maintenance, Ineffective

Health Seeking Behaviors

Home Maintenance Management, Impaired

Hopelessness

Hyperthermia

Hypothermia

Identity, Disturbed

Incontinence, Bowel

Incontinence, Functional

Incontinence, Reflex

Incontinence, Stress

Incontinence, Total Urinary

Incontinence, Urge Urinary

Incontinence, Risk for Urge

Infant Behavior, Disorganized

Infant Behavior, Readiness for Enhanced Organized

Infant Behavior, Risk for Disorganized

Infant Feeding Pattern, Ineffective

Infection, Risk for

Injury, Risk for

Intracranial Adaptive Capacity, Decreased

Knowledge, Deficient

Latex Allergy

Latex Allergy, Risk for

Loneliness, Risk for

Memory, Impaired

Mobility, Impaired Bed

Mobility, Impaired Physical

Mobility, Impaired Wheelchair

Nausea

Noncompliance

Nutrition, Imbalanced: Less Than Body
Requirements

Nutrition, Imbalanced: More Than Body
Requirements

Nutrition, Risk for Imbalanced: More Than Body
Requirements

Oral Mucous Membranes, Impaired

Pain, Acute

Pain, Chronic

Parental Role Conflict

Parent/Infant/Child Attachment, Risk for Impaired

Parenting, Deficient

Parenting, Deficient, Risk for

Perioperative-Positioning Injury, Risk for

Peripheral Neurovascular Dysfunction, Risk for

Poisoning, Risk for

Post-Trauma Syndrome

Post-Trauma Syndrome, Risk for

Powerlessness

Powerlessness, Risk for

Protection, Ineffective

Rape-Trauma Syndrome

Rape-Trauma Syndrome, Compound Reaction

Rape-Trauma Syndrome, Silent Reaction

Relocation Stress Syndrome

Relocation Stress Syndrome, Risk for

Role Performance, Ineffective

Self-Care Deficit, Bathing/Hygiene

Self-Care Deficit, Dressing/Grooming

Self-Care Deficit, Feeding

Self-Care Deficit, Toileting

Self-Esteem Disturbance

Self-Esteem, Chronic Low

Self-Esteem, Situational Low

Self-Esteem, Risk for Situational Low

Self-Mutilation

Self-Mutilation, Risk for

Sensory Perception, Disturbed (specify: visual,
kinesthetic, auditory, gustatory, tactile, olfactory)

Sexual Dysfunction

Sexuality Pattern, Ineffective

Skin Integrity, Impaired

Skin Integrity, Impaired, Risk for

Sleep Deprivation

Sleep Pattern, Disturbed

Social Interaction, Impaired

Social Isolation

Sorrow, Chronic

Spiritual Distress

Spiritual Distress, Risk for

Spiritual Well-Being, Readiness for Enhanced

Suffocation, Risk for

Suicide, Risk for

Surgical Recovery, Delayed

Swallowing, Impaired

Therapeutic Regimen: Individual, Ineffective
Management of

Therapeutic Regimen: Community, Ineffective
Management of

Therapeutic Regimen: Families, Ineffective
Management of

Thermoregulation, Ineffective

Thought Processes, Disturbed

Tissue Integrity, Impaired

Tissue Perfusion, Ineffective (specify: renal, cerebral,
cardiopulmonary, gastrointestinal, peripheral)

Transfer Ability, Impaired

Trauma, Risk for

Unilateral Neglect

Urinary Elimination, Impaired

Urinary Retention

Ventilation, Impaired, Spontaneous

Ventilatory Weaning Response, Dysfunctional

Violence, Risk for

Walking, Impaired

Wandering

Injury Prevention Resources

Emergency Nurses Association Injury Prevention
  Institute/Emergency Nurses CARE
915 Lee Street
Des Plaines, IL 60016
800/900-9659
www.ena.org/encare/

American Academy of Pediatrics (AAP)
141 Northwest Point Boulevard
Elk Grove Village, IL 60007-1098
847/228-5005
www.aap.org

The American Trauma Society
8903 Presidential Parkway
Suite 512
Upper Marlboro, MD 20772
800/556-7890
www.amtrauma.org

Arthritis Foundation (Sports Injury Prevention)
P.O. Box 7669
Atlanta, GA 30357-0669
800/283-7800
http://www.arthritis.org/resources/SIP/intro.asp

Center for Children with Special Needs
Children's Hospital and Regional Medical Center
P.O. Box 50020
Mail stop: S-219
Seattle, WA 98145
http://www.cshcn.org/resources/injuryprevention.htm

Consumer Product Safety Commission (CPSC)
National Injury Information Clearinghouse
4330 E West Highway, Room 504
Bethesda, MD 20814
301/504-0424
www.cpsc.gov

Emergency Medical Services for Children (EMS-C)
National Resource Center
111 Michigan Avenue, NW
Washington, DC 20010-2970
202/884-4927
www.ems-c.org

Farm Safety 4 Just Kids
110 South Chestnut Avenue
P.O. Box 458
Earlham, IA 50072
800/423-KIDS (5437)
www.fs4jk.org

Harborview Injury Prevention and Research Center
Box 359960
325 Ninth Avenue,
Seattle, WA 98104-2499
206/521-1520
http://depts.washington.edu/hiprc/

Injury Prevention Web
http://www.injuryprevention.org/links/links.htm

National Center for Injury Prevention and Control
Centers for Disease Control and Prevention
1600 Clifton Road
Atlanta, GA 30333
404/639-3311
www.cdc.gov/ncipc

National Highway Traffic Safety Administration (NHTSA)
400 Seventh St., SW
Washington, DC 20590
800/424-9393
www.nhtsa.dot.gov/

National Program for Playground Safety
School of HPELS, WRC 205
University of Northern Iowa
Cedar Falls, IA 50614-0618
800/554-PLAY
http://www.uni.edu/playground

National SAFE KIDS Campaign
1301 Pennsylvania Ave., NW, Suite 1000
Washington, DC 20004-1707
202/662-0600
www.safekids.org

National Safety Council (NSC)
1121 Spring Lake Drive
Itasca, IL 60143-3201
630/285-112
www.nsc.org

MANAGEMENT OF THE ILL OR INJURED PEDIATRIC PATIENT SKILL STATION

Principles of Pediatric Initial Assessment and Interventions

The care of the ill or injured pediatric patient is based on performance of a systematic assessment and initiation of the appropriate interventions. The management priorities are based on the life-threatening compromises found in the primary assessment and other abnormalities found during the secondary assessment, as well as the pediatric patient's age and the resources available for providing care.

The primary assessment consists of assessment of the airway with cervical spine stabilization or maintenance of spinal stabilization when trauma is suspected, breathing, circulation, disability or neurologic status, and exposure with environmental control. Life-threatening conditions are identified and treated before the assessment continues. The secondary assessment is a systematic approach to identifying additional problems and determining priorities of care.

Simultaneous assessment, diagnosis, and intervention may be required for the pediatric patient who is critically ill or injured. The priorities of intervention will depend on the complexity of the pediatric patient's condition and the availability and qualification of the emergency care providers. Those conditions that have the greatest potential to compromise the airway, breathing, circulation, and/or disability are given the highest priority.

The pediatric patient must be re-evaluated after any interventions that have an immediate effect on him or her to determine their effectiveness. The evaluation and ongoing assessment begin at the completion of the secondary assessment. These include primary reassessment and a re-evaluation of vital signs.

The systematic assessment can be remembered as follows.

A = Airway with simultaneous cervical spine stabilization

B = Breathing

C = Circulation

D = Disability—brief neurologic assessment

E = Exposure and environmental control

F = Full set of vital signs and family presence

G = Get comfort measures

H = Head-to-toe assessment and history

I = Inspect posterior surfaces

The template for Management of the Ill or Injured Pediatric Patient provides guidelines for conducting the primary and secondary assessments and identifying the appropriate interventions.

Summary

During evaluation, the learner must demonstrate all critical steps designated with one (*) or two (**) asterisks, and 70% of the total number of points. Each learner will be evaluated using a new and different scenario. Therefore, concentrate on understanding the principles of the station and not memorizing the specific case scenarios. Learners will not be evaluated on the ability to perform spinal stabilization during this station.

Certain critical steps must be demonstrated or described in order during the primary assessment. These are designated with ** on the evaluation form. The total number of critical steps (**) in any scenario is 6 to 8. Critical steps designated with ** may include

- Assessing airway patency.
- Identifying one appropriate airway intervention.
- Assessing breathing effectiveness.
- Identifying one appropriate intervention for ineffective breathing.
- Assessing perfusion status.
- Stating one appropriate intervention for ineffective circulation.
- Assessing the level of consciousness (AVPU).

Additional critical steps that must be demonstrated or described during the remainder of the station are designated with an asterisk (*) on the evaluation form. All of these steps must also be performed to successfully complete the station.

- States one measure to prevent heat loss

- Identifies appropriate diagnostic studies and interventions
- Identifies appropriate evaluation and ongoing assessment

At the end of the primary and secondary assessments the learner will be asked the following three questions.

- What additional diagnostic studies or interventions may be completed? If the learner has identified any appropriate diagnostic studies or interventions as he or she progressed through the primary and secondary assessments these will be counted toward the total of five that is necessary to complete this step.

- What is the evaluation and ongoing assessment of this patient? At a minimum the learner should identify the need to reassess the components of the primary assessment and vital signs. In addition the learner should identify the need to reassess the additional problems/injuries found during the secondary assessment.

- Is there anything that the learner would like to add or revise related to the assessment of this patient? Although the learner may not add to or revise any of the ** steps, it does allow the learner to identify additional components of the secondary assessment criteria or interventions that may have been overlooked.

Management of the Ill or Injured Pediatric Patient Template

PRIMARY ASSESSMENT	
Assessment	**Potential Interventions**
Determines patient's level of consciousness	Positions the patient **AND** demonstrates manually opening the airway while considering spinal stabilization
A=Airway	
Assess at least three of the following.(**)	Must identify at least one of the following interventions.(**)
• Vocalization	• Open the airway with jaw thrust or chin lift
• Tongue obstruction	• Repositions head to neutral position
• Loose teeth or foreign objects	• Suction or remove foreign objects
• Vomitus or other secretions	• Insert an oropharyngeal/nasopharyngeal airway
• Edema	• Prepare for endotracheal intubation/rapid sequence intubation
• Preferred posture	• Prepare for needle or surgical cricothyroidotomy
• Drooling	
• Dysphagia	
• Abnormal airway sounds	
B=Breathing	
Assess at least three of the following.(**)	Must identify at least one of the following interventions.(**)
• Level of consciousness	• Maintain position of comfort
• Spontaneous respirations	• Provide supplemental oxygen
• Rate and depth of respirations	• Provide bag-mask ventilation
• Symmetric chest rise and fall	-Reassessment of breathing effectiveness should occur prior to proceeding with primary assessment (**)
• Presence and quality of breath sounds	
• Skin color	• Prepare for endotracheal intubation/rapid sequence intubation
• Work of breathing	-Assessment of tube placement should be done prior to proceeding with primary assessment (**)
- Nasal flaring	• Insert gastric tube to reduce abdominal distention
- Retractions	• Prepare for needle thoracentesis
- Head bobbing	
- Expiratory grunting	
- Accessory muscle use	
• Jugular vein distention and tracheal position	

Management of the Ill or Injured Pediatric Patient Template (cont.)

C=Circulation

Assess at least two of the following.(**)	Must identify at least one of the following interventions. (**)
• Central **AND** peripheral pulse rate and quality	• Perform cardiopulmonary resuscitation and advanced life-support measures
• Skin color **AND** temperature	• Control any obvious bleeding
• Capillary refill	• Prepare for defibrillation/synchronized cardioversion
	• Obtain intravenous or intraosseous access
	• Administer 20 ml/kg fluid bolus of isotonic crystalloid solution
	• Administer medications
	• Administer blood or blood products
	• Correct electrolyte and acid-base imbalance

D=Disability

• Level of consciousness (AVPU)(**)	• Perform further investigation during secondary assessment
• Pupils	• Administer pharmacologic therapy

E=Exposure and Environmental Control

• Obvious skin abnormalities	Must identify at least one of the following. (*)
• Sources of heat loss	• Apply warm blankets
	• Provide overhead warming light
	• Provide radiant warmer or approved warming device
	• Maintain warm ambient environment
	• Increase room temperature as needed
	• Administer warm intravenous fluids
	• Administer warm humidified oxygen

SECONDARY ASSESSMENT

F=Full Set of Vital Signs

• Rate and depth of respirations	• Place on cardiorespiratory monitors
• Rate and quality of pulse	• Trend vital signs
• Blood pressure	-Estimate weight using length-based resuscitation tape (e.g., Broselow® tape)
• Temperature	
• Weight (Kg)	

F=Family Presence

• Identification of family members and their relationship to the child	• Facilitate and support family involvement
• Needs of the family	• Assign health care professional to liaison with family and provide explanation of procedures, plan of treatment
• Need for additional support and desire to be in resuscitation room	• Assign a staff member to provide family support

G=Give Comfort Measures

• Presence and level of pain	• Facilitate family presence for support of the child
	• Initiate pain management measures.
	-Use age-appropriate nonpharmacologic methods to facilitate coping
	-Administer analgesics and other appropriate medications
	-Initiate physical measures (splints, dressing, ice)

Management of the Ill or Injured Pediatric Patient Template (cont.)

H=Head-to-Toe Assessment

- Head-to-toe assessment using inspection, palpation, and auscultation techniques for signs and symptoms of illness or injury such as rashes, lesions, petechiae, edema, ecchymosis, or tenderness
- Reassessment of airway, breathing, and circulation status once head-to-toe assessment is completed

- Initiate appropriate interventions based on findings

H=History

- MIVT
- Complete history (CIAMPEDS)
- Specialized history
- Social history
- Family history

- Initiate social service consult as needed

I=Inspect Posterior Surfaces

- Inspect and palpate posterior surfaces for signs and symptoms of illness or injury such as rashes, lesions, petechiae, edema, ecchymosis, or tenderness

- Logroll patient to maintain airway patency and spinal alignment

PEDIATRIC CLINICAL INTERVENTIONS SKILL STATION

Principles of Pediatric Clinical Interventions

A variety of interventions are performed during the care of pediatric patients in the emergency department and in other emergency care settings or situations. An essential aspect of providing these interventions is the availability of equipment in the appropriate sizes for all age groups—newborns through adolescents. Determining the correct equipment size for a specific patient can be a challenge. Formulas and charts have been developed to assist in this process. Products such as the Broselow™ tape and color-coded equipment storage systems are valuable tools in assisting with rapid selection of the appropriate-sized equipment.

The priorities of intervention depend on the complexity and acuity of the pediatric patient's illness or injury. The approach to these interventions is governed by the pediatric patient's development and psychosocial needs as well as the physiologic status. Integrating the priorities of intervention with a developmentally appropriate approach is essential in planning and implementing care that meets the needs of children and their families. Although emergency interventions include an array of procedures, many pediatric interventions include one or more of the following components: stabilization and positioning techniques, vascular access, pain management and medication administration, respiratory interventions, and rhythm disturbances.

Summary

Pediatric Clinical Interventions is a teaching station in which the learner has an opportunity to integrate the principles of growth and development with priorities of intervention. The case scenarios provide the learner with an opportunity to incorporate multiple components of care into the planning and implementation of specific interventions.

A minimum of three of the following seven stations will be presented during the course. Respiratory Interventions and Spinal Stabilization are mandatory teaching stations. The Rhythm Disturbances station must be used for PALS renewal participants.

Medication Administration

Case 1

Cindy is an 18-month-old brought to the emergency department via ambulance because she was seizing. Attempts at vascular access are unsuccessful.

- What additional route can be used for administration of diazepam or lorazepam?

Procedure for Medication Administration

- Draw the calculated dose into a tuberculin or 3 cc syringe.
- Attach the plastic portion of an over-the-needle catheter; can also cut off the needle tip of a butterfly needle and use the tube attached to a syringe for insertion.
- Lubricate the syringe and catheter.
- Introduce the syringe and catheter into the rectum approximately 2 inches (5 cm).
- Inject the medication then remove the syringe and catheter.
- Hold or tape the buttocks together for 10 seconds.

Medication Administration

Case 2

Mackenzie is a 4-year-old child who presents following the development of a fever and rash. Her vital signs are pulse 190 beats/minute; respirations 36 breaths/minute; blood pressure 90/48 mm Hg; and temperature 38.6°C (101.4°F). Capillary refill is 3 seconds; her skin is cool and pale. A petechial rash is noted on her chest, abdomen, and extremities. Appropriate isolation precautions have been initiated. An intravenous line is established in the left hand with a 22-gauge catheter. A rapid bolus of crystalloid solution, such as 0.9% normal saline, is ordered. The patient's weight is 18 kg.

- How many ml/kg should be administered for the fluid bolus?
- What is the total volume of fluid to be administered?
- Describe and demonstrate the use of a stopcock to rapidly infuse the intravenous fluid.
- What are the other methods to rapidly infuse fluids?

Fluid bolus = 20 ml/kg; 20 x 18 = 360 cc

Refer to Chapter 10, *Medication Administration,* for a description of rapid intravenous fluid administration.

Medication Administration

Case 3

Jennifer is a 2-year-old toddler who presents to the emergency department with difficulty breathing and wheezing. Her mother reports one previous wheezing episode about 6 months previously. Jennifer is alert and interactive. She is tachypneic, with labored respirations, nasal flaring, and subcostal and intercostal retractions. Her color is slightly pale; capillary refill is 2 seconds. Her pulse is 132 beats/minute, her respirations are 48 breaths/minute, her blood pressure is 90/60 mm Hg, and her axillary temperature is 36.6°C (97.8°F).

- What strategies may assist in gaining the child's cooperation for administration of oxygen or inhaled medications?

- Describe your initial interventions for this patient.

Strategies for Administration of Oxygen or Inhaled Medications

Children may be frightened and/or resist the application of an oxygen mask directly on their face. It is important to gain the child's cooperation through explanation and a nonthreatening approach. Refer to Chapter 10, *Medication Administration,* for a description of strategies.

Pain Assessment and Management

Case 1

Patty, a 7-day-old infant, is brought to the emergency department by her parents. Her mother states that she won't stop crying. The infant is inconsolable in her mother's arms. She exhibits facial grimacing and tightly clenched fists and eyes. Her mother has attempted to feed her but the infant only nurses for a couple of minutes.

- Using the FLACC pain assessment tools calculate the patient's score.

- Describe appropriate nonpharmacologic interventions that may be implemented with this patient.

Refer to Chapter 12, *Pediatric Pain Assessment and Management,* for a description of FLACC and nonpharmacologic interventions for pain.

Pain Assessment and Management

Case 2

Sean is an 8-year-old who is brought in by his parents after he fell from a trampoline. He is holding his right arm against his body and grimaces with every step. He states that he flipped off the trampoline, landing on his right arm, on the grass. He is alert, oriented, and cooperative. He rates his pain as 7 on the Oucher® scale. He has an obvious angulated deformity to his right forearm. Neurovascular status is intact distal to the injury.

- Name three nonpharmacologic interventions that may be initiated to assist in reducing the pain associated with the injury.

- Review appropriate pharmacologic interventions.

Refer to Chapter 12, *Pediatric Pain Assessment and Management,* for specific information.

Pain Assessment and Management

Case 3

Steven is a 12-year-old who presents with partial-thickness burns to his right arm. His shirtsleeve caught on fire when he was lighting a fire in the fireplace. His parents wrapped the arm in a moist towel. He rates his pain as a 9 on a numeric pain scale.

- Describe pain management measures appropriate for this patient.

Refer to Chapter 12, *Pediatric Pain Assessment and Management,* for related information.

Procedural Preparation and Positioning

Case 1

David is a 4-week-old infant with a fever who is brought to the emergency department by his parents. As part of his workup for possible sepsis, a lumbar puncture will be performed. Standard and isolation precautions have been initiated.

- Demonstrate, with the infant manikin, how to position and hold the infant for the procedure.

- Describe the appropriate assessment during the procedure.

Procedure for Lumbar Puncture

A lumbar puncture involves the placement of a spinal needle in the subarachnoid space of the lumbar area to obtain a sample of cerebrospinal fluid. Refer to Chapter 17, *Procedural Preparation and Sedation,* for information related to this procedure.

Procedural Preparation and Positioning

Case 2

Jimmy is a 5-year-old who presents to the emergency department with a 4-cm laceration to the forehead, requiring sutures for subcutaneous and skin closure. The procedure for the laceration repair has been explained to him.

- Demonstrate a method to restrict his movement during the laceration repair.
- In addition to preparation for the procedure, what other strategies may you use to gain cooperation?

Procedure for Use of Physically Restrictive Devices During Procedures

The least restrictive methods of controlling the child's movement should be used. Distraction and other non-pharmacologic pain management techniques should always be used with all restrictive devices. Refer to Chapter 17, *Procedural Preparation and Sedation,* for a description of positioning for comfort and the use of physically restrictive devices. Refer to Chapter 12, *Pediatric Pain Assessment and Management,* for a description of nonpharmacologic interventions.

Procedural Preparation and Positioning

Case 3

Jenny is a three-year-old who was brought in by her parents after falling off the top bunk bed. Her right thigh is very swollen and ecchymotic. The physician orders a radiograph of the right leg. Upon entering the radiology suite, Jenny begins crying and screaming and will not cooperate to complete the x-ray. The physician recommends IV sedation for the child.

- Describe the standards that should be met when administering sedation to pediatric patients.
- Review sedation discharge criteria.
- Describe the most common complications to assess for.

Refer to Chapter 17, *Procedural Preparation and Sedation,* for related information.

Respiratory Interventions

Case 1

James is a 3-month-old brought into the emergency department by his mother after she noted that he tired easily when offered the bottle. On initial assessment you notice that his lips are blue tinged. His primary assessment reveals a patent airway; his respiratory rate is 32 breaths/min with no accessory muscle use or retractions. His nares are crusty. The tech is unable to obtain a pulse oximeter reading and states that the machine is not working.

- Demonstrate various locations for pulse oximeter readings.
- How would you assess the accuracy of the pulse oximeter reading?
- Demonstrate bulb suctioning.

Procedure for Pulse Oximeter[1]

1. When choosing a pulse oximeter for your pediatric patient consider the following.

   -Patient's body weight

   -Duration of use (long-term, short-term, or spot-check)

   -Patient activity

   -Infection control concerns

2. Refer to operational manual for pulse oximeter regarding sensor indicators.

   -When selecting a site, priority should be given to an extremity free of an arterial catheter, blood pressure cuff, or intravenous infusion.

   -Ensure that the optical components of the sensor are properly aligned as outlined in the directions for use.

   -Adhesive sensor sites must be checked at least every 8 hours and moved to a new site if necessary. Reusable sensors must be moved to a new site at least every 4 hours.

Tips for Bulb Suctioning

1. Suction the mouth before the nares. Avoid suctioning too deep into the mouth because it can result in bradycardia.
2. Instill saline drops to loosen secretions as necessary.
3. Occlude the nare with the bulb.

Respiratory Interventions

Case 2

Daniel is a 5-year-old who presents following an ingestion of an unknown medication. His primary assessment reveals that he is unresponsive and pale, with a sonorous respiratory pattern at an adequate rate. Manual positioning of the airway is required to maintain patency.

- Describe indications for use of nasopharyngeal versus oropharyngeal airways.
- Describe and demonstrate the insertion of nasopharyngeal airway.
- Describe and demonstrate insertion of an oropharyngeal airway.

Indications for Use[4,5]

Nasopharyngeal Airway

- Relief of upper airway obstruction due to tongue or soft tissue (except epiglottitis) in a conscious patient or an unconscious patient with an intact gag reflex
- Oropharyngeal airway placement is technically difficult or impossible due to massive oral trauma
- Copious nasal secretions, to facilitate atraumatic suctioning

Oropharyngeal Airway

- Impaired gag reflex and loss of tonicity to the submandibular muscles causing airway obstruction in the unconscious patient
- To facilitate bag-mask ventilation by elevating the soft tissues of the posterior pharynx
- In an orally intubated patient to prevent biting of the endotracheal tube
- To facilitate suctioning of oral secretions

Insertion of Nasopharyngeal Airway

- Sizes are available from 12F to 36F. The airway adjunct should not cause any blanching to the nares.
- An endotracheal tube can be used if the correct size of nasopharyngeal airway is not available.
- Measure from the tip of the nose to the tragus of the ear.

- Consider lubricating the tube prior to insertion.
- Begin with the bevel toward the septum advancing the tip along the nasal floor.

  -Right nostril: advance until phalange is seated against the outside of nare.

  -Left nostril: insert the airway with the curvature upward until resistance is felt, then rotate the airway 180 degrees and continue to advance until flange reaches the nare.

- Insertion should be gentle never forced.
- Contraindications: nasal obstruction preventing easy insertion, suspected basilar skull fracture, or facial trauma.

Insertion of Oropharyngeal Airway

- Determine size by placing the airway next to the face with the flange at the level of the central incisor, the bite block parallel with the hard palate, and the tip of the airway at the angle of the jaw. An airway that is too small may push the tongue into the oropharynx; an airway that is too large may obstruct the trachea.
- Insert the oropharyngeal airway, using a tongue blade to depress and displace the tongue forward. Insert the airway, curve down, over the tongue.

  -Do not insert the airway inverted and rotate it, as in the adult, because this may cause soft palate injury.

Respiratory Interventions

Case 3

Sarah is a 9-year-old brought to your emergency department by EMS. She was found floating face down in a swimming pool. EMS has been assisting ventilation with a bag-mask device. The Pediatric Assessment Triangle reveals a child who is limp and unresponsive, cyanotic, and does not exhibit any respiratory effort.

- What would be your next step for definitive airway management?
- Describe patient assessment and nursing interventions during intubation.
- Demonstrate appropriate bag-mask ventilation.
- Describe two methods for determining endotracheal tube size and depth.
- Demonstrate two methods to confirm endotracheal tube placement.
- Demonstrate one method for securing the tracheal tube.

Preparing for Endotracheal Intubation

- Place the child on a cardiac monitor, pulse oximeter, and noninvasive blood pressure monitor if not already completed.
- Ensure that the child is well oxygenated prior to the intubation attempt.

  -Ventilate using a bag-mask device with reservoir and 100% oxygen prior to the intubation attempt.
- Ensure suction and appropriate-sized catheters are available.
- Administer medications if rapid sequence intubation is being used.
- Apply cricoid pressure, as indicated.
- Monitor the child's heart rate, oxygen saturation, and color continuously during the intubation attempt.

  -Avoid prolonged intubation attempts. Intubation attempts lasting longer than 30 seconds can result in profound hypoxia.

  -If the heart rate or oxygen saturation begins to drop, or pallor or cyanosis are observed, interrupt the intubation attempt and ventilate the child with the bag-mask device and 100% oxygen.

Choosing Correct Size and Type of Endotracheal Tube

- Use the uncuffed endotracheal tubes in children younger than 8 years of age. In these children, the cricoid ring is the narrowest portion of the airway and acts as a natural cuff.
- Use a length-based resuscitation tape (i.e., Broselow® tape) that lists tube and equipment sizes that correspond to the child's length to estimate tube size.
- Use the following formula to estimate the appropriate tube size.

  (16 + patient's age in years) / 4
- Optional sizing techniques

  -The width of the endotracheal tube should be no wider than the width of the nail bed of the small finger (5th digit).

  -The circumference of the endotracheal tube should be no larger than the circumference of the nare.
- An endotracheal tube that is 0.5 mm smaller and one that is 0.5 mm larger than the estimated tube size should also be available.

Depth of Endotracheal Tube Insertion

The following methods may be used to estimate the appropriate depth of endotracheal tube placement in the child. Endotracheal tube position and depth should be evaluated by radiograph and adjustments of depth of insertion made, as appropriate, based on the tube's position in the trachea.

- Formula for estimating oral endotracheal tube depth (length of tube at the lip)

  -Newborn (2 kg to 5 kg in weight):   8 to 10 cm

  -6 months of age: 11 cm

  -1 year of age: 12 cm

  -Older than 1 year of age: 12 + ½ age in years = cm length at the tip
- The length-based resuscitation tape includes information on estimated depth of endotracheal tube insertion for each weight grouping.
- Record the position of the tube at the level of the lip or teeth.

Confirming Endotracheal Tube Placement

Once intubated, hold the tube firmly at the level of lip and evaluate placement.

- Observe the chest for bilateral, symmetric chest rise.
- Listen for equal breath sounds bilaterally at the apices, midaxillary lines, and sternal notch. Compare pitch, intensity, and location of the sounds.
- Listen for low-pitched gurgling and observe for distention of the epigastrium with ventilation that indicates esophageal intubation.
- Observe the child for clinical signs of improvement, such as color, perfusion, and oxygen saturation.
- When available, use an exhaled CO_2 detector to confirm tube placement. It is not useful for the child in cardiopulmonary arrest because CO_2 may not be detected even when the tube is correctly placed in the trachea because of the lack of pulmonary circulation.

  -The exhaled CO_2 detector may need to be changed if it gets wet, i.e., copious secretions.

  -Color indicator[6]
  Y = Yellow—Mellow (or Yes the tube is in)
  T = Tan—Think (about a problem after 6 more breaths and reassess)
  P = Purple—Problem (No CO_2 detected–pull it); may also remain purple during CPR in a patient with a nonperfusing rhythm.
- Obtain a chest radiograph to confirm tube position as soon as possible.

Securing the Endotracheal Tube

The following is one suggested method for taping the endotracheal tube.

- Cut two pieces of 1-inch-wide tape (approximately 6 inches in length). Cut or tear the pieces in half lengthwise for approximately 4 inches (leave a 2-inch length of tape that remains the full width).

- Lightly paint the upper lip, cheeks, and endotracheal tube with tincture of benzoin. Avoid contact with mucous membranes.
- Apply the intact piece of adhesive tape to the cheek and adhere one length of the torn portion across the upper lip.
- Wrap the second length of the torn portion around the tube at least two or three times.
- Apply the second strip in a similar fashion from the opposite direction.
- Document the location of endotracheal tube at the lip or gum line.

Rhythm Disturbances

Case 1

A 10-month-old is brought in by her mother who states that the child has been irritable for the past 2 days and has been breathing faster than normal. Today the mother noted that the infant's heart seemed to be "pounding in her chest."

Your primary assessment reveals the following.

- Appearance: Color pink, infant sitting on mother's lap.
- Airway: Patent and maintainable. No abnormal airway sounds noted. Infant babbling.
- Breathing: Respiratory rate of 30 breaths/minute, lungs clear, good aeration bilaterally, no increased work of breathing.
- Circulation: Peripheral pulses present and strong although difficult to count due to rapid rate.
- Disability: Awake, alert, intermittently irritable and playing with toy.

Describe the appropriate interventions for this patient.

Interventions

- Place on cardiac monitor which shows a narrow complex tachycardia at a rate of 240 beats per minute.
- Place the infant on supplemental oxygen as tolerated.
- Obtain cardiology consult.
- Obtain a 12-lead ECG; reading is consistent with supraventricular tachycardia (SVT).
- The cardiologist recommends the use of vagal maneuvers.

-The vagal maneuver most often used in infancy is placing a small bag of ice water over the infant's eyes and face for ten to twenty seconds, while running a continuous strip on either the monitor or 12-lead ECG machine (preferred). This is effective in about

25% of cases.

-Ocular pressure is not recommended in children.

-Older children are taught to perform a Valsalva maneuver.

- The infant immediately gasps when the bag of ice water is placed on her face, and her heart rate slows to 120 beats per minute, sinus rhythm.
- Obtain venous access using a saline lock.
- Prepare for admission for a cardiac work-up.
- If the vagal maneuver had not worked, the next treatment choice would be adenosine.

-Adenosine, an endogenous nucleoside producing acute AV node blockade, is now the first drug of choice for terminating SVT, and is effective in about 90% of cases.

-Electrical cardioversion with 0.5 to 1 joule/kg is also a treatment choice for SVT with critical hypotension.

Rhythm Disturbances

Case 2

You are attending a local elementary school baseball game being played by children 9 to 10 years of age. As the ball is thrown, you note that the batter is hit in the chest and falls to the ground. You immediately respond.

Initial assessment:

- Appearance: Child is unresponsive and cyanotic
- Airway and breathing: Child is unresponsive, airway is open and patent with chin lift, but no spontaneous respirations are noted; skin color is cyanotic
- Circulation: No central pulses are palpable; skin diaphoretic.
- Disability: Child is unresponsive to voice and painful stimuli
- Age & eight: 9 years old and 27 kg (per father)

Describe the appropriate interventions that should be initiated on this patient.

Interventions

- Instruct someone to obtain the AED from inside the school and to call the emergency medical services ambulance.
- Begin ventilation (mouth-to-mouth or mouth-to-barrier device); assess for adequate chest expansion with ventilations.
- Begin chest compressions.
- When AED arrives, place pads on child (dry chest off first) and follow AED commands.
- The AED indicates that a shock is advised.

- Following the AED command, making sure that everyone is clear, and deliver the shock.
- As the AED is doing the repeat analysis, you note that the child is moving and breathing.
- The AED indicates that a repeat shock is not advised.
- The child is now awake, with adequate breathing and strong central pulses.
- EMS arrives; the child and his father are transported to the closest hospital.

Rhythm Disturbances

Case 3

A father rushes into the emergency department carrying his 5-year-old son who was playing with some loose wires that were sticking out of a lamp pole in front of the house. The child was thrown backwards approximately 10 feet. He was motionless when his father got to him. They live only a block away so the father put the child in his car and drove him here.

Your primary assessment reveals the following.

- Appearance: Child is unresponsive and cyanotic
- Airway and breathing: Child is unresponsive, airway is open and patent with chin lift, but no spontaneous respirations are noted; skin color is cyanotic
- Circulation: No central or peripheral pulses are palpable
- Disability: Child is unresponsive to voice and painful stimuli
- Weight: 20 kg (per father)

Describe the appropriate interventions that should be initiated on this patient.

Interventions

- Ventilate child with appropriately sized bag-mask device, using 100% oxygen. Assess adequacy of chest expansion with ventilation. Prepare for endotracheal intubation.
- Assess for a pulse – if no pulse, begin compressions. Assess for central pulses with compressions.
- Simultaneously, place child on cardiac monitor, which shows ventricular fibrillation (v-fib) with compressions paused.
- Defibrillate once at 2 joules/kg and immediately resume CPR for 5 cycles (about 2 minutes).
- If no change in rhythm, defibrillate once at 4 joules/kg and immediately resume CPR.
- Administer epinephrine during chest compressions
-IV/IO: 0.01 mg/kg (0.1 ml/kg of 1:10,000 solution).

-If unable to obtain IV or IO access, may give epinephrine 0.1 mg/kg (0.1 ml/kg of 1:1000 solution) via the endotracheal tube.

- Circulate epinephrine for 5 cycles (about 2 minutes).
- If no change in rhythm, defibrillate once at 4 joules/kg and resume CPR immediately.
- If no change in rhythm, administer amiodarone (5 mg/kg) or lidocaine (1mg/kg) IV or IO, if amiodarone is not available, and circulate for 5 cycles (about 2 minutes).
- If no change in rhythm, defibrillate once at 4 joules/kg and resume CPR immediately for 5 cycles (about 2 minutes).
- Monitor shows sinus rhythm at a rate of 120 beats/minute with a palpable central pulse, but no peripheral pulses. Capillary refill 3 to 4 seconds.
- Patient does not have spontaneous respirations – ventilation continues at age-appropriate rate with good chest expansion.
- Administer fluid bolus of 20 ml/kg of appropriate crystalloid solution.
- Reassess circulation. Heart rate 110 beats/minute, peripheral pulses present but weak, capillary refill 3 seconds. Consider another fluid bolus.
- Prepare for admission or transfer.

Spinal Stabilization

Case 1

Debbie is an 8-month-old infant involved in a motor vehicle collision. She was alert and stable at the scene and was transported, immobilized in her car seat, to your emergency department for evaluation. The Pediatric Assessment Triangle reveals an alert, interactive infant.

- Demonstrate transferring the infant from the car seat to a backboard while maintaining spinal immobilization.

Procedure for Removing a Child from a Child Safety Seat While Maintaining Spinal Stabilization

- Remove towel rolls, if present, and manually stabilize the head and cervical spine.
- Remove or cut the shoulder harness and move the safety bar out of the way as much as possible.
- Position the child safety seat at the foot of a backboard. Tip the child safety seat back and lay it down onto the backboard.
- One person should slide his or her hands along each side of the child's head until the hands are behind the child's shoulders. The head and neck are then supported laterally by the person's arms. A second person should take control of the child's body.

- On the instruction of the person at the head, slide the child out of the child safety seat onto the backboard and proceed with immobilizing the child.

Spinal Stabilization

Case 2

Now that Debbie, our 8-month-old, has been transferred from her car seat to the backboard

- Demonstrate correct cervical and spinal stabilization.
- Describe techniques to keep the infant calm and/or distracted during this process.

Cervical and Spinal Stabilization in the Infant

- Secure the child's body to the backboard or immobilization device. The leader should maintain manual stabilization of the cervical spine until the body and then the head are secured to the backboard.

-Consider placing padding under the child's shoulder blades to keep the spine in anatomical alignment and decrease flexion of the neck because of the larger occiput.

-Place three straps across the child's body. One strap is placed across the chest, one across the hips, and one above the knees.

-In infants and small children, towel or blanket rolls are placed along the side of the body to secure the patient and restrict the movement of the hips and knees. If there is a space between the edge of the backboard and the child's body, the child will be able to move beneath the strap. This space is filled with a blanket or towel roll.

- Secure the head to the board after the child's body is secured to the board.

-Apply a lateral head support device to either side of the head to prevent lateral and anterior movement. Towel or blanket rolls or a commercially available cervical immobilization device should be used to provide lateral stabilization. If lateral stabilization cannot be achieved with available devices, manual stabilization is continued.

- Instruct caregivers to replace the car seat when involved in a crash. In some areas, auto insurance may cover the cost of replacing the car seat.

Providing Comfort Measures

Comfort measures that are effective for an infant include sensorimotor soothing techniques, such as providing a pacifier and stroking the skin. Keep the caregiver in the infant's line of vision and encourage him or her to participate in comforting strategies.

Appropriate distraction techniques in this situation include playing soothing music; speaking quietly in soothing, rhythmic tones; and using soap bubbles, glitter wand, or puppets to engage the infant's attention.

Spinal Stabilization

Case 3

Steven is an 8-year-old brought to the emergency department after reportedly falling on the playground. He presents complaining of head and neck pain. The Pediatric Assessment Triangle reveals an alert, oriented, cooperative child. The primary assessment is within normal limits. It is decided to apply cervical and spinal stabilization.

- Demonstrate sizing the cervical collar.
- Demonstrate the application of cervical and spinal stabilization. (Resource for PALS verification—Spinal Stabilization video)
- Discuss alternatives for infants to adapt cervical stabilization (refer to Case 1).

Proper Sizing and Application of Cervical Collar

Always follow the manufacturer's directions for correct application of the cervical collar. The Stifneck® collar is one type of rigid collar and its application will be described here.

- Determine the appropriate size by measuring from the patient's chin to the top of the shoulder. Place your fingers on top of the shoulder where the collar will rest and measure the distance to the point of the chin (not the angle of the jaw). Compare this distance on the collar by placing the same number of fingers below the black fastener. The correct size collar is equal to the measurement between the black fastener and the edge of the rigid plastic at the bottom of the collar (not the foam portion of the collar).

Procedure for Cervical and Spinal Stabilization

- Leader approaches the patient in patient's line of vision, takes position at head of the patient and positions hands on each side of head, with thumbs along mandible and fingers behind the head on the occipital ridge. Maintain gentle but firm stabilization of the neck throughout the entire procedure. The leader briefly explains to the patient what to expect and not to move the head or neck.
- Leader asks patient to wiggle his or her toes and fingers, **OR** gently lift an arm and a leg, and determines if sensation is present.
- While maintaining firm control of patient's head, the leader assigns the assistants to locations beside the patient's body.

-Assistant 1—near the patient's head and upper body

-Assistant 2—beside Assistant 1, near the patient's hips and legs

-Assistant 3—opposite side of patient

- Leader directs Assistant 1 to remove any jewelry (earrings, necklace).
- Leader directs Assistant 1 to apply and secure an appropriate-sized rigid cervical collar. A properly fitted collar will fit between the point of the chin and the suprasternal notch, resting on the clavicles and supporting the lower jaw.

-Assemble the collar by moving the chin piece up and snapping the black fastener into the hole on the side of the collar.

-Preform the collar.

-Slide the back portion of the collar under the patient's neck until the Velcro® can be seen on the patient's other side.

-Slide the collar up the sternum until the chin piece fits snugly under the chin.

-Secure and fasten the Velcro.

- Leader directs Assistant 2 to straighten patient's arms at patient's side and to straighten legs.
- On the count of three, the leader directs Assistants 1 and 2 to roll the patient as a unit towards them onto the patient's side. Leader monitors the alignment (nose with umbilicus) continually rather than watching backboard placement.
- Leader directs Assistant 3 to position backboard on its side up against the patient's back.
- Leader uses mnemonic "Ready, Steady, Roll" or "1, 2, 3" to guide logroll procedure. On "Roll" or the count of "3", the leader directs Assistants 1 and 2 to gently roll the patient as a unit onto the backboard as Assistant 3 guides the board.
- Leader maintains stabilization of head until the straps are correctly placed. Leader directs assistants to place straps to encircle the patient and backboard at the shoulders, hips, and proximal to the knees.
- Leader directs assistants to place head support devices (i.e., towel rolls or rigid foam blocks) on either side of head. Secures the head to the backboard with tape to prevent movement of head. Tape is not placed across chin.
- Leader continually maintains manual stabilization of the head and neck until the head is immobilized. Once the head is immobilized, leader may remove hands from patient's head.
- Leader reassesses motor and sensory function.

Vascular Access

Case 1

A 6-month-old with a 3-day history of vomiting, diarrhea, and decreased oral intake is brought to the emergency department by her parents. She is clinically dehydrated but stable. The physician orders intravenous fluids for rehydration.

- What intravenous sites would be most appropriate for this infant?
- How would you secure the catheter?

Refer to Chapter 8, *Vascular Access*, for related information.

Vascular Access

Case 2

Denise is a 9-year-old who presents to the emergency department with a possible infection of her peripherally inserted central catheter (PICC).

- What are the indications for a PICC?
- What signs and symptoms would you assess to determine if an infection was present?

Peripherally Inserted Central Catheters (PICC line)

PICC lines are usually placed in the antecubital fossa, either in the median basilica or cephalic vein by a specially trained nurse or doctor. They are used for long-term IV access for purposes of long-term antibiotic therapy, chemotherapy, or IV nutrition.

Signs and symptoms of infection include redness, swelling, tenderness, drainage, pain, and/or fever.

Vascular Access

Case 3

Mary is an 8-week-old infant who arrives by ambulance in full cardiopulmonary arrest. She is orally intubated and cardiac compressions are in progress. An intraosseous needle was placed in the left tibia by the paramedic.

- What are the indications for intraosseous insertion?
- Name two preferred sites for intraosseous insertion in the infant.
- Locate landmarks and sites for intraosseous insertion in the tibia and the femur.
- What fluids and medications may be infused through an intraosseous needle?
- Describe how to evaluate patency of the intraosseous access and the signs of intraosseous infusion site infiltration or extravasation.

- If the intraosseous access is not functional, can another intraosseous needle be placed in the same bone?

Intraosseous Insertion and Infusion

- Intraosseous access is indicated when immediate vascular access is needed for the critically ill or injured pediatric patient who requires intravenous fluid, medication, and/or blood administration for resuscitation (i.e., cardiopulmonary arrest, decompensated shock).

- Obtain intraosseous access by inserting a rigid needle into the medullary cavity of a bone, providing access to a noncollapsible venous plexus.

  -The tibia is the preferred site; the distal femur is an alternate site.

  - Anterior medial portion of the tibia; 1 to 3 cm below the tibial tuberosity.

  - Distal tibia, medial surface proximal to the medial malleolus.

  -A commercially available intraosseous needle or a bone marrow aspiration needle is the most commonly used needle.

  -18-gauge, 16-gauge, 15-gauge, and 12-gauge needles are generally available. 18-gauge needles are usually used in infants younger than 3 months of age.

- Limit insertion attempts to one attempt per bone. Multiple sticks in the same bone will result in leaking of fluids and medications into the tissues.

- Intraosseous access is usually only short-term (less than 4 hours or until other routes of access are obtained).

- Any fluid or medication that can be given intravenously can also be given via intraosseous access.

- Closely observe the site for extravasation of fluids. Monitor the insertion site and the posterior surface of the extremity (calf or lower thigh) for swelling, tension, or fullness. Discontinue the infusion if extravasation is suspected.

- The properly placed intraosseous needle should be taped and secured. The extremity should be immobilized to avoid movement of the leg or kicking which may dislodge the intraosseous needle.

- If an intraosseous site is not functioning, the needle should be removed and the site marked. This will alert providers to the fact that an intraosseous needle was placed in that bone and further attempts in that bone are to be avoided.

- When the intraosseous needle is removed, apply manual pressure for several minutes, then apply a pressure dressing. Label dressing as an intraosseous site.

References

1. Nellcor sensors basic principles and tips for use. (1999). St. Louis, MO: Mallinckrodt, Inc.
2. York, D. (1999). Laryngeal mask airway. In J. Proehl (Ed.), *Emergency nursing procedures* (2nd ed., pp. 15–17). Philadelphia: Saunders.
3. Brain, A. I. J., Denman, W. T., & Goudsouzian, N. G. (1996). *Laryngeal mask airway instruction manual.* San Diego, CA: Gensia Automedics, Inc.
4. Knight, S. B. (1999). Nasal airway insertion. In J. Proehl (Ed.), *Emergency nursing procedures* (2nd ed., pp. 14–15). Philadelphia: Saunders.
5. Knight, S. B. (1999). Oral airway insertion. In J. Proehl (Ed.), *Emergency nursing procedures* (2nd ed., pp. 12–13). Philadelphia: Saunders.
6. Hazinski, M. F. (2002). Airway, ventilation, and management of respiratory distress and failure. In *Pediatric advanced life support provider manual* (pp. 81–126). Dallas, TX: American Heart Association.

TRIAGE SKILL STATION

Principles of Triage

Observation of the pediatric patient's status should occur before the pediatric patient is touched. This is referred to as the Pediatric Assessment Triangle ("across-the-room assessment") and includes

- General appearance—What is the general impression the triage nurse perceives when initially looking at the child? Does the child look well or look ill, or is the triage nurse not sure?
- Airway status—What is the position of comfort to facilitate air entry? Are there audible upper airway sounds, such as stridor or snoring? If stridor is present, what is the potential for a foreign body to be the cause? If the pediatric patient is coughing, what does the cough sound like? Is it productive, is it dry, or does it have a barking quality?
- Breathing status—Is the respiratory rate within normal limits for this pediatric patient's age, or is the rate too slow or too fast? Are the respirations shallow or deep? Are signs of accessory muscle use evident (with clothing on)? Is the pediatric patient's skin color normal, pale, or dusky?
- Circulatory status—Is the pediatric patient flushed, normal color, mottled, or dusky? Is there any obvious bleeding?
- Disability (brief neurologic assessment)—Is the pediatric patient running, walking, requiring assistance to ambulate, or being held? Is the pediatric patient alert, irritable, or sleepy? Is the muscle tone good or are the extremities flaccid?

The triage assessment starts with a rapid evaluation of the primary assessment. If the pediatric patient has life-threatening alterations, the pediatric patient is immediately taken to a resuscitation area. The components of the initial assessment are listed in the Management of the Ill or Injured Pediatric Patient skill station (pp. 277)

The history is obtained from the caregiver of the infant or young child or from both the caregiver and older child or adolescent. The CIAMPEDS mnemonic (Table 4-8) organizes the components of the basic pediatric history.

The following findings are emergent or urgent findings.

- Signs of airway obstruction
- Signs of moderate or severe respiratory distress
- Pallor or mottled skin color with delayed capillary refill

- Lethargy; decreased response to environment; decreased response to pain
- "Paradoxical irritability" (inability to comfort the child)
- Bulging or sunken anterior fontanel in infants
- Fever higher that 38°C (100.4°F) in any infant younger than 3 months of age
- Hypothermia in the neonate
- History inconsistent with illness or injury
- History of existing illness such as sickle cell disease, cystic fibrosis, or congenital heart defect

Summary

- During evaluation, learners are evaluated individually, not as a group as in the teaching station.
- During evaluation, pencil or pen and paper will be provided for the learner to record his or her findings.
- Each learner will be evaluated for his or her ability to correctly prioritize the order of treatment for three patients. Therefore, learners should concentrate on understanding the principles of the station and not memorizing the specific case scenarios.
- Learners may ask as few or as many questions as needed to determine the appropriate priority. Learners will be provided with only the information they ask for.
- The learners should be reminded that once they have asked all of their questions for one patient and have begun assessment of another patient, they may not return to the previous patient.

Triage Teaching Scenarios—Set #1

Case A: An 8-year-old boy, accompanied by his parents, walks in cradling his obviously deformed left arm. His skin color is normal; he complains of numbness and tingling of the left hand. There is no obvious respiratory distress.

Case B: A mother carries in a 2 ½-year-old girl. A strong odor of petroleum is present. The child is alert, pale, and quiet.

Case C: A mother walks up to the triage desk with a 1-year-old infant and says, "Please help me—my baby was shaking all over." The baby is flushed; no obvious respiratory distress is noted.

Triage Teaching Scenarios—Set #2

Case A: A 14-year-old adolescent is brought in by wheelchair, accompanied by his wrestling coach. The adolescent appears pale and is slouched in the wheelchair.

Case B: A mother walks up to the triage desk carrying a 2-year-old boy. The toddler has normal skin color, watery eyes, clear nasal drainage, and a barky cough.

Case C: A father approaches the triage desk carrying a 2-week-old infant wrapped in a blanket. The infant's skin color is normal. As the father unwraps the infant, she begins to cry.

Triage Scenarios Sample

A 5-year-old boy is sitting in his father's lap while his mother waits in the triage line. He is pale, does not appear to be in respiratory distress, and has a dressing on the side of his head with a small amount of bloody drainage.

Chief complaint: "He fell and hurt his head 1 hour ago."			
Physical		**History**	
A	Clear.	I	Has completed the recommended vaccine series for age. No exposure to communicable diseases.
B	Respiratory rate of 24 breaths/minute, not labored; breath sounds clear to auscultation	A	None
C	Skin color is pale, cool, and moist; capillary refill 2 seconds. Pulses regular with rate 110 beats/minute and strong. Heart sounds normal.	M	None
D	Pupils equal and reactive. Unable to sit up—leans on Dad or against back of chair; opens eyes when name is called but is not answering questions. Able to move all extremities.	P	Previously healthy with no underlying illness. Mom is concerned because he is not as active as usual.
E	Scalp laceration is 4 cm long and begins to ooze blood when the dressing is removed. No other noticeable injuries.	E	About 1 hour ago he tripped at school and hit his head against a metal fence. No reported loss of consciousness. According to his mother, there is a laceration under the dressing.
F	Pulse–110 beats/minute Respiratory rate–24 breaths/min Blood pressure–100/60 mm Hg Temperature–37.1°C (98.8°F) Weight–18 Kg	D	Ate a large lunch about 4 hours ago. Last void was several hours ago at school.
G-I	(G) Unable to assess presence of pain (H, I) There are no additional findings on focused secondary assessment.	S	No loss of consciousness. Has vomited twice since he hit his head. Mom says that he is now acting sleepy and is just not himself. She states that he seemed confused at home.

CASE A

Chief complaint:	
Physical	**History**
A	I
B	A
C	M
D	P
E	E
F	D
G-I	S

CASE B

Chief complaint:	
Physical	**History**
A	I
B	A
C	M
D	P
E	E
F	D
G-I	S

CASE C

Chief complaint:	
Physical	**History**
A	I
B	A
C	M
D	P
E	E
F	D
G-I	S

CASE A

Chief complaint:	
Physical	**History**
A	I
B	A
C	M
D	P
E	E
F	D
G-I	S

CASE B

Chief complaint:	
Physical	**History**
A	I
B	A
C	M
D	P
E	E
F	D
G-I	S

CASE C

Chief complaint:	
Physical	**History**
A	I
B	A
C	M
D	P
E	E
F	D
G-I	S